DRY THOSE TEARS WITH THESE DOCTOR-TESTED REMEDIES. . . .

ATTENTION PROBLEMS: Getting your child to focus on homework can be easy if you just "frame" the problem. Page 26.

NIGHTMARES: Keep those imaginary bogeymen at bay by monster-proofing your child's bedroom. Page 303.

CANKER SORES: Find out about the over-the-counter digestive aid your child can chew to oust that ouch. Page 81.

GROWING PAINS: These mysterious aches that strike youngsters between ages four and nine just might take a hike if you "go camping" in the bedroom. Page 229.

BAD POSTURE: Encourage your youngster to straighten up by allowing him or her to "barefoot it." Page 330.

STOMACHACHES: Use this simple method of "hands-on" TLC and chances are your child will stop bellyaching. Page 379.

THE DOCTORS BOOK OF HOME REMEDIES FOR CHILDREN

THE DOCTORS BOOK OF
HOME REMEDIES
FOR
Children

From Allergies and Animal Bites to Toothache and TV Addiction, Hundreds of Doctor-Proven Techniques and Tips to Care for Your Kid

By Denise Foley, Eileen Nechas, Susan Perry,
Dena K. Salmon
and the Editors of
PREVENTION Magazine Health Books

BANTAM BOOKS
New York   Toronto   London   Sydney   Auckland

This edition contains the complete text
of the original hardcover edition.
NOT ONE WORD HAS BEEN OMITTED

THE DOCTORS BOOK OF HOME REMEDIES FOR CHILDREN

A Bantam Book / published by arrangement
with Rodale Press

PUBLISHING HISTORY
Rodale Press edition published 1994
Bantam edition / February 1995

All rights reserved.

ISBN 0-553-56985-6

Published simultaneously in the United States and Canada

PRINTED IN THE UNITED STATES OF AMERICA

0 9 8 7 6 5 4 3 2

Contributing Editors and Writers:
   Douglas Dollemore, Marcia Holman, Ellen
   Michaud, Elisabeth Torg
Research Chief:
   Ann Gossy Yermish
Researchers and Fact Checkers:
   Susan E. Burdick, Carlotta B. Cuerdon, Christine
   Dreisbach, Sandra Salera-Lloyd, Deborah Pedron,
   Sally A. Reith, Anita Small, Bernadette Sukley

Contents

D

E

F

INTRODUCTION

Here's Help for Your Child's Health

If you're a parent, you've probably been wishing to have a book like this at your fingertips since your child came into the world uttering that first, infantile, give-me-something-I-don't-know-what-it-is cry of alarm.

Sometimes it seems as if all childhood is a series of crises interrupted only occasionally by blissful periods of calm. First come the problems with nursing or bottlefeeding. Then the diaper rash, the little coughs, sneezes and intestinal upsets.

As your child grows, her health may seem less fragile, but inevitably new questions arise. What's to be done about thumb-sucking? Or what about bed-wetting? If your child doesn't want to go to school—why? What are those red blotches on her skin—the beginning of a new rash or the first signs of chickenpox? Why is my child sneezing—does he have allergies or a cold? This aggressive behavior—what can I do about it? And how can I unglue my kids from the TV screen?

Of course, all parents compare notes. And before long, you're an amateur expert on food, fever, eczema, earaches, crying, hiccups, colds, croup and many other problems that kids always have. But parents also need authoritative answers to common questions about their children's health.

The book that you hold in your hands is meant to provide those answers. Like *The Doctors Book of Home Remedies*—a 10-million-copy bestseller published in 1990—this book emerged from thousands of hours of interviews with hundreds of health professionals. Once again, we asked doctors to recommend safe, simple, practical tips and techniques for healing everyday health problems. But this time, we asked them to give advice about *children's* health.

In *The Doctors Book of Home Remedies for Children*, you'll find more than 1,100 tips from pediatricians, researchers, nurses, dietitians and child psychologists for children from infancy through age 12. True, this book is no substitute for a doctor's care, but it's the best reference you can have on hand to supplement your doctor's advice.

This book is filled with extra-clear, easy-to-find information on the most effective treatments for dozens of minor complaints that you can take care of at home. Here you'll find the techniques that really do clear up diaper rash; tips for dealing with sibling rivalry; advice on how to treat bee stings, bug bites and minor scrapes and scratches; ways to make your child more comfortable when she gets poison ivy and dozens of tactics for preventing everyday injuries.

Also, this book will tell you when you *should* call the doctor—information clearly highlighted in boxes titled "Medical Alert: When to See the Doctor." You'll know the signals that tell you when emergency medical care is absolutely essential.

In the second section, you'll find "Accidents: Prevention and First Aid," with advice based upon the procedures recommended by the American Red Cross and by leading emergency-care physicians. Under "Prevention," you'll find out how to create an injury-free home for your infant and toddler—and safety tips on bicycle riding, playground activities and many other subjects. Under "First Aid," you can look up emergency procedures to use in case of poisoning, near-drowning, snakebite, severe bleeding and other catastrophes that you hope will never happen (but you always want to be prepared for).

Yes, this is a book that belongs on every parent's shelf, but not a book that's meant to *stay* on the shelf. It's our hope that this will be the book that you refer to any time you have a question about your child's health—from acne to warts, bad breath to stuffy nose, canker sores to temper tantrums. Just take down your copy of *The Doctors Book of Home Remedies for Children* and look up the answer. At last, it's at your fingertips.

Edward Claflin
Managing Editor
Prevention Magazine Health Books

ACNE

Steps to a Clearer Complexion

So you thought acne only struck during the teenage years? Not so, says Sidney Hurwitz, M.D., clinical professor of pediatrics and dermatology at the Yale University School of Medicine in New Haven, Connecticut. "It's not uncommon for children as young as nine to begin to show signs of acne," he says.

Although most kids outgrow acne by the time they reach their early twenties, self-conscious youngsters can worry a lot about their skin condition. For this reason alone, even a mild case of acne should get some helpful attention from parents, says Dr. Hurwitz.

Experts agree there's not much you can do to prevent acne from occurring in the first place, but there's plenty you *can* do to help control flare-ups. Fortunately, the ingredient benzoyl peroxide, found in many anti-acne medications, is effective. And some of these medications can be purchased without a prescription. So the first thing to do if you're going to treat the acne at home is:

Head for the drugstore. Look for lotions or gels containing benzoyl peroxide in any drugstore, suggests Dr. Hurwitz. Gels are the most effective at delivering the medicine where it's needed—just below the surface, he says. There are also soaps containing benzoyl peroxide on the market, but they are not as effective as gels or lotions.

Before your child uses the medication, however, make sure she isn't allergic to that product. "Take a tiny amount and rub it on the inside of your child's forearm," says Dr. Hurwitz. "Then wait a day to make sure no redness or irritation appears." If it does, you'll need to consult your child's doctor for another remedy.

Once your child starts using the medication, make sure she applies the medicine to the whole face (and chest and back, if those areas are also breaking out). Benzoyl peroxide not only helps heal existing pimples, it helps keep new pimples from forming. So your child should apply medica-

MEDICAL ALERT

When to See the Doctor

It can be a painful world for a child suffering from unsightly pimples.

But it doesn't have to be. Today there are numerous medications and treatments that can help even the most stubborn and severe cases of acne, says Sidney Hurwitz, M.D., clinical professor of pediatrics and dermatology at the Yale University School of Medicine in New Haven, Connecticut. If your child's skin doesn't improve after two or three months of home treatments, it's time to schedule a trip to a dermatologist.

A dermatologist can prescribe stronger medications, such as the more potent benzoyl peroxide gels, vitamin A derivatives such as Retin-A, and various topical or internal antibiotics. These can, in most cases, help clear your child's complexion and help make a happier and less stressful childhood.

tion even if the skin appears clear. "Usually once a day is adequate, but for a more severe case, your child can try it twice a day," says Dr. Hurwitz. "In fact, this should become a daily habit, like brushing your teeth to prevent cavities."

Wait for bedtime. An unfortunate "side effect" of benzoyl medication is that it can bleach material it comes in contact with. To limit the potential damage, make sure your child uses only a tiny amount and rubs it in gently. Ask your child to take care not to spill or drip medication onto towels, bedding, carpeting or upholstered furniture while applying it. Applying the medication only at bedtime can also help avoid ruining school clothes, advises Dr. Hurwitz. If your child does apply the medication in the morning, it's best to either apply a thin coating *after* getting dressed or apply the medication and wait for it to dry thoroughly before getting dressed.

Start with a low dosage. You'll find that over-the-counter benzoyl peroxide products come in concentrations of 2.5 percent, 5 percent and 10 percent. The lower the concentration, the less irritating to the skin it is likely to be, says Dr. Hurwitz, so start with the 2.5 percent product. If the lowest dosage doesn't work, you can then try a stronger one.

Be patient. Acne medications (even prescription ones) take from six to eight weeks or more to bring real improvement in your child's complexion, says Dr. Hurwitz. Of course, if the opposite occurs and your child's skin becomes worse, stop using the medication and consult your child's doctor.

Acne Myths

There are two common myths that persist about acne, despite medical evidence to the contrary. Experts have long tried to put these myths to rest—and here's what they say.

Myth #1: Acne is caused by excessive dirt and poor hygiene. There's no truth to this, says Sidney Hurwitz, M.D., clinical professor of pediatrics and dermatology at the Yale University School of Medicine in New Haven, Connecticut. "Dirt and hygiene have nothing to do with acne. It's not dirt on the face nor the oils coming to the surface that cause pimples to break out," he says.

The problem occurs under the surface of the skin, says Dr. Hurwitz. "Hormones trigger glands to produce oil, and because clogging of the oil ducts occurs about an eighth of an inch below the surface of the skin, no amount of scrubbing and cleansing will help," he explains.

Myth #2: Chocolate and fried foods cause your face to break out. Doctors used to believe this, says Dr. Hurwitz. But studies have proven conclusively that except in a few cases—people who are sensitive or allergic to certain foods—there is no particular type of food that causes acne. It is true, however, that high levels of iodine (common in many fast foods) might produce more pimples.

Don't put pressure on pimples. Pressure aggravates existing outbreaks, says Alfred Lane, M.D., associate professor of dermatology and pediatrics at Stanford University School of Medicine in California. Be sure to let your child know this—and point out some ways to avoid putting pressure on these areas. Wearing a sweatband or a beloved old baseball cap or just resting the chin in the hands while gazing at the blackboard can make pimples worse.

Steer around the fast food. While the burger, fries, chocolate shake and apple turnover themselves don't *cause* acne, these foods may have a high iodine content because of the way they're processed. According to the Food and Drug Administration, the average iodine content of a burger and milkshake alone may exceed the recommended daily intake by more than 50 percent. And high iodine may make breakouts worse, says dermatologist Harvey Arbesman, M.D., of the State University of New York at Buffalo School of Medicine. So if your youngster is a fast-food freak, you might suggest that he slow down on the burgers and fries and maybe try a trip to the salad bar instead.

Screen skin care products. You want to make sure that any soaps, sunscreens, moisturizers or makeup you buy for your child won't irritate the skin or make the acne worse, says Dr. Hurwitz. Some products will specifically state that they are *nonacnegenic* or *noncomedogenic*—which means that they don't promote acne. Others, however, won't specifically say so.

Good choices include Dove or Neutrogena soap; PreSun, Photoplex or Neutrogena Sunblock sunscreen; and Purpose, Neutrogena Moisture or Moisturel moisturizers. Any brand of makeup is okay, says Dr. Hurwitz, as long as it is nonacnegenic or noncomedogenic. When in doubt, check with your child's dermatologist.

Be gentle. Don't pick or squeeze pimples, says Dr. Hurwitz, and avoid hard scrubbing. Acne is not the result of poor hygiene, he says, so gentle cleansing is all that's needed. Remember, too much pressure on pimples just makes the problem worse.

Let your child have the shaggy look. If your child wants to wear her bangs long to cover up blemishes, you may as well let her have her way, says Dr. Lane. "Bangs, even naturally greasy ones, do not cause pimples to break out," he explains. "That's because it's not oils from outside that cause acne, it's the oils under the skin that cause it." And your child will feel a lot better if she can hide the blemishes.

You should not let your child use greasy pomades such as Dax Pomade or Ultra Sheen on hair that will touch the face. These products contain man-made oils such as petroleum jelly that can block oil glands and make acne worse, Dr. Lane says. Gel and mousse, however, are okay.

Reduce those stress levels. Yes, even preteens can be stressed out these days, and there's no question that stress can cause acne flare-ups, says Dr. Lane. "Stress raises the levels of the hormone testosterone," he says, "which in turn increases the activity of the oil glands." Take a look at your child's lifestyle: Is he or she struggling in school? Having problems with friends? Involved in too many after-school activities? You may want to cut back on activities and encourage your child to talk out problems. You can also teach your child relaxation techniques such as deep-breathing exercises.

AGGRESSIVENESS

Taking the Menace Out of Dennis

M any children go through a period—between the ages of two and four—when hitting, kicking and biting are forms of communication, often their only way of saying, "I'm angry" or "I want that." Without the language or social skills to get what they want, they're likely to express their frustration with flying fists or sharp baby teeth.

Although it's a normal developmental stage, aggression

can become a way of life. Kids who don't learn to replace their violent eruptions with more civilized behavior, such as sharing, turn-taking and verbal negotiating, often go on to become full-time bullies, says James Bozigar, a licensed social worker and coordinator of community relations for the Family Intervention Center at Children's Hospital of Pittsburgh. Fighting gets them the things they want but makes them feared and unpopular.

If your child is going through this phase, he'll probably get over it before long. But just to nudge his progress a bit (and help protect others!), here are a few techniques to help your child curb his aggressive tendencies.

Love that victim. If you witness your preschool child striking another, make your first move toward his victim, advises pediatrician Robert Mendelson, M.D., clinical professor of pediatrics at Oregon Health Sciences University in Portland. "Pick up the victim. Say, 'Jimmy didn't mean to hurt you.' Give the victim a big hug and kiss and take him out of the room."

What you are doing is depriving your child of attention, a playmate and you, all at the same time. Suddenly, his fun is gone and he's alone. "It usually doesn't take more than two or three responses like that until the aggressor realizes that being the aggressor isn't in his best interest," says Dr. Mendelson.

Lay down the law. Early on, get your toddler used to the idea of rules. "Just say, 'We don't hit, we don't hurt,'" says Lottie Mendelson, R.N., a pediatric nurse practitioner in Portland, Oregon, and coauthor of *The Complete Book of Parenting*, with her husband, Robert. With children aged four and over, the law can be a little more detailed. "You can say, 'In our house, the rule is: If you want a toy, you ask for it, and if the person doesn't give it to you, you wait,'" suggests Bozigar.

Be their guardian angel. Children who strike out physically often cannot control their tempers. For example, when another child has a toy he wants, a hot-tempered child is likely to act impulsively and wrestle it away. He may need to be reminded frequently about the rules you've set.

"Be his adjunct ego or guardian angel," says William Sobesky, Ph.D., assistant clinical professor of psychiatry at the University of Colorado Health Sciences Center and research psychologist at Children's Hospital, both in Denver. "When a child's aggression starts to escalate, point out to him what he is doing and give him alternatives. Say, 'In this situation you may feel like hitting, but that's not okay. You can tell me you're angry. You can tell me you feel like hitting, but it's not okay to do it.' "

Beware the mouth that roars. Don't overlook verbal aggression—it's often the start of something bigger. "A child can have a mouth that 'pushes a button,' causing a playmate to strike back," says Lottie Mendelson. When that happens, be careful not to blame the hitter and allow the instigator to go free. The child who speaks aggressively and starts throwing "verbal punches" should also be reprimanded, she notes.

Call a time-out. A cooling-off period is often the most effective way to change bad behavior. Bozigar says younger children should be placed on a chair away from all distractions for two to three minutes, and older children should be sent to their rooms.

"Just don't do it in a punitive way," he says. "Make it clear you're taking this action because you want things to work out and you want everyone to be happy. Say, 'You can't stop hitting, and I want you to have control of that. So I'm going to help you. I'm going to give you time-out for two or three minutes until you're in control on the inside.' "

Praise good efforts. When children respond in an appropriate way, make sure to reinforce it. "Tell them, 'I like the way you did that,' " says Bozigar. Kids respond better to praise that reflects how their behavior makes their parents feel.

"Saying 'good boy' or 'good girl' is often lost on children," he says. "It's better to say, 'It made me feel so great on the inside when I saw you sharing with your little brother instead of hitting him. It made me feel I could trust you with him.' That kind of praise is very meaningful to children. It makes them feel that they've had an impact on you."

Create scenarios for success. A child who bullies others learns very quickly that physical aggression has only limited success. It may get him the toy he wants or a turn on the swing, but he's likely to find himself friendless and lonely. He may be very motivated to work on other alternatives.

"You want kids to develop critical thinking skills," says Bozigar. First, talk about what happens when the child uses aggression. "If your child is always beating up other kids at the playground, you can say, 'What happens to you when you do that?' He may say, 'I get into trouble with the playground monitor, the principal calls me into his office and I have detention.' Then you can say, 'That's not a success for you. What can we do to give you a success?' Kids really respond to that."

Once the child realizes he's getting in trouble, you can start him thinking about possible solutions, Bozigar points out. For example, if he's being aggressive on the playground, you might want to practice different ways of getting involved in activities. Urge him to ask nicely whether he can join in—or to toss a ball back from out-of-bounds until the other kids ask him to play.

Use a scrapbook to scrap bad behavior. With a younger child who's beginning to show signs of aggressiveness, Bozigar recommends that you make up a little storybook with the child as the hero. Using pictures cut from magazines or photographs of the child himself, show situations where the child uses verbal or other problem-solving skills to deal with his frustration. Talk with him about these options. "Do it at a time when the child is not in the midst of emotional turmoil," he says. "When those emotions are up, it's hard to bring them down."

Share the fantasy. One technique that is often effective in helping children gain a new perspective on their behavior is to grant in fantasy what you can't in real life, says Bozigar. "A child who thinks he should have the playground all to himself can have it—in fantasy. Say, 'Okay, for the rest of the week, Tommy is the only one who is allowed on the playground. No one is allowed on the swings but Tommy, and everyone is going to have to stand around and applaud.' "

Once Tommy sees that his wildest dreams are just that—and funny, to boot—bring him back to earth. "Say, 'Yeah, that sounds cool, but in real life you have to *share* the playground. So let's talk about another way we can make this a success for you,' " says Bozigar.

Use force as the last resort. Forceful restraint should be used only when a child is putting himself or someone else in danger, says Dr. Sobesky. "If you must use physical restraint, approach the child from behind, pulling his arms down. Wrap your legs around his legs and keep your chin away from his head."

Be aware that restraint may increase rage in some children. "But others may find it reassuring that you can control them," he says. "Just make sure you hold your child in a comforting, nonaggressive way so he doesn't feel he's being attacked."

ANAL ITCHING

Strategies to Stop the Scratching

Kristie is dressed in her Sunday best for a visit to Aunt Gert. You're so proud of how sweet she looks ... until you notice what part of her anatomy she's scratching. Again.

One of the most frequent causes of anal itching in preschoolers is pinworms. (See page 320 for more information on pinworms.) Other common causes include chafing, hemorrhoids and a yeast infection. The irritating itch may also follow a bout of diarrhea, or it may simply be the result of poor hygiene, says Paul M. Fleiss, M.D., a pediatrician, lecturer at the University of California, Los Angeles, School of Public Health and assistant clinical professor of pediatrics at the University of Southern California School of Medicine.

Some of these causes may require a doctor's intervention. But others are more easily remedied. Once a doctor has ruled out anything serious, you can try some of these tips at home to help your child find relief.

Keep the area dry. "It's important to keep your child's bottom dry," says Dr. Fleiss. Moisture can cause irritation as well as create an ideal environment for yeast infection, he says.

Have your child change his underwear several times a day. "For a persistent itch, change your child's underpants frequently (three or four times a day), and don't let your child wear them to bed," he says.

MEDICAL ALERT

When to See the Doctor

You should take your child to a doctor for a diagnosis if the anal itching is accompanied by weight loss, diminished appetite or constant stomach upset, says Paul M. Fleiss, M.D., a pediatrician, lecturer at the University of California, Los Angeles, School of Public Health and assistant clinical professor of pediatrics at the University of Southern California School of Medicine. These could be signs of a more serious problem. You'll also need to check with a physician if there's a raw, oozing rash or if there are other symptoms of infection such as fever or nausea.

Pinworms, yeast infections and hemorrhoids are other causes of anal itching that may require a doctor's attention, according to Dr. Fleiss. The doctor can prescribe medication that will reduce the itching and speed your child's recovery from these conditions.

Take a powder. "A cornstarch powder may be helpful for keeping the anal area dry," says Dr. Fleiss. When you apply it to the child, be sure to shake the powder into your hand and then spread it on his bottom. Don't shake it all over, because it could be irritating if inhaled.

Always come clean. "Itching could be due to the child's not cleaning himself well," says Dr. Fleiss. So teach your child to wipe himself properly. "Dry toilet paper cannot get the anal area completely clean," he points out. But some children can easily learn to clean themselves with moistened toilet paper.

"Show your child how to wet the toilet paper and use it after each bowel movement," Dr. Fleiss suggests. "It's a good idea to bathe after a bowel movement. Or have a supply of moistened wipes near the toilet for him to use," he says. Afterward, he should use dry toilet paper to finish wiping.

Serve fiber-rich foods. Hemorrhoids are rarely the cause of anal itching in children. But if your child has been diagnosed with a case of these bulging veins, it's time for some diet changes.

"Be sure your child eats more high-fiber foods such as vegetables, fruits and whole grains and cuts down on low-fiber items such as cake, candy, cookies and potato chips," says Dr. Fleiss. "A low-fiber diet can cause constipation. When a constipated child strains to have a bowel movement, that can result in hemorrhoids or aggravate those already there." When increasing dietary fiber, it's also important to see that your child drinks more water and eats more fruits and vegetables, he says.

Sitz 'em down. In a bathtub, dissolve three to four tablespoons of baking soda in a couple of inches of warm water and have your child sit in it for 15 minutes or so, suggests Howard Jeffrey Reinstein, M.D., a pediatrician in Encino, California, and clinical assistant professor of pediatrics at the University of Southern California School of Medicine, Children's Hospital of Los Angeles. "Sitz baths are very soothing to itchy bottoms, regardless of the cause," he says.

Add oatmeal where he sitz. For some extra relief, try putting one packet of Aveeno Bath Treatment containing colloidal oatmeal, a finely powdered form of oatmeal, into your child's bathwater. "It's especially soothing," says Dr. Reinstein.

Smooth on something soothing. Though it's mainly intended for insect bites, Itch-X Gel is an over-the-counter anti-itching medication that can be useful for anal itching, too, says Dr. Reinstein. It's for external use only. He also suggests trying petroleum jelly (Vaseline) or a soothing over-the-counter ointment such as Desitin to coat and protect the itchy area.

Look out for lingering laundry soap. "Traces of laundry soap in your child's clothing can sometimes cause an itch," says Susan Aronson, M.D., a pediatrician at The Children's Hospital in Philadelphia and clinical professor of pediatrics at the University of Pennsylvania. "To get the last traces of soap out, put your child's clothes through an extra rinse," she says.

Get the softness out. Some kids are also sensitive to fabric softeners, adds Dr. Aronson. If you've been using them in your laundry, stop for a while and see if that reduces the itching.

ANEMIA

Upping the Energy Level

Your two-year-old has just spent the morning drifting from sofa to chair and back again with hardly enough energy to lift his head. He picks up a toy, lets it fall, picks up a book, lets it fall, then lets himself fall—bottom-first, thank heavens—to the floor. Now he sits on the rug looking up at you in mute appeal. He's thoroughly exhausted—even though he's had a full night's sleep.

Healthy children—particularly healthy two-year-old children—bounce through life like Super Balls. They do not stop unless it's to attack the cat, clear the bookshelf or throw pots and pans on the floor. So when any child slows to a walk—particularly a listless, lethargic, blankie-dragging-behind kind of walk—it's time to check with your child's doctor.

Sometimes the problem is iron-deficiency anemia, says Fergus Clydesdale, Ph.D., head of the Department of Food Science at the University of Massachusetts—Amherst. It's especially likely if your child is experiencing the growth spurt that occurs between the ages of 9 and 18 months or, in girls, around the age when menstruation begins. Children of those ages may frequently demand more iron than they get in a normal, balanced diet.

The National Research Council reports that children need anywhere between 6 and 12 milligrams of iron every day to build the red blood cells that will carry food and oxygen to hard-working organs throughout the body. So if you suspect your child is not getting even the Recommended Dietary Allowance of iron, here are a few tips to boost his intake and help battle anemia.

Use C as a mixer. "Increase your child's vitamin C intake when she's eating something rich in iron and she'll absorb more of the iron," suggests Lisa Licavoli, R.D., a dietitian in Newport Beach, California. Broccoli, green peppers and citrus fruits are good sources of vitamin C.

Strive for variety. Other iron-rich foods include pinto or kidney beans, almonds, enriched cereals and enriched whole-grain breads, says Licavoli. Beans are not usually the favorite of most kids—but you can include them in soups and salads, suggests Dr. Clydesdale. And make whole-grain breads the standard in your household.

Toss that Teflon. "When you use a cast-iron skillet instead of a Teflon-coated or aluminum one, you increase the iron content of foods, particularly when you cook acidic foods like tomato sauce," says Licavoli.

MEDICAL ALERT

When to See the Doctor

"If your child is pale, lethargic and listless, it's time to see a doctor," says Paul M. Fleiss, M.D., a pediatrician, lecturer at the University of California, Los Angeles, School of Public Health and assistant clinical professor of pediatrics at the University of Southern California School of Medicine. Although these symptoms in children are possibly signs of iron-deficiency anemia, other causes need to be ruled out.

In very rare cases, children may be suffering from blood loss or other blood problems that would affect their behavior. So be sure to check with a doctor before assuming that your child just needs more iron.

Snack and grow. "Give your kids dried fruit," Licavoli adds. "When you dehydrate fruit and get rid of the water, it concentrates nutrients like iron. Children especially like apricots, figs and raisins"—all of which are rich in iron.

Note: Dried fruit is sweet and sticky and may cause dental problems if kids don't brush their teeth after eating it, according to Dr. Clydesdale.

Hold the tea. If your child loves iced tea, be aware that the tannic acid in tea hinders iron absorption, says Gregory Landry, M.D., staff pediatrician at the University of Wisconsin Sports Medicine Clinic in Madison and associate professor in the Department of Pediatrics at the University of Wisconsin-Madison Medical School. A glass once in a while isn't going to hurt. But Dr. Landry says you shouldn't let children substitute iced tea for water on a hot summer day. In addition to interfering with iron absorption, several glasses of tea provide a large amount of caffeine for a child.

Breastfeed. To help prevent iron-deficiency anemia in infants, all doctors should recommend breastfeeding, according to Los Angeles pediatrician Paul M. Fleiss, M.D., a pediatrician, lecturer at the University of California, Los

Angeles, School of Public Health and assistant clinical professor of pediatrics at the University of Southern California School of Medicine. "Breast milk supplies almost all the nutrients your baby needs," he says.

Teach. "Give your children nutrition lessons, especially when your daughters begin to menstruate," suggests Dr. Landry. Help them identify various iron-rich foods as "good," "better" and "best" choices. Occasional praise when they select iron-rich foods may also be helpful.

Skip the supplements. You might assume that extra iron in supplement form is a cost-effective way to prevent anemia. Not so, according to Dr. Landry. "Vitamin supplements with iron are a waste of money for most children," he says. Unless the doctor specifically recommends supplements for your child, they are usually unnecessary, he says.

ANIMAL AND HUMAN BITES

Tactics When Teeth Bring Tears

I t can happen in the blink of an eye. Your toddler hollers out "Kitty!" as he grabs at a fluffy tail. An irate Kitty spins around and sinks her teeth into your toddler's hand.

The same thing can happen with Bowser or Fido, of course. Even the mildest-mannered pet can turn feisty or excited when overwhelmed by kid irritations.

And sometimes it's another *child* that takes a bite. Small children tend to try out their teeth on anything within reach. With older children, the hard bite that breaks the skin is usually the result of anger and frustration—a down-and-dirty kids' battle that gets out of hand.

Whether your child is bitten by a pet, a wild animal or an intolerant playmate, you should call a physician as soon as possible. In the meantime, here's what you can do before you get to the doctor's office.

Stop the bleeding. "Apply continued pressure until the bleeding stops, which should be two to five minutes," says Ellie J. C. Goldstein, M.D., clinical professor of medicine at the University of California, Los Angeles, UCLA School of Medicine. Never, however, use a tourniquet, he says: A tourniquet cuts off blood flow to the injured area and can lead to permanent damage.

Clean it up. "Bites should immediately be cleansed with

MEDICAL ALERT

When to See the Doctor

Physicians recommend that all bite wounds, whether animal or human, be seen by a doctor if the skin is broken.

If your child has been bitten by a wild animal or a pet that has rabies, he will need a series of shots to prevent rabies, says Ellie J. C. Goldstein, M.D., clinical professor of medicine at the University of California, Los Angeles, UCLA School of Medicine. And even if there's no chance the pet is rabid, your child could get tetanus from an animal or human bite. Tetanus can be fatal—so the doctor needs to know about the bite in case your child needs a tetanus booster shot.

Aside from rabies and tetanus, the main concern about bites—both human and animal—is that the child could get an infection from bacteria that have been driven into the skin. Cat bites in particular become easily infected, says Joseph Hagan, M.D., clinical assistant professor of pediatrics at the University of Vermont College of Medicine in Burlington and a pediatrician in South Burlington. "A cat's jaw is small, but its teeth are like hypodermic needles," he comments.

Even after a doctor has tended to the bite, if it later becomes painful, red or swollen, you should contact your child's doctor again as soon as possible.

AVOIDING DOG ATTACKS

About three million dog bites are reported each year, and nearly 60 percent of those bitten are children, says Marc Paulhus, vice president for companion animals at the Humane Society of the United States in Washington, D.C. Some of those bites could be prevented, he says, if children knew the proper procedures to follow when they are threatened by a dog.

Here's what you should tell your child to do when he is approached by a dog.

Don't run—stay still. When someone runs, a dog will tend to chase—even a nonaggressive dog. Your child should stop in his tracks and not move.

Don't stare in the dog's eyes. This can be threatening to the dog, who will likely attack.

Try a command. Many dogs will respond to a simple command such as "Sit" or "No." Your child should say the command in a firm but low voice, and if the dog obeys the command, the child can back slowly away.

Flop to the ground. If the dog is charging or attacking—or the child is too frightened to try the command-and-walk-away routine—your child should quickly lie face down and cup his hands behind his neck, with his forearms and elbows over his ears. This covers the sensitive areas, and the dog may just sniff and walk away.

soap and water," says Joseph Hagan, M.D., clinical assistant professor of pediatrics at the University of Vermont College of Medicine in Burlington and a pediatrician in South Burlington. "Wash the wound carefully, then soak it for 10 to 15 minutes in warm, soapy water."

Cover it. To keep the area clean, use a simple adhesive bandage or gauze pad, says Dr. Hagan. Apply it loosely.

Use ice. Some bites just leave deep imprints without actually breaking the skin. But the pressure of the teeth leads to swelling around that area. "In these cases, ice would be

HOW TO SOOTHE CHEEK AND TONGUE BITES

Everyone has done it—bitten the inside of the mouth or the tongue by accident while chewing. It's painful, and if it was done with any force, it can bleed.

But the home remedy is simple, not to mention tasty, according to Joseph Hagan, M.D., clinical assistant professor of pediatrics at the University of Vermont College of Medicine in Burlington and a pediatrician in South Burlington. "In the Hagan household," he says, "we keep a Popsicle in the back of the freezer for emergencies. If children won't put ice in their mouth—most of them won't—they will suck on a Popsicle."

Caution: While most tongue bites are minor and will heal on their own, if the bite is gaping or is about ¼ inch wide, take your child to see the doctor.

helpful," says Dr. Goldstein. "Remember not to apply ice directly. Wrap the ice (or an ice-pack) in a clean towel, to avoid freezing the skin."

And elevate limbs. While the ice is on, you should also elevate the limb above the level of the heart to help avoid or get rid of swelling, says Dr. Goldstein. "In the case of leg injuries, the child should lie down and place the limb on a pillow," he says. For hand injuries, either use the pillow arrangement or rig a sling that holds the hand at shoulder level.

Check tetanus shots. Find your child's immunization records. Because tetanus bacteria in an open wound can cause a fatal infection, your child will need a tetanus shot if hers isn't up-to-date, says Dr. Goldstein.

Note: Children should have had a series of tetanus shots as part of their DTP—diphtheria, tetanus, pertussis (whooping cough)—inoculations from the time they're about two months until they're five. A booster shot is needed every ten years thereafter.

Check rabies records. Any unvaccinated animal *could* be carrying rabies, even if it appears healthy, says Dr. Hagan.

Check records of pets to see that vaccinations are up-to-date.

Keep tabs on the animal. Any animal that has not been vaccinated against rabies who bites your child should be impounded by an animal control authority for ten days, says Marc Paulhus, vice president for companion animals at the Humane Society of the United States in Washington, D.C. Animals infected with rabies can only pass on the virus when they are near death themselves. "Any animal shedding the virus will die within ten days," Paulhus says. The animal may not *look* like it is near death, however. The animal can be active and alert even up to its last day.

ASTHMA

Managing the Wheezing

Cases of childhood asthma are on the rise, which can be pretty frightening for parents. But the rise in asthma has been accompanied by much research on the subject, and today many doctors can recognize the early symptoms of asthma and help children with this condition.

It's not always easy for parents to recognize that a child has asthma. "About half of those with asthma never wheeze," says Ted Kniker, M.D., professor of pediatrics, microbiology and internal medicine in the Division of Pulmonology, Allergy and Critical Care Medicine in the Department of Pediatrics at the University of Texas Health Science Center in San Antonio. "Coughing is the most common symptom, and especially coughing at night. Your child may also complain of tightness in the chest and a general feeling of tiredness, particularly after exercise."

What happens during an asthma flare-up? The airflow becomes reduced as the airways become inflamed and swell. Muscle contractions and thick mucus further impair breathing. A number of things can trigger asthma: pollen, a viral respiratory infection, pollution, dust, animal dander, mold or even exercise.

If you think your child may have asthma, take him to the doctor as soon as possible. If asthma is diagnosed, your physician may prescribe a medication to prevent the inflammation of airways and a bronchodilator, a drug to be used during flare-ups to help open tightened airways. These medications are administered by devices called inhalers and nebulizers. Your physician may also prescribe regular use of a peak flow meter, a hollow tube with a built-in numbered gauge that measures how much air is getting to the airways.

Here are tips from the experts to help you manage your child's asthma.

Make it part of a routine. Daily peak flow meter readings eliminate the guesswork when you're trying to estimate how well your child is breathing. Have your child use the peak flow meter at a specified time every day, such as right after he gets up. If the reading is lower than usual—indicating that less air is getting through the airways—check with your doctor to see if extra medication can be given to head off a full-blown flare-up, says Thomas Irons, M.D., professor of pediatrics and senior associate dean at East Carolina University School of Medicine in Greenville, North Carolina.

Practice peak-flow blowing. To produce an accurate reading on a peak flow meter, your child needs to take a deep breath of air, close her lips around the mouthpiece and then blow as fast and as hard as she can. This may take some practice. To help your child develop her blowing technique, place a cotton swab inside one end of a straw, suggests Nancy Sander, president and founder of the Allergy and Asthma Network/Mothers of Asthmatics in Fairfax, Virginia, and author of *A Parent's Guide to Asthma*.

"Make a game of it. Have your child take a deep breath, then place the other end of the straw in her mouth and tell her to blow out as hard and as fast as she can. The object

MEDICAL ALERT

When to See the Doctor

While asthma is a chronic condition that is usually successfully managed at home with the help of your child's physician, there can be flare-ups so acute that they're life-threatening.

Unfortunately, there's no clear-cut line designating when medical help is required, says Thomas Irons, M.D., professor of pediatrics and senior associate dean at East Carolina University School of Medicine in Greenville, North Carolina. "But there are definite symptoms that would indicate that your child is in danger and requires immediate attention by your doctor or emergency room personnel." You should seek medical help if your child is:

- Struggling to get air. He may have flaring nostrils or a pinched-in look at the ribs or at the collarbone.
- Too busy trying to breathe to talk.
- Sitting up and leaning forward in an effort to get air.
- Grunting with each breath.
- Sitting very quietly and attempting to get his breath (won't get up and walk around).
- Refusing to eat or drink
- Not feeling better within 15 minutes after medication is given.

Because of the life-threatening nature of this disease, you should immediately consult your doctor if you have any doubts, says Dr. Irons.

is to make that cotton swab pop out of the straw and sail across the room. That gives your child a sense of the amount of effort needed to use the peak flow meter," says Sander.

Keep an asthma diary. "Keep a record of symptoms and what triggered them, daily peak flow meter readings and medications," says Gary Rachelefsky, M.D., clinical professor of pediatrics and associate director of the allergy and immunology training program at the University of California, Los Angeles, and director of the Allergy Research Foundation in West Los Angeles. This information may help you avoid things that trigger symptoms and will help your doctor adjust your child's medication as needed.

Be knowledgeable about your child's medications. "That includes the benefits and side effects," says Sander. Ask your pharmacist to include the package inserts with any medications you are getting. Ask your doctor or pharmacist any additional questions you may have about the medications, and write down the information so there's no confusion later.

Call a conference. Everyone involved with a child with asthma—from parents to day-care workers to school personnel—needs to appreciate the seriousness of this condition and know the details of your child's treatment, says Dr. Kniker. Arrange where your child's asthma medication will be kept during school hours and what plans are to be followed if symptoms develop.

Supervise practice sessions. Your physician may recommend a metered-dose inhaler for an older child to take asthma medications—but these devices are tricky to use and require practice. "It takes a bit of coordination and timing to use them properly," says Dr. Kniker. "Kids can start to use it adequately by the time they are 7, but not until they're 10 or 12 do most of them do it well." Many children find a metered-dose inhaler more comfortable to use with the help of a "spacer." This collects the cloud of medication, which makes inhaling easier. If your child is just beginning to use an inhaler, watch closely to make sure he is following the doctor's instructions. Later on, check up from time to time to make sure he's following the correct procedure.

Encourage visualization. Sometimes kids breathe the medication from their inhalers too quickly or not deeply enough, depositing most of the medicine in their mouth and throat. To help your child use the inhaler properly, help her understand what the medicine is going to do and visualize where it should go, says Sander. "Explain to your child that her lungs are injured, and you want the medicine to go where the injury is, which is deep down in the lungs. And then show her how to breathe in slowly by having her say—in her mind—a silly phrase or line of a rhyme as she takes her breath in. Then she should hold her breath as long as possible to let the medicine go as deeply as possible." This will help her prolong the breathing in.

Reach out for support. The Allergy and Asthma Network/Mothers of Asthmatics offers a monthly newsletter, *The MA Report,* which provides coping strategies, medical update information, tips and moral support for families affected by asthma and allergies, says Sander. For more information, send a business-size envelope with two first-class stamps to the Allergy and Asthma Network, 3554 Chain Bridge Road, Suite 200, Fairfax, Virginia 22030-2709.

Allergy-proof your home. Over 90 percent of children under age 16 who have asthma also have allergies, according to the National Institute of Allergy and Infectious Diseases in Bethesda, Maryland. "That means that if your child with asthma is diagnosed as allergic to cats, dust mites or whatever, you need to allergy-proof your house," says Dr. Kniker. Encase your child's mattress, box spring and pillows with plastic covers, for example, and consider removing carpets from your child's bedroom. Ideally, cats and other pets to which the child is allergic should be removed from the house. If not, the pet should be washed regularly to reduce allergen shedding and should be kept out of the child's bedroom. (See page 238 for more allergy-proofing tips.)

Make your house a smoke-free zone. Smoke from tobacco, fireplaces and wood-burning stoves can trigger an asthma flare-up, says Dr. Kniker. No one should be allowed to smoke in a house where a child with asthma lives. And if your house has a wood-burning stove, it would be best to install some other kind of heating system.

Teach breathing from the belly. Breathing slowly in and out for ten times twice a day can help your child learn to use a metered-dose inhaler. And knowing how to breathe deeply and slowly can help calm him during an asthma attack, says Dr. Irons. But the *kind* of breathing makes a difference. Help your child practice diaphragmatic breathing—which means holding the upper chest still while taking a deep breath by moving the abdomen.

To do this, have your child lie on the floor and put a book flat on his belly, suggests Dr. Irons. Tell him to make the book move up and down as he breathes. "Have him purse his lips and breathe in as deeply as possible. Then show him how to tighten his lips and let the air out very slowly."

Make breathing exercises fun. To build lung power and exercise the airways, your child can take up a musical instrument or help you blow up balloons, says Sander. For both, the child should be encouraged to do diaphragmatic breathing rather than "chest breathing."

Keep extra inhalers around. In case of an asthma emergency, you want to have medication immediately available, says Sander. "Always have one more inhaler than you think you'll need. Keep the extra taped to an inside cupboard door in the kitchen." But don't store a metered-dose inhaler over a hot stove and don't keep it in the glove compartment of a car in the summer, because heat can break down the valves in the canister, allowing small amounts of medication to escape. Extreme heat can also cause metered-dose inhalers to explode. These medicines are generally good for about two years, so keep a check on the expiration date, says Sander.

Consider medicine before exercise. "If your child has exercise-induced asthma, he can prevent an attack by simply taking a dose of prescribed medicine from an inhaler a few minutes before he begins exercise or sports activity," says Dr. Kniker.

Determining the correct pre-exercise dose will require some trial and error, which should always be done in consultation with your doctor. "Most kids need two puffs on their inhaler for adequate protection," says Dr. Kniker. "Sometimes the child may have to repeat whatever dose she used within an hour or so. The weather may also affect the amount needed. Warm weather is easier on asthma than cold days."

Keep calm during flare-ups. When an attack does occur, remain calm and speak in soothing tones. "An asthma attack is distressing to parents," says Dr. Irons, "but it will help the child to stay calm if you don't lose your cool." If your child is excited or coughing or crying, your nervousness or panic will make the wheezing worse.

Talk your child through it. During an asthma attack, talk to your child calmly, says Sander. "Tell him, 'I'm here and I'm going to help you. First we're going to use your inhaler. Now let's use it together. Now the medicine is inside you, and very soon you will start to feel better. So now, let's relax while the medicine does the work. Hey, wasn't that a great vacation we took last summer?' " Talking about fun times you've had together as a family helps divert his feelings of panic as the attack subsides, she explains. If your child's asthma episode does not respond to medicines as your doctor has instructed, seek immediate medical attention.

Reach for a tape or book. "A child who starts to panic during an asthma flare-up can often be calmed with a favorite tape—either video or audio," says Dr. Rachelefsky. "Concentrating on the music or show takes their minds off the attack." Reading a favorite storybook aloud can also help.

ATTENTION PROBLEMS

A Matter of Focus

Your son sits down to start his homework, but his attention is distracted by the rustling of a tree outside his window. So he stares out the window awhile. Then he jumps up to play with a toy truck. On the way back to his desk, he stops to tickle his little brother.

So why can't he sit still long enough to finish a task? His short attention span may seem like an unconquerable problem. But experts say there are things you can do to help your child focus better.

Confer with the teacher. "If your child's attention problems occur only at school, there may be a teacher problem," says Cynthia Whitham, a licensed clinical social worker and staff therapist at the University of California, Los Angeles, Parent Training Clinic and author of *Win the Whining War and Other Skirmishes*. If this is the case, arrange a conference with the teacher to discuss the problem and possible solutions.

Arrange a hearing check. If your child is inattentive and easily distracted, but not overactive or impulsive, consider having him screened for hearing problems or auditory processing problems, suggests Sam Goldstein, Ph.D., a child psychologist who is a clinical instructor at the University of Utah School of Medicine and codirector of the Neurology, Learning and Behavior Center in Salt Lake City. "Though he may hear you, it's possible that all the information he's hearing isn't reaching his brain effectively," he says.

Check out home stressors. If the problems occur only at home, they could be a reaction to home stressors. "If you see distractibility, overactivity and impulsiveness in your child, and you're going through separation, divorce or other troublesome times, the behavior might be temporary," says Whitham. She suggests increasing time with your child to give her opportunities to express her feelings to you.

MEDICAL ALERT

When to See the Doctor

Most young children are naturally active and may be unable to pay attention to a single task for a long period of time. However, some children who are consistently hyperactive should be evaluated by a mental health professional for possible Attention Deficit Disorder (ADD), according to Sam Goldstein, Ph.D., a child psychologist who is a clinical instructor at the University of Utah School of Medicine and codirector of the Neurology, Learning and Behavior Center in Salt Lake City.

The following behaviors, if they occur excessively, may indicate the early signs of an ADD problem.

- Fidgets with his hands or feet
- Talks frequently and loudly
- Has difficulty remaining seated
- Is easily distracted
- Has a short attention span and flits from activity to activity
- Has trouble awaiting his turn
- Intrudes and acts bossy with other children
- Acts impulsively

Some ADD traits, such as impulsiveness, hyperactivity and difficulty paying attention to routine activities, are not always liabilities, points out Dr. Goldstein, and can be effectively managed by parents and teachers, with guidance from a professional. In severe cases, stimulant medication may be prescribed for a child with ADD.

Heighten the fun level. Build the following elements into as many of your child's activities as possible: movement, novelty, variety, color, skin contact and excitement. When helping with spelling, for example, have your child print the words with crayons onto three-by-five-inch cards rather than merely spelling them out loud. The cards can be used for drill and review. To sustain attention during chores, play lively music and join the child in dance-like move ments. "If the activity has an intrinsic appeal to a distractible child, his attention span will be longer," says John F. Taylor, Ph.D., a family psychologist in Salem, Oregon, and author of *Helping Your Hyperactive Child*.

Turn the desk. A child who's easily distracted will be able to focus on homework and other tasks more easily and for longer periods if his desk chair faces a wall rather than an open room or a window, says Dr. Taylor.

Frame and focus. Cut a large piece of cardboard into a shape like a picture frame and place it around the "attention area" on your child's desk, suggests Dr. Taylor. Tell her to look inside the picture frame to do her work. This will help her concentrate, according to Dr. Taylor.

Tell, don't ask. Get in the habit of using statements, not questions. "A short series of commands is much easier to follow," says Whitham. For example, don't say, "Can't you find your jacket, honey?" Instead, say, "Go find your jacket now, and come back and show me."

ENSURE A GOOD NIGHT'S SLEEP

To reduce bedtime hassles and ensure your child gets enough sleep, John F. Taylor, Ph.D., a family psychologist in Salem, Oregon, and author of *Helping Your Hyperactive Child*, suggests that half an hour before bedtime, you give your child a glass of milk or a slice of turkey. Both these snacks are high in protein and contain tryptophan, which can help induce sleepiness. Then follow these bedtime rituals or similar ones.

- Bath
- Gentle skin contact, such as a back rub
- Bedtime story
- Warm, friendly tuck-in
- Night-light
- Tape-recorded bedtime stories the child can play to help soothe him to sleep after you leave the room.

Make eye contact. To improve communication with your inattentive child, always make eye contact with her before you speak, suggests Whitham.

Be specific. "Provide positive directions," says Dr. Goldstein. Instead of telling your child what *not* to do, tell him what *to* do. Don't say "Take your feet off that chair." Instead, say "Put your feet on the floor." Otherwise, your child may remove his feet from the chair but do something equally distracting, such as putting his feet on the bookcase.

Make a list. Make and post a list or chart of tasks your child can check off or cross out when completed, says Whitham. "That way, you won't have to repeat yourself, because the chart gives the reminder," she explains. If the tasks aren't getting done, calmly tell your child to go check his list.

Give credit for trying. Have patience with your inattentive child: She may be doing her best. "Many children

---

CUT DOWN ON ADDITIVES

A number of studies indicate that there is a connection between childhood attention problems and the chemical additives in processed food. According to one study, the behavior of more than half of a group of hyperactive children deteriorated markedly when they were exposed to artificial flavorings, colors and preservatives. Their behavior improved when the additives were removed.

While some authorities disagree about the exact role of additives with respect to attentional difficulties and hyperactivity, "it certainly can't hurt and very possibly may help to eliminate chemical additives as much as possible from your child's diet," says John F. Taylor, Ph.D., a family psychologist in Salem, Oregon, and author of *Helping Your Hyperactive Child*.

For information on common additives and how to avoid them, contact the Feingold Association, P.O. Box 6550, Alexandria, Virginia 22306.

have trouble starting a task and sticking to it," says Dr. Goldstein. "This is not behavior that they can easily control or stop just because you repeatedly tell them to."

Choose your battles. Child development experts often recommend ignoring your child when his behavior is something you don't like but can tolerate. Eventually, your child will stop the troublesome behavior because he's not getting any attention for it. "The trick is to *always* pay attention to your child when he stops the behavior you don't like and starts the behavior you *do* like," says Dr. Goldstein.

Be consistent. "Set up and stick to schedules and routines," suggests Dr. Goldstein. "Children with attention problems often benefit from consistent routines, including specific time periods for watching television, doing homework, playing, performing chores and eating dinner." Minimize disruptions. When interruptions are unavoidable, however, try to warn your child ahead of time that there's going to be a change of schedule.

Supply a release. To keep your child on a task longer, Dr. Taylor suggests you allow ways she can incorporate some movement into her work. For instance, give her a sponge rubber ball, a ball of colorful yarn or a colorful shoelace to squeeze or fiddle with while working.

Consider the sugar connection. While research findings don't thoroughly condemn sugar, according to Dr. Taylor, he believes parents should consider cutting down on their child's intake. "After diagnosing and treating about 1,400 children, I've found that somewhere around a third of the parents have told me that food with high sugar content causes their child's behavior to deteriorate significantly," says Dr. Taylor.

He adds that some research has shown that giving a high-protein food can block the effect of sugar in children sensitive to it. So if your child eats a sugary meal such as pancakes and syrup, supply a protein source such as yogurt, peanut butter, eggs or cheese.

BAD BREATH

The Less Scent, the Better

Most children hate garlic, shrink from the sight of onions and steer a wide course around smelly Roquefort cheese. So why do so many kids wake up with breath that smells like the odorous memory of a garlic-and-onion gourmet gala?

There's a good reason why classic "morning mouth" is prevalent among many children as well as adults. "During the day, normal muscle action and saliva wash all the debris out of the mouth. But bacteria counts go way up during the night," says Timothy Durham, D.D.S., assistant professor of dentistry at the University of Nebraska Medical Center College of Dentistry in Omaha. Because of that bacterial action, a child's morning breath is likely to smell . . . well . . . a bit yucky.

Other causes of bad breath could be infections or dental problems. So if your child's breath is consistently offensive, you should take him to the doctor. But, often, bad breath can be sweetened with consistent toothbrushing and a few other strategies suggested by dentists and physicians. If your child's breath has you wincing, here are some ways to make those telltale whiffs go away.

Lend a hand. The better a child's toothbrushing technique, the less likely he is to have bad breath. But learning to brush correctly takes longer than most parents suspect. "We suggest parents help kids brush their teeth until they're about eight years old," advises Eric Hodges, D.D.S., a pediatric dentist and assistant professor of pediatric dentistry at the University of Nebraska Medical Center in Omaha.

Time the toothbrushing. "Most kids don't brush their teeth nearly long enough," says Dr. Durham. To get your kids to brush longer, Dr. Durham suggests making brushing into a game. Place an egg-timer by the side of the sink and have your child set the timer for two to five minutes. When the timer goes off—but not before—he's done brushing.

MEDICAL ALERT

When to See the Doctor

"Chronic bad breath in children is distinctly uncommon unless there's something wrong," says Ronald S. Bogdasarian, M.D., an otorhinolaryngologist at the Catherine McAuley Health Center and clinical assistant professor in the Department of Otolaryngology at the University of Michigan, both in Ann Arbor. The problem could be caused by something stuffed up the nose.

If you have a toddler with bad breath, also check for a bad-smelling yellowish nasal discharge. "A little child sometimes stuffs an object up his nose and then forgets about it," says Dr. Bogdasarian. If your child has that telltale discharge, you should seek medical help.

Many young children habitually breathe through their mouths, resulting in dry mouth tissues and bad breath, says Eric Hodges, D.D.S., a pediatric dentist and assistant professor of pediatric dentistry at the University of Nebraska Medical Center in Omaha. Since mouth-breathing may be caused by a stuffy nose, allergies, blocked sinuses or enlarged tonsils or adenoids, your child may need the attention of a pediatrician to help correct the problem.

Also, chronic bad breath may be caused by an infection in the tonsils, adenoids or nose and sinuses, according to Dr. Bogdasarian.

And you should take your child to a doctor any time you detect bad breath accompanied by fever, weight loss, increased urination, diarrhea or abdominal cramping, says Timothy Durham, D.D.S., assistant professor of dentistry at the University of Nebraska Medical Center College of Dentistry in Omaha. "Also, see a doctor if your child has bleeding gums or loose permanent teeth," says Dr. Durham.

Make after-meal brushing a habit. "Your child has to brush after she's eaten to remove food debris from around the tooth and other areas of the mouth," says Dr. Durham. An older child can learn to carry a portable toothbrush with her for after-lunch brushing. Or, if she absolutely refuses, encourage her to rinse her mouth with water after she eats.

Go for high tech. "Get your child a rotary-type electric tooth-cleaning device," suggests Dr. Durham. "Their action is similar to that of dental instruments. They typically do a little better job than regular toothbrushes," he says.

Tidy up the inside debris. Even with the best tooth-brushing technique, your child may be missing the areas of the mouth that produce plaque—that infamous film of mucus harboring bacteria that produce bad odors as well as tooth decay. Plaque-holding areas, including the tongue and insides of the cheek, deserve special brushing attention.

"Roll the brush gently from the back to the front of the tongue, and take a swipe across the back," says Dr. Durham. "Then roll the toothbrush across the inside of the cheek—or take a washcloth and wipe down the inside of the cheek," he suggests. After you've shown your child how, she should be able to do it herself.

Moisten cotton mouth. Excessive stress can cause dry mouth, and dry mouth leads to bad breath. "When you lose the natural lubricant of the saliva, any debris that's in your mouth cakes to the teeth and the soft tissue and doesn't get washed away," Dr. Durham explains. If your child tends to get stressed-out about tests, homework or daily problems, remind her to drink water now and then to keep her mouth moist.

Offer something sour. More salivation can mean less bad breath, since saliva helps to wash away bacteria and debris. Using sugarless sour candy (or chewing sugarless gum) can get the saliva moving.

But beware breath mints and candies made with sugar: These only create fertile ground for more bacteria to grow and produce plaque, which results in bad breath, says Donna Oberg, R.D., a registered dietitian and public health nutritionist for the Seattle–King County Department of Public Health in Kent, Washington.

Hold the mouthwash. Many adults rely on mouthwash

to eliminate bad breath, but that's not the best solution for kids. "Fluoride mouth rinses and mouthwashes are not recommended for kids under age five because these children may swallow some of the liquid," says Oberg.

And researchers advise caution in using antibacterial rinses that contain a lot of alcohol, such as Listerine, according to Ronald S. Bogdasarian, M.D., an otorhinolaryngologist at the Catherine McAuley Health Center and clinical assistant professor in the Department of Otolaryngology at the University of Michigan, both in Ann Arbor.

For the older child who does want to use mouthwash, Dr. Bogdasarian recommends diluting it to one-half or one-third strength by mixing it with water.

Pic and floss around braces. "With any type of orthodontic treatment, you'll have increased plaque retention and food debris," says Dr. Hodges. "Teach your child to use an irrigation device, such as Teledyne WaterPik, to get around the braces," suggests Dr. Hodges. He also recommends a floss threader—a flossing device that allows the patient to thread floss through the orthodontic wires to clean between each tooth. This is a time-consuming procedure, but highly effective. You can get a floss threader from your dentist or at most pharmacies.

BED-WETTING

For Sheets Like the Sahara

S ally, age four, routinely wakes up in the mornings with a wet bed. Joe is five years older. But even at age nine, he tries to stay awake all night whenever he sleeps over at a friend's house. He's still terrified he will wet the bed in his sleep.

Sally and Joe share a common childhood problem: bedwetting. About one in five 4- and 5-year-olds wet the bed, and as many as one in ten boys still has a problem by age 12. (For some reason, it's more common in boys than girls.)

"It's not unusual for children not to be dry at night at age four and five, and some of us really don't consider it something that should be treated until a child is at least six," says George Sterne, M.D., clinical professor of pediatrics at Tulane University Medical School and a pediatrician in New Orleans.

There may be some kind of physical problem or health condition that's causing your child to wet the bed. If you're concerned about that, you should definitely discuss your child's bed-wetting with a doctor. But usually bed-wetting can be cured without medical intervention, given enough time along with a healthy dose of patience. Here are the techniques the experts recommend.

Rid yourself—and Junior—of guilt. Realize that you're not a bad parent because your child wets the bed, and make it clear to your child that he isn't a bad child because he wets. "Bed-wetting is a biological problem. It occurs in a child who, during sleep, has not learned bladder-control skills," says Barton D. Schmitt, M.D., professor of pediatrics at the University of Colorado School of Medicine, director of consultative services at the Ambulatory Care Center at Children's Hospital of Denver and author of *Your Child's Health*.

"I think it's so important to tell parents of bed wetters that this is *rarely* a psychological problem," says Dr. Schmitt. "There's a lot of unnecessary guilt imposed on some very good parents because they see themselves as being somehow to blame."

Ban punishments. One study found that nearly three-fourths of parents punished their children for bed-wetting. Never punish or scold your child for a wet bed, says Thomas Bartholomew, M.D., a pediatric urologist and assistant professor of surgery and urology at the University of Texas Health Science Center at San Antonio. "Parents should understand that this is not going to help their child," says Dr. Bartholomew. "I've never met a child who *wants* to wet the bed."

MEDICAL ALERT

When to See the Doctor

Bed-wetting is usually a normal, harmless condition of childhood, but there could be a serious physical reason such as a urinary tract infection, diabetes or a physical abnormality.

These are rare, but it's still worth a visit to the pediatrician to rule out such possibilities, says George Sterne, M.D., clinical professor of pediatrics at Tulane University Medical School and a pediatrician in New Orleans. You should always see the pediatrician if your child:

- Complains of abdominal pain, backache or fever.
- Wakes up at night regularly with an intense thirst.
- Wets during the day as well as at night.
- Has pain during urination.
- Has urine with an unpleasant odor.
- Is suddenly wetting again after months of staying dry.

Also, if your child is over age two and shows no sign of bladder control, you should bring this to the attention of your doctor. Some children take longer than others to begin potty training, but your pediatrician should be aware of your child's progress at this age.

Protect with plastic. A zip-up plastic mattress cover should be standard equipment on any bed wetter's bed. It protects the mattress, of course. But also it means there's less of a "crisis" when the child wets the bed, Dr. Schmitt points out. Both parents and kids will stay calmer if they know there's not much clean-up to worry about.

Encourage clean-up duties. You should, however, matter-of-factly tell the child he is expected to clean up the wet bed or at least help. "Even at age four and five a child can take the sheets off the bed and put them in the laundry room," says Lottie Mendelson, R.N., a pediatric nurse practitioner in Portland, Oregon, and coauthor of *The Complete Book of Parenting*. "It should not be punitive, just an acknowledgment that this is the child's responsibility. It also helps you. That way, you don't feel the child is doing this *to* you."

Check out your child's motivation. Before taking active steps to cure bed-wetting, make sure your child *wants* to stop, says Jeffrey Fogel, M.D., a pediatrician in Fort Washington, Pennsylvania, and staff physician at Chestnut Hill Hospital in Philadelphia. "When a parent asks me how to cure bed-wetting I ask, 'Does your child want to be dry?' If they say 'no,' I say, 'You can try all you want, but you probably won't be successful.'" If a child wants to stop, she'll not only cooperate, but her conscious mind will also work on her subconscious to help her awaken at night, explains Dr. Fogel.

Recognize the signs. A child often becomes motivated to stop wetting when it begins to interfere with his social options, says Dr. Bartholomew. When the child starts to refuse invitations to spend the night away from home, or doesn't go to camp because of bed-wetting fears, you can point out the benefits of being able to do these things. Then suggest some ways your child can help himself get through the night with a dry bed.

Pick a good time. Before starting, choose a relatively peaceful period—not, for example, just before an exciting holiday or vacation, advises Cathleen Piazza, Ph.D., assistant professor of psychiatry at Johns Hopkins University School of Medicine and chief psychologist of the neurobehavioral unit at Kennedy Krieger Institute in Baltimore. "You should pick a time when you're not having multiple stressors at work and in the household," she says.

Keep bedtimes calm. Lots of rough-housing or even an exciting television program close to bedtime can increase the risk of bed-wetting, says Patrick Holden, M.D., associate professor of psychiatry at the University of Texas Health Science Center. "When kids are excited, they tend to produce more urine," he explains. Instead of letting your child watch television before bedtime, give him a book to read, have a quiet conversation or read a story to him.

Put the child in charge. You want your child to understand from the outset that staying dry at night is his responsibility. That means *don't* wake your child at night to take
him to the bathroom.

"Waking the child doesn't teach him anything about
bladder control, and it's probably counterproductive," says
Dr. Schmitt. "If the child goes to bed thinking his parent
is going to wake him up at night, that's teaching the child
that the parent is going to take care of his bladder and that
he doesn't have to worry about it. Your child has to go to
bed just a little bit worried to stay dry."

Reward dry nights. Consistently reward or congratulate
your child when she has made it through the night with
a dry bed. "You'll get a lot further if you give positive
psychological support such as hugs and warm congratula-
tions," says Dr. Bartholomew. Some kids might like happy
faces drawn on a calendar or special stickers, says Dr. Piazza. Whatever reinforcement you use, do it first thing in
the morning.

Mum's the word. But if your child wakes up with wet
sheets, be careful not to grimace or say something like, "Oh,
no, your bed is wet this morning." Instead, say nothing, says
Dr. Piazza. "You only want to focus on success," she says.

IS YOUR CHILD SLEEPING ENOUGH?

Setting an earlier bedtime for your child may help solve a
bed-wetting problem, says Ronald Dahl, M.D., director of
the Children's Sleep Evaluation Center at Western Psychiatric
Institute and Clinic in Pittsburgh and associate professor of
psychiatry and pediatrics at the University of Pittsburgh Medical Center. A sleep-deprived child may sleep so deeply that
the need to urinate doesn't awaken her.

"Increase the total amount of sleep for the child," suggests Dr. Dahl. "Get on a regular schedule with a set bedtime. Often this can have a big effect."

"If we give as much attention to failure as success, we're defeating the purpose."

Make getting up easy. Some kids are reluctant to leave their beds, and others have been ordered by parents never to get up after they've been tucked in, says Dr. Schmitt. "So you need to give your kids permission to get up to go to the bathroom. They need a flashlight or a night-light, and they need to be asked if they want a potty chair next to their bed. Some kids who don't want to go to the bathroom are perfectly willing to use the potty chair and go back to sleep."

Give your child an alarm clock. If the child has a regular pattern of wetting the bed at the same time every night, furnish an alarm clock and explain how it works, says Barbara Howard, M.D., assistant clinical professor of pediatrics at Duke University Medical Center in Durham, North Carolina. "The child can set the alarm clock to wake him up 20 minutes to half an hour before he usually wets the bed so he can get up and go the bathroom," she explains.

Encourage a dry run. This is a "dress-rehearsal" technique your school-age child can do during the day. "I have the child lie in bed, close his eyes, pretend it's the middle of the night and give himself a little pep talk," says Dr. Schmitt. "It goes something like, 'I'm in a deep, deep sleep, my bladder is full, my bladder is starting to feel pressure and is trying to wake me up. It's saying *get up* before it's too late.' "

The child should then practice getting up, walking to the bathroom and going to the toilet. "I have them actually walk from bedroom to bathroom, so they know exactly how many paces it is," says Dr. Schmitt.

Avoid caffeine. Caffeine is a diuretic, a substance that *encourages* urination, explains Dr. Howard. It's in many sodas and in chocolate as well as in coffee and tea. Avoiding these foods and drinks may help your child avoid wetting, she says.

Encourage bladder-control practice. Explain to your

child that she can help "train" her bladder by practicing during the day. Have your child drink a lot, and then wait as long as she can to go to the bathroom. "Have her try to wait a little bit longer each time," says Dr. Piazza. "You want to train a child to associate the feeling of having a full bladder with having to go to the bathroom."

Stream-interruption exercises can also help, says Dr. Schmitt. Have the child begin to urinate and then stop briefly before starting up again. She should try to do this several times each time she urinates. "Those exercises build up the bladder sphincter," says Dr. Schmitt.

Buy a bed alarm. Most experts agree that moisture-activated bed alarms are the most effective treatment for bed-wetting. "When moisture hits the pad, an alarm goes off and wakes the child," explains Dr. Sterne. "It conditions the child to recognize the sensation and wake up before they have to urinate." Alarms are battery-operated, cost around $40 and are available from several companies without a prescription. Ask your pediatrician to recommend a brand or type. Use the alarm until your child is dry every night for one month. In most alarms, wetting triggers a loud sound that awakens the child. A silent, vibrating alarm is also available for children who don't respond to sound.

Dr. Schmitt recommends portable, transistorized alarms that are worn on the body rather than the bell and pad devices. And he says parents shouldn't insist on using the alarm if the child is opposed to it.

Stick with it. Be understanding and patient with your child, and stick with your efforts to stop the bed-wetting. "Conditioning requires time," says Dr. Bartholomew. He compares it to piano lessons: "Children might not get any results in the first month or two, but if they continue to practice, they'll be able to improve."

BEE STINGS

This Season, Be Ready

I t's a lovely spring day. You're sitting on the patio, a
magazine on your lap, an iced drink nearby, enjoying
the outdoors and listening to the shouts and laughter
of your children at play nearby. Suddenly a scream pierces
the air.

You rush to the rescue to find a sobbing child pointing
to a swelling on her arm. Your youngster has run afoul of
a flying insect of the stinging variety. Whether honeybee,
wasp, hornet or yellow jacket, the result is similar—your
child is in pain.

So here's some advice from experts on how to ease the
pain if your child gets stung. But there are ways that children can avoid getting stung, so you can pass along the
experts' advice on how not to get stung in the first place.

Treatment

Remove the stinger. If your child is stung by a honeybee
or bumblebee, the stinger will be left behind. The stinger
has a venom sac attached, so you'll want to remove it. But
don't try to pull it out, cautions John Yunginger, M.D.,
professor of pediatrics at Mayo Medical School and pediatrics consultant at the Mayo Clinic in Rochester, Minnesota.
Pulling the stinger can squeeze the venom sac and release
more venom. Instead, take a blunt-edged object such as a
credit card, knife or fingernail and gently scrape the stinger
and whisk it out.

Try a "high-tech" venom remover. After removing the
stinger, you can use a product called Sting X-Tractor—
which is sold in many outdoor and camping stores—to
remove the venom, says Gary Wasserman, D.O., a pediatric
emergency medicine specialist, chief of the section of clinical
toxicology and director of the Poison Control Center at
The Children's Mercy Hospital in Kansas City, Missouri.
"It looks like a big syringe without the needle. You stick

MEDICAL ALERT

When to See the Doctor

In children who are allergic, a bee sting can be fatal, warns wilderness medicine specialist Kenneth W. Kizer, M.D., M.P.H., professor of emergency medicine and medical toxicology at the University of California, Davis, School of Medicine. And you shouldn't assume that because your child has been stung before with little or no ill effects that he's immune from having a severe allergic reaction.

If your child exhibits any of the following symptoms, seek *immediate* medical assistance.

- Swelling over a large area of the body
- Shortness of breath or difficulty breathing
- Tightness in the throat or chest
- Dizziness
- Hives
- Fainting
- Nausea or vomiting
- Pain and swelling for more than 72 hours

Doctors also recommend that you seek immediate medical care if your child gets stung in the mouth or nose, which can cause swelling that blocks the airways.

If you know from previous experience that your child is prone to severe reactions, your doctor will likely recommend a prescription emergency kit to be carried with you everywhere. This will contain either antihistamine pills, injectable adrenaline or both, says Dr. Kizer. Stay close to younger children when you're outdoors, and train older children to administer the emergency measures themselves.

it against the skin and it works by creating a vacuum that sucks out the venom liquid. If you spend a lot of time outdoors, it's the thing to have." It can also be used for spider bites or any venomous insect bite or sting, he points out.

Keep the area clean. "Clean the wound with soap and water," says Dr. Wasserman. "What's going to cause infection is not the bite or sting, but the child's own germs getting into the wound." He advises that the area be washed several times that first day and a few days after, until the skin heals. When infections occur, it is usually three to four days after being stung.

Cool it. For bee stings, put ice in a cloth and apply to the site for 10 to 30 minutes, says Dr. Wasserman. Be sure to keep the ice from direct contact with the skin, to avoid the chance of freezing. If your child objects to the ice, use a washcloth rinsed in cold water and then wrung out. "This may help with itching, pain and tenderness. Repeat as needed," he says.

Make a paste. A paste of baking soda and water applied directly to the stung area for 15 to 20 minutes can help relieve pain, says Claude Frazier, M.D., an allergist in Asheville, North Carolina, and author of *Insects and Allergy: And What to Do about Them.*

Apply antiperspirant. Another handy remedy is one you'll find in your medicine cabinet. "Take underarm deodorant that contains aluminum chlorohydrate—it doesn't matter if it's spray or roll-on—and work that in. It will relieve pain and itching," says Dr. Wasserman. "If the child is itchy again an hour later, do it again." Why this works isn't clearly understood, says Dr. Wasserman. Probably an ingredient in the antiperspirant chemically neutralizes part of the venom.

Swab with ammonia. Carefully dab a bit of household ammonia on a cotton ball and swab the sting, suggests Herbert Luscombe, M.D., professor emeritus of dermatology at Jefferson Medical College of Thomas Jefferson University in Philadelphia and senior attending dermatologist at Thomas Jefferson University Hospital. Or you can try a product called After Bite, which comes in towelettes that contain ammonia. Rub the disposable towelette on the sting to soothe the pain.

Try an antihistamine. An antihistamine such as Benadryl may lessen some of the unpleasant side effects of a bee sting, such as local swelling, inflammation, itching, pain and allergic reaction. "Benadryl is a really safe medicine, and you can buy it without a prescription in liquid, tablet or capsule form," says Dr. Wasserman. Be sure to read package directions to make certain the product is recommended for your child's age. For the correct dosage, follow package directions or consult your physician. Some doctors don't advise Benadryl cream or spray because it could cause a reaction.

Give pain relief. If your child over the age of two is in pain from the sting, you can give acetaminophen (Children's Tylenol), says Kenneth W. Kizer, M.D., M.P.H., professor of emergency medicine and medical toxicology at the University of California, Davis, School of Medicine. Check the package directions for the correct dosage for your child's age and weight. If your child is under age two, consult a physician.

Use meat tenderizer with caution. Meat tenderizer made into a paste with water and applied to a sting may relieve the itch and pain, says Dr. Wasserman. The enzyme in meat tenderizer breaks down and inactivates the protein in the venom that causes the itch and pain. But if tenderizer is used, it should not remain on the skin for more than 30 minutes. In some cases, the ingredients may actually burn children's tender skin or cause allergic reactions.

Preventive Care

Pretend to be a statue. Bees are generally docile creatures who only attack when they feel threatened, say the experts. "Your child shouldn't swat at them," says Dr. Wasserman. "Tell your child to get stiff like a statue. If a bee lands, it should fly right off because it has no reason to sting."

Dress them in light colors. Your kids may love neon colors and flashy patterns, but those aren't the right hues if they're out picnicking or frolicking in bee territory. "Clothing in bright colors or with patterns like flowers attracts bees," Dr. Wasserman explains. Tell your child you don't want her to be mistaken for a flower patch, and encourage her to wear plainer clothing on summer outings.

Don't smell sweet. Bees and wasps tend to be attracted to smells such as perfume, cologne and scented soaps, says Dr. Kizer. So be sure your child avoids these products, at least when she'll be playing outdoors.

Repel them. A bath oil from Avon called Skin-So-Soft helps repel insects and is safe to use even on young children, says Dr. Wasserman.

Cover up the sweet drinks. Bees like sweet things, so they're drawn to soft drink cans. "It's not unusual for a bee to get inside a soft drink can. When the child takes a drink, it stings her on the lips or inside the mouth," says Dr. Wasserman. Keep soda cans and glasses covered, or use bottles or thermoses that have caps, and replace the cap immediately after each drink.

BLACK EYES

Ways to Soothe a Shiner

J ohnny reaches for a fly ball, but instead of falling cleanly into his glove, the ball smacks him in the eye.

Judy's bike skids on wet leaves and down she goes, banging her head on the ground. Accidents do happen, and tomorrow both Judy and Johnny will be wearing testimony to their mishaps: dark, swollen, black eyes.

While you shouldn't panic at the sight of a shiner on your child, don't laugh it off either. Your child could have suffered a concussion or serious damage to the eye, so it's important that you check with your doctor.

But once your doctor has reassured you that the damage is only superficial, it's time for tender, loving home care. Here's what the experts recommend to help soothe the hurt.

Chill out first. "Use cold compresses during the first 24 to 48 hours after the injury," says Alvina M. Janda, M.D., assistant clinical professor of ophthalmology at the University of Minnesota School of Medicine in Minneapolis. She suggests using crushed ice in a plastic bag covered by a towel.

But when you use it, be sure it doesn't come directly in contact with the eye. "The skin of the eyelid is the thinnest on the body and the most delicate, so you don't want to place ice right up against it," says Eugene Helveston, M.D., professor of ophthalmology at Indiana University School of Medicine in Indianapolis.

Off and on. "You should gently apply the cold intermittently to your child's eye—5 to 10 minutes on, 10 to 15 minutes off, and then on again, and so on," says Dr. Helveston. The cold shrinks blood vessels and decreases bleeding into the surrounding tissues, he says.

"If you're at a ball game or picnic and don't have ice handy, a can of cold soda will do the job," says David Smith, M.D., attending physician at Wills Eye Hospital in Philadelphia, consulting ophthalmologist for the New Jersey State Athletic Commission and director of the Division of Ophthalmology at the Atlantic City Medical Center.

Switch to warm. Forty-eight hours after the injury, apply a warm compress—a towel or washcloth soaked in hot water and then wrung out. "Apply these on an intermittent basis, too," says Dr. Smith. "Warm compresses help the body reabsorb the leakage of blood that has occurred." This means the discoloration will vanish a bit more quickly, which can be a comfort to your child.

Give acetaminophen. If your child is in pain, reach for the acetaminophen (Children's Tylenol). Check the package directions for the correct dosage for your child's age and weight. If your child is under age two, consult a physician. "And don't substitute aspirin or ibuprofen, even though those are used for pain relief, too," says Dr. Smith. "That's because both of those drugs have some anticlotting properties and can lead to increased bleeding."

MEDICAL ALERT

When to See the Doctor

Medical professionals recommend that every black eye be seen by a doctor because of the possibility of concussion or injury to the eye. "This is one injury that should *always* be taken seriously," says Eugene Helveston, M.D., professor of ophthalmology at Indiana University School of Medicine in Indianapolis. "If your child is hit hard enough to cause a purple, swollen-shut eye, there's a real possibility of serious, even permanent damage." Only an ophthalmologist can determine if your child's eyesight is in jeopardy, he says, or if the injury is merely cosmetic.

But even after an all-clear from your doctor, complications could occur. If your child experiences any of the following symptoms, say the experts, it's time to return to the doctor.

- Increasing redness of the eye
- Any drainage from the eye
- Complaints of blurred or double vision
- Irregularly shaped pupil
- Hazy or clouded pupil

Sleep heads-up. When your child goes to bed the first night, prop up his head with a few pillows, suggests Dr. Janda. "This could help keep the pressure and swelling to a minimum."

Turn the other cheek. "Encourage your child not to sleep on the injured side of his face. Pressure on the swollen area will not only hurt but could make the swelling worse," says Dr. Smith.

Help avoid future injury. If your child is active in a sport with a high possibility of getting a ball or elbow in the eye, invest in protective goggles, says Michael Easterbrook, M.D., associate professor of ophthalmology at the University of Toronto and consultant to Canadian and American squash, badminton and racquetball clubs and associations.

For high-risk activities such as racquetball or doubles tennis, protective goggles with unbreakable polycarbonate lenses are a must, he says. Or if your sports-loving child wears glasses, have them made with unbreakable polycarbonate lenses.

BLADDER CONTROL PROBLEMS

Wet No More

In midafternoon comes the call from your daughter's school: She says she doesn't feel well and you must come get her. Worried, you rush to the school. Only when you get your ashen-faced daughter in the car does she admit that she's not ill at all—she just wet her pants.

It's a humiliating experience for a child who's past the toilet-training years. But accidents do happen. Sometimes a child will wet her pants during a fit of shrieking laughter; sometimes she's so engrossed in an activity that she puts off going to the bathroom until it's too late. Even constipation can lead to daytime wetting accidents.

It may not happen again, if your child and you can work out ways to prevent it. But before you attempt a home remedy, see your pediatrician or family physician to rule out physical causes or health problems, such as urinary tract infections and bladder abnormalities. Then try these approaches.

Treat constipation. Constipation can indirectly cause daytime wetting, says Joseph Hagan, M.D., clinical assistant professor of pediatrics at the University of Vermont College of Medicine in Burlington and a pediatrician in South Burlington.

A constipated child who has had a painful bowel movement wants to avoid the pain she associates with going to the bathroom, says Dr. Hagan, so she tries to "hold it

---

MEDICAL ALERT

When to See the Doctor

When a child past the diaper years has a wetting problem during the day, it's best to see a physician to rule out anything serious, says Barton D. Schmitt, M.D., professor of pediatrics at the University of Colorado School of Medicine, director of consultative services at the Ambulatory Care Center at Children's Hospital of Denver and author of *Your Child's Health*. Daytime wetting could be a symptom of a urinary tract infection, diabetes or bladder abnormalities.

And it's imperative that you visit the doctor if your child:

- Is over five and wets regularly.
- Has had previous urinary tract infections.
- Experiences pain or burning when urinating.
- Has constantly damp underwear.
- Has a weak or dribbling urine stream.
- Wets while running to the toilet.
- Is thirsty all the time.

---

in." This is where the problem starts. "Some kids who are plugged up with stool develop sphincter confusion. They think they're holding onto stool, but they're also holding onto urine," explains Dr. Hagan. When the child just can't hold the urine any longer, accidents occur.

If your child is constipated, encourage her to drink plenty of fluids and serve her fruits, vegetables and whole grains. If the problem persists, ask your pediatrician for advice.

Turn off the tube. Kids can get so engrossed in a television show or video game that they don't take a break to go to the bathroom. "When they wet during an activity, that activity should halt immediately and not be turned back on for half an hour," says Barton D. Schmitt, M.D., professor of pediatrics at the University of Colorado School of Medicine, director of consultative services at the Ambulatory Care Center at Children's Hospital of Denver and author of *Your Child's Health*. Explain to your child that if he can't remember to stop to relieve himself, you'll have to limit video or TV time.

Put your child in charge. It should be your child's responsibility to remember to go to the bathroom, says Dr. Schmitt. Reminding the child only makes the problem worse: If you take charge, then your child doesn't have to. "It's also very intrusive to tell a child to go to the bathroom when he doesn't need to go or when his bladder's only half full," points out Dr. Schmitt. "The only one who knows when the bladder is full is the child."

Reward dry days. Be sure to compliment your child when she *doesn't* wet, says Patrick Holden, M.D., associate professor of psychiatry at the University of Texas Health Science Center at San Antonio—and avoid punishment when she does. Encouragement can come in the form of hugs or positive statements, says Dr. Holden. It helps to put a calendar in the child's room and mark it with stars or stickers for dry days.

Have short-range goals. If you're going to reward your child for staying dry, make sure it's a goal the child can attain in the near future, says Dr. Schmitt. Don't make the mistake that one mother did, who promised her son a treat if he could stay dry five days in a row. "The child had rarely been dry *one* day," says Dr. Schmitt. "There's no value in setting a five-day goal that he can never achieve."

Empty the bladder. Parties or sleepovers are high-risk activities for kids prone to lose bladder control when they're laughing hysterically. Remind them to empty their bladders immediately before the event, says Dr. Schmitt.

Cut back on excess fluids. Never restrict what your child drinks to quench his thirst, says Dr. Holden. The drinks to watch out for aren't really thirst-quenchers—they're just sweet and tasty. "It can help to restrict access to sodas and soft drinks," he says. "Your child might drink them *not* because he's thirsty, but because they taste good," he says.

You can make a simple rule that the child may drink only a certain amount of juice or soda daily, although he can drink as much water as he wants.

Help your child practice control. Deliberately stopping and starting while urinating helps improve bladder control, says Dr. Schmitt. Explain to your child how to do this, and ask him to practice every time he urinates.

Change her stance. When a girl is in a hurry to go to the bathroom, she may not take the time to pull her pants all the way down. If she ends up urinating with her knees together, this can push urine up into the vagina, explains Thomas Bartholomew, M.D., a pediatric urologist and assistant professor of surgery and urology at the University of Texas Health Science Center. And when she stands up, the pooled urine runs out, leaving an embarrassed child with wet underwear.

Remind your daughter to urinate with her knees apart. If she can't remember, ask her to sit on the toilet *backward*, says Dr. Bartholomew. That position makes sure that her knees remain apart while she's urinating.

Beware of tights. In girls, tight-fitting clothing can cause inflammation that leads to wetting problems, says Dr. Hagan. Warm winter tights can cause perspiration, then vaginal irritation and painful urination. If your daughter begins to have problems, ditch the tights and have her wear loose, long pants instead.

Avoid bubble baths. These can cause an inflammation of the genitals in girls, which can in turn cause incontinence, says Dr. Schmitt.

BLISTERS

Pinwork and Prevention

I t's a sure sign that something is rubbing your child the wrong way: She has a puffy, water-filled sac just under the top layer of skin. To her it's a curiosity—something to poke and prod. To you, that blister is a signal that there's been too much friction between your child's foot and shoe—or hand and tennis racket.

Your biggest dilemma with a blister is whether to leave it be or drain it. If it's small and not likely to burst on its own, most doctors advise only cushioning it with moleskin, a soft adhesive-backed product you can find at most drugstores.

But if the blister is large or painful and the child can't avoid putting pressure on it, it's better to drain it, as long as the child is not frightened by the idea. Some studies have shown that blisters heal faster when drained, and it's preferable to drain the blister under sterile conditions rather than let it burst on its own. That's because burst blisters *can* become infected, cautions Suzanne Levine, D.P.M., a podiatric surgeon, clinical assistant professor at the New

---

MEDICAL ALERT

When to See the Doctor

A blister that becomes infected needs to be seen by a doctor immediately for treatment. Here are possible signs of infection.

- Extensive or prolonged pain
- Redness beyond the immediate area of the blister
- Oozing pus
- Yellow crusting around the blister
- Red lines away from the blister
- Fever

York College of Podiatric Medicine in New York City and author of *My Feet Are Killing Me*. (*Never*, however, puncture a blister caused by a burn.)

Here's how to proceed, for blisters large or small.

Treatment

Protect them with moleskin. Cut the moleskin into a circle about ¾ inch bigger in all dimensions than the blister itself, says Morris Mellion, M.D., clinical associate professor of family practice and orthopedic surgery (sports medicine) at the University of Nebraska Medical Center and medical director of the Sports Medicine Center, both in Omaha. "Just leave it on for about two days, until the fluid has been reabsorbed into the skin," says Dr. Mellion. Be gentle when you remove it, so the adhesive backing doesn't disturb the tender skin underneath.

Explain the draining process. If your child has a large blister you believe should be drained, first explain calmly why it's a good idea to puncture the blister—and that it won't hurt. "A child old enough to get a blister will probably be able to understand that the process will be painless because the skin is dead—just as there is no feeling when you cut your hair or nails," says Douglas Richie, D.P.M., a practicing podiatrist in Seal Beach, California, and clinical professor at the California College of Podiatric Medicine, southern campus, at Los Angeles County–USC Medical Center. If your child is afraid, however, don't proceed—just pad the blister with moleskin instead.

Don't waste time. If your child is agreeable to having the blister drained, do it now. "A blister will heal faster if you drain it during the first 24 hours after it has formed," says Dr. Richie.

Clean the scene. Before you puncture the blister, paint it with an iodine solution such as Betadine Solution, says Dr. Mellion. After you've disinfected the area with iodine, wait at least 90 seconds before you proceed, he advises. (Iodine stings on an open wound.)

Sterilize the needle. While waiting, sterilize the needle or pin with isopropyl alcohol or Betadine Solution. Holding it over a flame also sterilizes it, but it's also likely to frighten the child and isn't necessary, says Dr. Richie.

Prick with care. Press the fluid in the blister to one side and then gently insert the needle sideways (not straight up and down) into the fluid-filled part of the blister, advises Dr. Richie. Some of the fluid will come out at once.

Press it out. Gently press out the rest of the fluid with a sterile gauze pad. "Most important is to leave the roof of the blister intact," says Dr. Levine. That flap of dead skin acts as protection for the raw skin underneath. "Think of it as nature's bandage," adds Dr. Richie. If the blister fills up again after 24 hours or so, carefully drain it again.

Battle infection. After the blister has been drained, apply an antibiotic ointment or cream such as Neosporin Ointment or an ointment containing bacitracin, and put a Band-Aid over the area. Better yet, cover the blister with a product called 2nd Skin, which is 96 percent water and looks like jelly, says Dr. Richie. You can find it at most drugstores: It comes in large sheets and can be cut to fit. Whatever covering you use, change it twice a day.

Cover torn blisters. If the blister has already burst and the protective layer of skin is torn, you need a "replacement skin." First clean the exposed wound and apply an antibiotic, says Dr. Richie. Then use the over-the-counter 2nd Skin product to protect the exposed area.

"The 2nd Skin creates a moist environment for healing, covers open nerve endings, provides a cushion and protects the area from dirt," he says. He recommends changing the dressing twice every 24 hours. A dressing should be used until the wound starts to heal on its own and your child says it feels better.

Make removal a snap. Before you change the 2nd Skin dressing, moisten it if it has dried out. "That way, you'll save your child's newly healed skin from damage and prevent some unnecessary pain," says Dr. Levine.

Preventive Care

Shop for shoes that fit. One of the best ways to avoid heel, toe and arch blisters in the first place is to buy your child shoes that fit well, says Dr. Levine. Take your child shoe shopping when he's rested—*not* after he's been walking around the mall all day, when his feet are tired and he's irritable, says Robin Scanlon, owner and manager of Scanlon Stride Rite Bootery in Whitehall, Pennsylvania.

Scanlon recommends allowing no more than ½ inch of growing room at the toe of slip-on shoes, and no more than an inch for lace-up shoes. Check the heels to make sure they don't slip up and down easily. But if the shoes seem a bit snug, try another pair. "Never depend on a tight shoe stretching," Scanlon says. "It should be comfortable when first worn."

Get special footwear for the athlete. Although it can be tough on your pocketbook, you may want to invest in specific shoes for certain sports, to help avoid blisters. You don't want your child to play tennis or racquetball in running shoes, for example, because the foot twists inside the shoe during the quick stop-and-go action—and that twisting motion can cause blisters, says Dr. Mellion.

Go acrylic. If your child has blister-prone feet, choose acrylic socks rather than cotton, says Dr. Richie. His research shows that acrylic fiber socks are half as likely to cause blisters as cotton socks.

"Cotton stays wetter and it doesn't wick moisture off the foot and allow it to evaporate through the shoe," he explains. "Instead, it traps moisture against the foot, and moisture increases friction and rubbing and hence blisters."

Also, cotton can become rough and abrasive after many washings, while acrylic socks do not. "Wool is better than cotton but not as good as man-made fibers for protection against blisters," says Dr. Richie.

Ban the tubes. Tube socks, which don't have a fitted heel, can contribute to blisters, says Dr. Richie. "These can creep down into the shoe, balling up at the toes, creating wrinkles and lumps that become a source of irritation," he says. For the same reason, don't buy socks that are too large.

Double up on socks. "When extra friction is bound to occur, as in a sport activity, wearing two layers of socks can prevent blisters," says Dr. Mellion. "The inner pair should be made of a wicking material, such as acrylic fibers, while the outer pair can be cotton."

Soothe with a sprinkle. "For kids whose feet sweat a lot, you can sprinkle talcum powder or cornstarch between the toes and all around the foot to reduce the friction that causes blisters," says Dr. Levine.

Or grease those piggies. "Rub a bit of petroleum jelly onto any red or irritated spots on your child's feet before putting socks on," says Dr. Levine. "That will help reduce any mild friction that may be occurring." That soothing lubricant may be especially helpful for those times when your child is participating in a sport where overuse can create a blister, she says.

Battle sweat. Sweaty feet can contribute to blisters. For this reason your child is always better off wearing socks, says Dr. Levine.

"If your child insists on going sockless, sprinkle talcum powder inside her shoes and on her feet," she suggests. And make sure your child has an extra pair of well-fitting shoes that she can wear on alternate days. That way, each pair can dry out completely between wearings.

BOILS

Getting Them to Simmer Down

There it sits. Smack in the middle of your child's neck, in the curve between fragile neck and sturdy shoulder. A few days ago, the skin was soft and baby-smooth.

MEDICAL ALERT

When to See the Doctor

If your child gets a boil on his face—especially around the nose or mouth—the bacteria it contains may spread into the blood, sinuses or possibly trigger meningitis, warns Paul Rehder, M.D., a pediatric dermatologist in private practice in Oxnard, California. That's why any facial boil should be examined by a doctor.

You should also check with your doctor if the boil has a deep red color around it or red streaks running from it toward other parts of the body. These could all be signs of infection.

If your child is having trouble moving the part of his body on which the boil is located, or if he complains that the boil "really hurts," you might also want to check with a physician.

Then you noticed a little redness, a little swelling. And today, you're looking at a big, fat, ugly, red boil.

Yuck.

Boils are a nasty skin infection in which bacteria—the highly infectious staphylococcus—invade an oil gland or hair follicle and cause it to swell with pus. The result is a red, swollen, painful bump on the surface of the skin that can appear without warning on any part of your child. Boils have no respect for anything private. And if they're not in a place where you can sight them soon and take steps to heal them, boils can assume awesome proportions.

Fortunately, a boil is usually so painful that a worried, uncomfortable child will bring it to parental attention fairly soon after its debut. Hopefully, he tells you about a telltale boil before he's had much chance to spread the infection by poking or prodding it.

"Children are more prone to boils than adults because their active lifestyle often puts their skin in contact with the environment in a way that gets them scratched," says Rodney S. W. Basler, M.D., assistant professor of dermatology at the University of Nebraska Medical Center in

Omaha. Even if it's just a haphazard fall on a pebble-strewn playground, the staph bug *can* sneak into the wound and under the skin.

Fortunately, unless the boil appears on your child's face, you can often treat it on your own, says Dr. Basler. "Hippocrates reported on how to treat a boil 5,000 years ago, and there hasn't been much new since then."

Updated by modern doctors, here are some old Hippocratic methods plus a few new ones besides.

Heat it up. "Apply hot, wet compresses with a moist towel to your child's boil for three minutes at a time, ten times a day," suggests Paul Rehder, M.D., a pediatric dermatologist in private practice in Oxnard, California. The idea is to bring the boil to a head so the pus can begin to drain. Continue with the compresses for three days after drainage begins.

The water in which you soak the towel should be somewhat warmer than body temperature, but not much.

Do not poke, squeeze or pinch. "Generally, the main thing is not to poke, squeeze or pinch a boil," says Dr. Rehder. That can spread infection and cause scarring.

Needle it a bit. "When you can actually see pus through a thin layer of skin over the top of the boil, that's the time you can very carefully put a flame-sterilized needle to it," says Dr. Basler. Just be sure there's no sign of redness or swelling anywhere around the boil before you prick gently.

Wash bacteria away. After the boil drains, "wash the boil and the area around it with soap," says Jane S. Wada, M.D., a dermatologist in private practice in Montrose, California. This will help prevent any further infection.

Avoid oil. As the skin heals, "Avoid oily products, which may plug up the skin," suggests Dr. Wada. And if your child is prone to boils, consider having him use an antibacterial soap on a regular basis.

BOTTLEFEEDING

Finding the Formula for Success

A rriving home from the hospital with your new baby, you mix the formula your doctor recommended. Then you happily settle down to feed the newest member of the family, anticipating a peaceful, fulfilling experience.

But for some reason it doesn't work out the way you planned. Your baby fusses or squirms or spits up or refuses the bottle. You're disappointed, frustrated and worried that your baby won't thrive.

What went wrong? There are a number of possible reasons—your baby could be allergic to milk products, for example. But chances are you just haven't smoothed out the process yet. To help you do that, here are some tips from our professional advisers to make bottlefeeding easier, more trouble-free and more rewarding for both parent and tot.

Make the mood mellow. Feeding your baby is an important comforting and bonding time. Get comfortable, and hold the baby so that the two of you can look at each other, advises Joan DeVito-Agins, R.D., a registered dietitian and nutrition consultant in Tarzana, California. Hold your infant securely, but not tightly. And try to focus your attention on the child. "It's important to give your baby uninterrupted time," says DeVito-Agins. Turn off the TV and turn on your telephone answering machine (or turn off the telephone ringer).

Pay attention to temperature. Babies have individual tastes: Some like their bottles the same temperature every day, and some don't care if you feed them warmed formula one day and chilled formula the next. If yours fusses when the temperature varies, keep it constant.

But what temperature should it be? As long as it isn't so hot it will burn your baby, it doesn't matter (test a few drops on your wrist). "For my daughter I ran warm water over the refrigerated bottle to take the chill off," says Alvin N. Eden, M.D., associate clinical professor of pediatrics at the New York Hospital–Cornell Medical Center, chairman of the Department of Pediatrics at Wyckoff Heights Medical Center, both in New York City, and author of *Positive Parenting* and *Dr. Eden's Healthy Kids*. Another alternative is warming the bottle in a saucepan of water—and it won't harm your baby if you feed formula straight out of the fridge.

Beware the microwave. It is a good idea to avoid microwaving formula, however. "Microwaving infant formula improperly may cause injury by either scalding or burning the tongue, lips, esophagus or cheeks," says Madeleine Sigman-Grant, Ph.D., R.D., assistant professor of food science at the Pennsylvania State University in University Park. "The plastic bag liners of the bottle may explode, or a hot spot in the formula may cause a mild burn."

If you *do* microwave formula, you should only use clean,

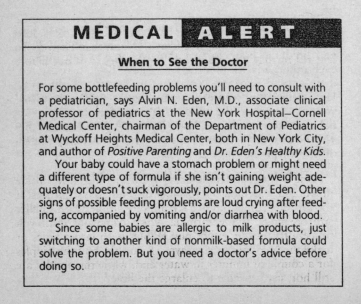

MEDICAL ALERT

When to See the Doctor

For some bottlefeeding problems you'll need to consult with a pediatrician, says Alvin N. Eden, M.D., associate clinical professor of pediatrics at the New York Hospital–Cornell Medical Center, chairman of the Department of Pediatrics at Wyckoff Heights Medical Center, both in New York City, and author of *Positive Parenting* and *Dr. Eden's Healthy Kids*.

Your baby could have a stomach problem or might need a different type of formula if she isn't gaining weight adequately or doesn't suck vigorously, points out Dr. Eden. Other signs of possible feeding problems are loud crying after feeding, accompanied by vomiting and/or diarrhea with blood.

Since some babies are allergic to milk products, just switching to another kind of nonmilk-based formula could solve the problem. But you need a doctor's advice before doing so.

clear plastic bottles—glass ones can crack—and never heat less than four ounces of formula at a time, to avoid overheating. You also must shake formula after heating so that hot spots mix with cooler spots, and test it by shaking a few drops on your wrist before serving. Don't simply check it by holding the middle of the bottle—you'll miss the hot spots.

Keep formula consistent. Mix your formula precisely the same way every time, says DeVito-Agins. Never dilute the formula any more than recommended on the label, because your child will end up being shortchanged of necessary nutrients.

Go for pure water. Because chemicals such as chlorine are added to tap water, you're better off mixing bottled water in your infant's formula, according to DeVito-Agins. Distilled water and bottled spring water are both fine for formulas. Filtered tap water may also be used: "But be sure you change the filter properly and frequently," says DeVito-Agins.

Boil new nipples. Brand-new nipples can have a plastic taste that your baby may not like, says Becky Luttkus, lead teacher at the National Academy of Nannies in Denver. To get rid of that new taste, boil the nipples in water before using them.

Consider the hole thing. It is important that the size of the hole in the nipple is neither too big nor too small, says Dr. Eden. If it is too large, formula will pour through too quickly and your baby may choke, and if it is too small, your baby may become frustrated and tired trying to get enough formula.

One way to check hole size is by turning the bottle upside down and watching the formula drip out, says Luttkus. If the formula comes out in a stream buy nipples with smaller size openings. If the formula won't come out until you squeeze the bottle, either buy nipples with larger holes or make the hole bigger, she says. To do this, boil the nipples for a couple of minutes in water and, while the nipples are still hot, use a needle to enlarge the hole.

You also need to keep aware of nipple hole size as your baby grows, says Luttkus. Nipples intended for newborns have smaller holes and are shorter than nipples for older infants, so if you're still using newborn nipples with your eight-month-old, it's time to make a change.

Replace aging nipples. Saliva and heat cause rubber to deteriorate. Change bottle nipples as soon as they begin to get rough or sticky, says Luttkus. Once a nipple starts sticking to itself or collapsing, your baby will have a much harder time feeding. "Most nipples have about a six-month life span," says Luttkus.

Hold on to the bottle. A parent with a million things to do may be tempted to prop up the bottle so that the baby can eat on her own. But babies need the cuddling and closeness that's a part of feeding, says Luttkus. "Look at your baby, talk to him," she advises. "It's important to have one-on-one time."

Also, a baby left alone with a bottle can choke if milk runs down her throat, cautions Dr. Eden. And when a baby lies flat on her back to drink, milk may back up into her throat and eustachian tube, possibly causing an earache or ear infection.

Get the right tilt. Start out holding your baby's bottle at a 45-degree angle, and raise the end as the baby feeds, recommends Luttkus. "Watch the neck of the bottle and keep it tilted so you don't get any air bubbles," she says.

Alter positions. If your baby tends to spit up more than once during feedings, a change of position may help. Pediatricians haven't found one "correct" way to hold your baby while you feed him. So you need to try out various angles until you find one that agrees with your baby. "The best position depends on each baby's esophagus and gastrointestinal tract," explains DeVito-Agins.

Go with the flow. Don't expect your child to drink a full bottle at noon today just because she took a full bottle at noon yesterday, says Dr. Eden. "Appetite varies from day to day," he explains.

You also shouldn't live by the clock. If it's half an hour before your baby's usual feeding time, and he's fussing and seems hungry, feed him. Or if he naps past his usual feeding time, let him sleep and feed him when he awakens.

Clue in to the signals. Your baby should be the one to decide how much he eats, says Dr. Eden. "When a baby stops sucking vigorously or starts squirming or looking around the room, that should signal the end of the feeding," he says. Never urge the rest of a bottle on a child who doesn't want it. "Don't force every last drop down your baby," says Dr. Eden. It's better to throw formula out than to have your baby overeat.

And don't hesitate to give more than the amount you measured out if your baby wants it, adds Dr. Eden: "If the baby drains the bottle in a few minutes, there wasn't enough in it in the first place."

Learn your baby's cries. "Babies cry for a lot of different

NIX THE BOTTLE AT NAPTIME

A bottle may seem like the perfect way to soothe a toddler to sleep—but pediatric dentists are strongly against it.

When a child falls asleep with a bottle in her mouth, the formula, milk or juice stays there and ferments, explains Heidi L. Hills, D.M.D., chief of the Section of Pediatric Dentistry, Preventive Dentistry and Behavioral Sciences at Columbia University School of Dental and Oral Surgery in New York City. If your baby's teeth have started to emerge, that naptime or nighttime bottle can cause the top front teeth to decay rapidly.

While your child sleeps, he doesn't manufacture much saliva or swallow very often, notes Dr. Hills. The sugars in juice or milk form an enamel-dissolving acid when they combine with bacteria present in the mouth, resulting in early tooth decay.

If you must put your baby to bed with a bottle, put only clear water in it, advises Dr. Hills. Or try a pacifier instead. Don't put a pacifier on a string around the baby's neck.

reasons: because they're hungry or cranky or gassy or lonely," says Dr. Eden. "Most parents can learn to differentiate the different types of messages from crying." Another clue is timing. If it has been less than two hours since the last full feeding, it isn't likely that the baby is hungry. There may be another problem that needs attention.

Give some attention without the formula. If you doubt that your child is hungry and can't find any other reason for her fussing, try cuddling her, smiling at her or taking her into another room for a change of scene, suggests DeVito-Agins. Your baby may just want attention. "Ask yourself if feeding time is the only contact the baby has with you," says DeVito-Agins. "If so, she may demand to eat more often, just because she needs more of your time."

Know when to switch to milk. At a year, children are usually ready to switch from formula to whole pasteurized milk, says Dr. Eden.

BREASTFEEDING

No-Problem Nursing

When Judy was breastfeeding, her friend Marta got the distinct impression that it was all fairly easy. Apart from slightly sore nipples at first, Judy had no problems—and Marta made up her mind that she, too, would breastfeed her baby when it was born.

But for Marta, things weren't so simple. Her baby fussed and refused to take her nipple. "Something must be wrong with me," a frustrated Marta told her husband.

Not so, according to doctors. Breastfeeding usually is trouble-free, but not always. And mothers shouldn't expect to automatically know what to do. Problems arise, but solutions are easily worked out. What makes breastfeeding easier for you usually makes it easier for your baby as well.

So here's some expert advice to make the breastfeeding experience go more smoothly for you *and* your baby.

Choose a good bra. A good nursing bra simplifies breastfeeding, says Ellen Petok, a certified lactation consultant in Woodland Hills, California, and an instructor at the Lactation Consultant Training Program at the University of California, Los Angeles. But don't go bra-shopping until the end of pregnancy. That's when your breasts are about the same size they will be when you are nursing. Look for a bra that will support your full breasts, with a trap-door flap that you can open with one hand (the other will be holding baby). When you're trying on the bra, make sure it is well-fitting but not tight.

Don't be passive about pacifiers. If your baby is satisfying his need to suck with a pacifier, you shouldn't be surprised if he's not breastfeeding well. "If you've noticed that your child seems uninterested, start putting him to the breast instead of giving him a pacifier. Judicious use—or, better yet, *no* use of a pacifier—may help," says Betty Crase, manager of the breastfeeding reference library and database of La Leche League International in Franklin Park, Illinois.

Watch your baby's movements. It's important to note the baby's body and eye movements to gauge if he's hungry, says Crase. For a new mother, you should notice if the baby gnaws on his fingers or turns his head back and forth. These are signs that the baby is interested in eating.

Give him a rub-down. Any skin-to-skin contact helps stimulate the baby. When he's stimulated, it comes out in a tendency to want to suckle, says Crase. Any rubbing of the arms, legs or back will help.

Try the football hold. If you're having trouble getting the baby to latch on to the breast, using the football hold will give you better control of his head, making the latch-on easier, suggests Petok.

Here's how: To feed the baby from your right breast, sit upright on a couch or wide chair and lay the baby on

MEDICAL ALERT

When to See the Doctor

If you have any concerns that your infant isn't getting adequate milk—if your child seems hungry after finishing nursing, persistently refuses to nurse or doesn't appear to be gaining weight—check immediately with your doctor or a lactation counselor, says Paul M. Fleiss, M.D., a pediatrician, lecturer at the University of California, Los Angeles, School of Public Health, assistant clinical professor of pediatrics at the University of Southern California School of Medicine and an adviser on the board of La Leche League International.

It's rare that an infant is unable to tolerate mother's milk or that a mother cannot produce adequate milk for her infant, notes Dr. Fleiss. (Most women can produce enough milk to satisfy even the appetite of twins.) More typically, he says, it's just a matter of refining your breastfeeding technique.

Or your child could be getting plenty of milk and you don't realize it. "Mothers who are new at breastfeeding are often nervous about whether their babies are eating enough," says Barry Herman, M.D., an obstetrician and gynecologist, director of the Southern California Women's Center in Encino and assistant clinical professor of obstetrics and gynecology at the University of California, Los Angeles, Medical Center. Your child's doctor can put your mind at rest by checking your baby's weight.

But if you have a red and tender area on one of your breasts along with flulike symptoms and a fever, you need to see *your* doctor, says Dr. Herman. Although you can continue to nurse, he says, you may have a breast infection called mastitis.

Mastitis is caused by bacteria entering the breast tissues through cracks in the nipples. Once it's diagnosed, your doctor can prescribe antibiotics to treat the infection, and the medication won't affect the quality of your milk. For the sake of your own comfort, however, you may want to encourage your child to drink primarily off the unaffected breast until the infection clears up.

a pillow, facing you, at your side. Hold the lower back of his head with your right hand. Support your breast with your left hand, thumb on top and other fingers beneath the breast. Bring the baby to the breast and tickle his lower lip with your nipple. When he opens his mouth wide, pull him in close so he latches on to the nipple and most of the areola. Adjust the pillow under the baby's backside (with your left hand) to help hold him up while he nurses.

Keep on moving. Vary the positions used at each feeding, suggests Petok. During one feeding you could use the usual cradle hold position, and the next feeding use the football hold. That way, you'll avoid putting pressure on the same parts of your nipples.

Time for a wake-up call. Some newborns are sleepier than others and need to be awakened to nurse. During the day, a newborn shouldn't go more than three hours without feeding, says Petok. To gently wake your baby, you can change her diaper or "walk up her spine" with your index and middle finger. If the baby seems awake but not interested in sucking, try letting her suck on your clean finger before putting her to the breast. This should stimulate your baby to become more interested in feeding.

This wake-up routine usually works, but if she is still disinterested, try again a little later.

Express yourself. "Express a little milk and the baby will smell it," says Petok. Better yet, dab a little bit of the expressed milk on the baby's lip to get him more interested in nursing.

Pump or hand express your milk first. It helps mothers to pump or hand express their milk before nursing, in order to make the suckling easier for the baby, says Crase. This encourages the milk to "let down," so as soon as the baby starts to suckle, there's a quantity of milk there. "This is particularly helpful for babies who have been receiving bottles. If you pump or hand express first, they get that instant gratification with your breasts that they get with the bottle."

You'll know the milk has "let down" when you experience a pins-and-needles sensation or tightening and then relaxation of the breast or even a dull or sharp pain (experienced by some mothers). When you see yourself go from drip to a spray, you're ready to nurse, according to Crase.

Aim for the bull's-eye. "The most common cause of sore nipples is incorrect positioning of the baby," says Dr. Herman.

The trick is to center your nipple in the baby's mouth and to place as much of the areola in the baby's mouth as possible. To encourage your baby to open his mouth wider, tickle his lower lip with your nipple.

"Make sure your fingers are well behind the areola so they're not in the way when the baby latches on," suggests Petok.

Straighten out tucked lips. The baby's lips should look like a wide-open fish's mouth on the breast. Make sure the lips are not tucked under or retracted, suggests Petok. That could interfere with his feeding. If the lips are tucked under, gently pull them out with the tip of your finger. That will help the baby maintain a proper latch-on at the breast.

Reduce suction. When your baby is finished nursing, gently break the seal between the nipple and his mouth with your finger before you move the baby away, says Dr. Herman. Otherwise, the pull on the nipple can contribute to soreness or can cause tiny cracks on the nipple, which can lead to infection.

Air-dry your nipples. The soreness women often feel during the early weeks of breastfeeding may be partly due to chapping of the skin because of the constant moisture, says Dr. Fleiss. Allow your nipples to dry in the air, or use a hair dryer set on low heat to dry them before you close the flaps of your nursing bra. If you have a sunny place, expose them to sunlight for a few minutes daily.

Eat garlic. When a mother eats garlic, her breastfeeding baby is likely to benefit, according to Julie A. Mennella, Ph.D., a biopsychologist who is the principal author of a

FOR WORKING MOTHERS: HOW TO HELP YOUR BREASTFEEDING BABY

It's possible to breastfeed your baby successfully even if you work outside the home—with some dedication and preparation. Here are some tips from Ellen Petok, a certified lactation consultant in Woodland Hills, California, and an instructor at the Lactation Consultant Training Program at the University of California, Los Angeles.

Prepare the baby for work. Get breastfeeding off to a good start but don't wait too long to introduce the bottle. It's a good time to introduce the bottle at three weeks. This lets Dad feed the baby and gives Mom a chance to practice expressing milk.

Try this two or three times a week. If you do not start the bottle early enough, the baby may not be ready to take it when you want to return to work.

Learn to express yourself. Before you return to work, practice expressing milk manually or with a breast pump. Once your maternity leave is over, you can express milk in advance and store it for the baby. Nurse whenever you can, and have a caregiver give your child expressed milk when you cannot.

Breast milk can be refrigerated for later use. It stays fresh in the refrigerator for 72 hours or for three to four months if stored in a separate-door freezer. It's only good for two weeks if stored in a freezer compartment located within the refrigerator. Previously frozen breast milk thawed in the refrigerator is good for 24 hours. Freshly expressed breast milk in a sealed container can stay unrefrigerated and is still good for 5 to 6 hours.

Keep the milk flowing. When you're with your baby before and after work, nurse often to help keep a steady milk supply. At work, pump two or three times a day during a regular 8-hour working day. (Some women can get good results with a hand-operated breast pump—and battery-operated pumps are also available. But Petok recommends a fully electric breast pump, available at some pharmacies and medical supply stores.)

study conducted at the Monell Chemical Senses Center in Philadelphia.

The Monell study showed that when mothers ate a diet high in garlic several hours before breastfeeding, their babies nursed longer. What's more, the babies tended to ingest more milk—without experiencing any additional cramps or other problems associated with spicy foods.

Apparently, the strong smell of garlic changes the flavor of mother's milk. "What this may do is help the infant learn what types of food the mother eats," says Dr. Mennella.

Skip the beer and wine. Folklore suggests that nursing women who drink beer and wine have an easier time breastfeeding, but that's not supported by research. When a mother drinks alcoholic beverages, it actually causes the baby to ingest less milk, according to Dr. Mennella.

"The alcohol tends to stay in mother's milk as long as it stays in her bloodstream—for two to three hours after drinking," she says. If you don't want your infant exposed to alcohol, you can time your nursing," she suggests.

Keep baby cool. Be sure your newborn is not too warmly dressed at feeding time. "If she gets too warm while she's up against your body, she'll get sleepy and may not nurse enough," warns Petok.

Prevent engorgement. If your baby is feeding frequently enough (at least every three hours), you may never suffer from breast engorgement, says Petok. If your breasts feel overfull and uncomfortable, however, you can relieve the engorgement by putting hot compresses on your breasts before feeding, then nurse until the baby is satiated. Repeat as often as necessary. Engorgement usually passes within 48 hours, according to Petok.

Avoid infant tooth decay. Nursing throughout the night and letting the baby sleep at the breast can also lead to cavities, warns Donna Oberg, R.D., a registered dietitian and public health nutritionist for the Seattle–King County Department of Public Health in Kent, Washington. When breast milk pools around the baby's teeth and stays there for hours, decay can occur.

That doesn't mean you have to wean the child early, says Oberg. "But once your baby has teeth, you should not let him sleep at the breast."

BRONCHITIS

Relieve the Chest Congestion

Just when your child is getting over a cold or the flu, his temperature starts to climb and he begins to have coughing fits and spit up mucus. When you take him to the doctor, you're likely to hear one of those "-itis" words, which means something is inflamed.

In this case, the -itis is bronchitis, and it means inflammation of the bronchial tubes, the two large tubes that branch off the windpipe. Bronchitis can be caused by wayward bacteria from the throat or by the same virus that caused the initial cold or flu. As the lining of those tubes swells, mucus builds up. The heavy coughing is a sign that your child is trying to clear that mucus from his bronchial passages.

If the bronchitis is caused by bacteria, your doctor may prescribe an antibiotic. If it's a viral infection, an antibiotic won't help, but there's a lot you can do to make your child more comfortable and maybe even get over it faster. Here are some home-remedy tactics that doctors recommend for both bacterial and viral bronchitis.

Give extra fluids. Water is best, but any liquid will do, says F. T. Fitzpatrick, M.D., a pediatrician in private practice in Doylestown, Pennsylvania. The fluids help thin the mucus, making it easier to cough up, and can also soothe a throat that's tickly from coughing. An eight-year-old child should drink at least four eight-ounce glasses of liquid a day.

Moisturize the bedroom. Humidity may help soothe the irritated bronchial membranes, says J. Owen Hendley,

M.D., professor of pediatrics and head of pediatric infectious diseases at the University of Virginia School of Medicine in Charlottesville. Close the door to your child's bedroom and turn on the vaporizer about a half-hour before he goes to sleep—and leave it on all night, he suggests. "That way you can get the humidity up to as much as 70 percent."

Encourage productive coughing. Since the mucus in the bronchial tubes is causing your child to cough, encourage her to clear her lungs, says Dr. Hendley. If a small child is having trouble coughing up the mucus, pat her gently on the back. Keep tissues available so that your child can use them if needed.

MEDICAL ALERT

When to See the Doctor

Most cases of bronchitis clear up in a week or two, with no repercussions other than lost sleep from coughing fits.

Complications such as pneumonia can occur, however, and certain symptoms should prompt you to seek immediate medical care, says William Howatt, M.D., professor of pediatrics in the Department of Pediatrics and Communicable Diseases at the University of Michigan Medical Center in Ann Arbor. If it's a weekend or evening and you can't get in touch with the doctor, visit an emergency treatment facility.

Seek medical care if the child who has bronchitis:

- Is an infant and is coughing often.
- Has a fever of 103° or higher.
- Has any trouble breathing.
- Has a change in color. (Especially look for a blue tint on the lips or tongue.)
- Seems unusually lethargic.
- Is wheezing.
- Has to visibly move her chest up and down as she tries to get air.

Use a prop. Use an extra pillow at night to help prop up your child while he sleeps, suggests Mary Meland, M.D., a pediatrician with HealthPartners in Bloomington, Minnesota. Propping up his head helps him breathe more easily.

Soothe with chicken soup. Mom's chicken soup is more than comforting to an ill child; it really does help clear congestion. "Some scientific evidence has shown that chicken soup helps clear secretions better than other liquids," says Dr. Meland. If your child likes it, now is the time to let her slurp her fill. You can use either store-bought or homemade.

Nix the smoking. Don't allow anyone to smoke in your house, says Dr. Fitzpatrick. If you smoke, go outside to do it. The smoke irritates the bronchial tubes and can make the infection worse.

Try an expectorant. Over-the-counter expectorants that contain guaifenesin such as Robitussin, Triaminic Expectorant and many others *may* help loosen the mucus so that coughing can work to clear the bronchial passages, says Dr. Hendley. There's no hard scientific proof that they work, he says, but there's no harm in trying one. Read the label carefully and give a dose suitable for your child's age.

Consider a cough suppressant. If your child is coughing so much she can't get any rest, it's okay to use a cough suppressant at night, says William Howatt, M.D., professor of pediatrics in the Department of Pediatrics and Communicable Diseases at the University of Michigan Medical Center in Ann Arbor. Robitussin Pediatric Cough Suppressant may help—and other over-the-counter suppressants for children are available at drugstores. Try to avoid giving the suppressants during the day if your child has productive coughing. That coughing is *needed* to help clear the bronchial tubes.

BRUISES

Treatments from the School of Hard Knocks

I was almost afraid to take my three-year-old in for his regular checkup," says a mother of an active pre-schooler. "He had so many bruises up and down his shins, he looked like we had beaten him."

For kids, bruises are an occupational hazard. Children run, jump, climb, skate, bike . . . and fall, crash, slam and bump. Jeffrey Fogel, M.D., a pediatrician in Fort Washington, Pennsylvania, and staff physician at Chestnut Hill Hospital in Philadelphia, says that bruises are so normal that

---

MEDICAL ALERT

When to See the Doctor

Some bruises require at least an evaluation by a physician before you begin any home remedies. And in very rare instances, bruises that appear spontaneously indicate serious diseases such as leukemia.

Seek professional help if:

- The eye or head is bruised.
- The blow is to the side of the head above the ear, an area at high risk for fracturing.
- Your child has trouble walking, talking or seeing, becomes drowsy or unresponsive or has one pupil that is larger than the other after receiving a bruising blow.
- Swelling occurs at a joint, particularly an elbow.
- Bruising occurs in abnormal places, such as the back, the calves or the backs of the arms.
- A minor blow results in a large bruise.
- A blunt or hard object, such as a bicycle handlebar, has struck your child's abdomen with significant force.
- A fever accompanies the bruising.
- Bruising appears with no apparent cause.

if he sees a young child *without* bruises on his legs, he wonders if the parents are being overprotective.

Most bruises require no medical attention and can be treated successfully at home with these simple techniques.

Ice the injured area. "If the skin is intact, apply ice for five minutes at least," says Grace Caputo, M.D., associate chief of the Division of Emergency Medicine at Children's Hospital and assistant professor of pediatrics at Harvard Medical School, both in Boston. You should never, however, apply ice directly to the skin.

If the skin is torn, cleanse the skin first, apply a clean covering and then apply ice to the *covered* skin. Wrap ice in a clean dish towel or washcloth or use an ice-pack. Ice the area continuously when the bruise first occurs, to minimize swelling. "Most children will tolerate only about 20 minutes of this," says Dr. Caputo. Reapply the ice until the swelling subsides.

Or apply cool compresses. If the injury seems minor and your child rebels at the freezing sensation of the ice, then use a cool compress instead, says Dr. Fogel. Just wring out a washcloth in cold tap water and place it on the injured area. If your child resists even that, don't push. It's not worth the trouble.

Elevate a limb. If a bruised arm or leg is swelling after applying ice, elevate the arm or leg with pillows, says Dr. Caputo. "This will minimize the swelling," she explains.

Switch to heat. After 24 to 48 hours, it's time to reach for warm compresses rather than ice or cold cloths. "Cold constricts blood vessels, which helps the bleeding stop quicker," explains Dr. Fogel. "After the blood vessel heals over, you want the bruise to go away. Heat dilates the blood vessels, encouraging blood flow, and the bruise gets better faster."

Wring out a washcloth in warm water and apply for five to ten minutes two or three times a day. Keep this up for two to three days or until the bruise begins to disappear. Explain to your child that the color change of the bruise— from red to purple to greenish-yellow—is the result of the bruise healing.

Kiss it and make it better. "I don't say that flippantly," says Joseph Hagan, M.D., clinical assistant professor of pediatrics at the University of Vermont College of Medicine in Burlington and a pediatrician in South Burlington. "A little sympathy and reassurance can help. Some bruises, even if they don't look bad, can really hurt."

Give a pain reliever. If a child is complaining of pain, you can give an appropriate dose of children's acetaminophen, says Dr. Caputo. (Check the package directions for the correct dosage for your child's age and weight. If your child is under age two, consult a physician.) "But in the case of bruises to the head and stomach, you don't want to give kids pain medications until you've seen the doctor," she cautions.

BURNS

Cool Ways to Treat Them

You're having coffee at the kitchen table with your best friend, listening with rapt attention as she describes her triumph over a rival at work, when your toddler suddenly darts up to the table, grabs a corner of your place mat and jerks. The coffee cup tips over and hot coffee cascades down your child's arm.

As your daughter's shrieks mount in a rising crescendo, so does your panic. You don't know whether to run for water, ice, butter or the doctor. What in the world should you do?

When your child is burned, you'll have to act quickly to control damage and ease the pain. Any serious burn requires immediate emergency care, but if the skin is just a bit red, the burn is usually minor and you can treat it at home. Here's how.

Cool it with water. "If your child has been burned or

scalded, apply cool compresses (using wet washcloths or paper towels) for 10 to 15 minutes," says Lynn Sugarman, M.D., a pediatrician with Tenafly Pediatrics in Tenafly, New Jersey, and an associate in clinical pediatrics at Babies Hospital, Columbia Presbyterian Medical Center in New York City. "The cool water helps stop the burn from extending and will help relieve the pain," says Dr. Sugarman.

Never mind ice. Don't apply ice to the burn, though, Dr. Sugarman warns, and don't add ice cubes to the cool water. Ice or ice water will further damage the skin. You can offer acetaminophen (Children's Tylenol) for the pain. Check the package directions for the correct dosage for your child's age and weight. If your child is under age two, consult a physician. But do not use topical anesthetic sprays, because these can cause an allergic reaction.

MEDICAL ALERT

When to See the Doctor

Serious burns need a doctor's attention, according to Lynn Sugarman, M.D., a pediatrician with Tenafly Pediatrics in Tenafly, New Jersey, and an associate in clinical pediatrics at Babies Hospital, Columbia Presbyterian Medical Center in New York City. She recommends that you take your burned child to the doctor or hospital under the following circumstances.

- Any burn that causes blistering or makes the skin turn white
- If oozing or redness persists for more than 24 hours or there is increasing pain
- All electrical burns
- All burns that involve the mouth, hands or genitals
- Any burn that covers 10 percent or more of your child's body
- A burn that completely encircles a leg or arm
- For smoke inhalation

Use gauze, not creams. "Never put butter, grease, oil or a cream ointment on a burn. They hold the heat in the burned tissue and make the burn worse," says Barbara Lewis, a burn technician and community burn educator at St. Barnabas Burn Foundation in Livingston, New Jersey. Instead, "gently cover the area with a clean, dry cloth such as a gauze pad," she advises.

Leave blisters alone. "If your child develops a blister at the burn site, leave it alone," says Dr. Sugarman. The surface of a blister acts as a protective covering for the healing skin underneath, and breaking it may lead to infection she warns. If the blisters should accidentally break, check with your doctor to make sure your child's tetanus immunization is up to date.

Watch for infection. "Keep an eye on your child's burn. If you notice any increase in swelling or redness, or if the area starts to smell or ooze, see your doctor," says Dr. Sugarman. "The burn may have become infected and will need to be treated with antibiotics."

BURPING

An Easy Exit for Excess Air

As a new parent, you are bound to be on the receiving end of a lot of information. So you've probably already discovered that the issue of burping is fraught with controversy. Your grandmother insists that if your little one doesn't burp before naptime, she'll wake up with colic. Your neighbor says you should burp your baby after every ounce of formula to make sure she won't have gas pain. Your sister says that your baby will burp by herself if you walk her after a meal.

But what if your own baby seems to be following the beat of a different drummer—and almost never burps at all? What's a parent to do?

Burping is no mystery, really. Every time your baby eats, she's bound to swallow some air along with the milk. The air collects in a bubble in her stomach, which may cause some discomfort. Burping your baby helps her release the air, so she'll feel more comfortable. And after a good, satisfying burp, she'll continue eating if she is hungry.

Older kids burp because of excess air in the stomach, too. But with them, the problem is a little different. You no longer need to encourage them to burp; you only wish they would stop.

It's not hard to deal with burping, say the experts. Here's what they suggest.

Let eating stop before burping begins. Your baby will let you know when he is ready to burp, says Abraham Jelin, M.D., assistant chairman of the Department of Pediatrics and director of pediatric gastroenterology at the Brooklyn Hospital Center. "When a baby's stomach is full and he starts to feel uncomfortable, he'll stop eating. A good burp at this point will make him feel better. If you interrupt his meal to burp him when he doesn't need it, though, you'll have a crying, frustrated baby on your hands," Dr. Jelin says.

Listen for "need-to-burp" cues. Some babies gulp their milk and swallow a lot of air while they are eating, while others are quiet, efficient eaters, notes Richard Garcia, M.D., a pediatrician and vice chairman of the Department of Pediatrics and Adolescent Medicine at the Cleveland Clinic Foundation in Ohio. "You can actually hear the difference between one baby's eating style and another," he says. "Babies who swallow a lot of air require a lot of burping. Babies who don't swallow a lot of air are very difficult to burp, and indeed, may not need to be burped."

Check out the bottle. If your baby seems to be sucking in a lot of air while he eats, see if the problem is related to a nipple hole that is too large or too small, suggests Dr. Garcia. "You can also try a few different types of bottles and nipples. One may suit your baby better than another," he says.

MEDICAL ALERT

When to See the Doctor

"If your child tends to burp and pass gas after eating a cheese pizza or drinking a glass of milk, he may have lactose intolerance, a common problem. Children with this condition don't have enough of the enzyme lactase, which is needed to break down lactose [milk sugar] in dairy products," says Betti Hertzberg, M.D., a pediatrician and head of the Continuing Care Clinic at Miami Children's Hospital.

Lactose intolerance may begin as early as infancy. It is easily diagnosed by a physician, Dr. Hertzberg says. Treatment usually doesn't require giving up foods containing lactose completely. These foods may be eaten and tolerated in small amounts, she says. Or the doctor may recommend an enzyme supplement to be given to the child prior to eating dairy foods.

Experiment with a variety of techniques. "A burping method that works well with one might not work with another," notes Dr. Garcia.

"Some babies burp more easily if you hold them against your chest and rub their backs," he notes. "Others may burp better if you sit them in your lap, and lean them forward against your hand while you pat the back. Still others do well being patted while they lie down on your lap."

If your baby tends to spit up a lot of milk after a feeding, he should be burped in an upright position, with his stomach against your chest, says Betti Hertzberg, M.D., a pediatrician and head of the Continuing Care Clinic at Miami Children's Hospital. "In the first year of life, the sphincter muscle around the esophagus may not be fully developed, which makes it easier for a bit of milk to come up with the air bubble," she says. While this is nothing to worry about, burping your baby in an upright position will make spitting up less likely.

Be suspicious of gum and soda. If you have an older child who's continually burping, investigate the diet connection. "Any food item that makes children swallow air can make them burp," says Dr. Jelin. The worst culprits are chewing gum and carbonated drinks, he says. If you find a link, encourage your child to cut back on the offending item.

Ignore show-off burping. Some kids learn how to swallow air to make themselves burp. "This can become an irritating habit, one that may drive you crazy," says Dr. Garcia. If the burping is intentional, he recommends that you try to ignore it. "If the behavior doesn't get a lot of attention, it will probably decrease," he says.

Blame it on the drip. If your child suffers with postnasal drip, the constant dripping and subsequent air swallowing may cause burping. "If this is the problem, treat the postnasal drip," says Dr. Jelin.

Make mealtime more leisurely. Your child may burp excessively if he tends to bolt down his food and dash out the door. "It helps if your child sits down to a leisurely meal and stops gobbling," says Dr. Hertzberg.

CANKER SORES

Ousting the Ouch from the Mouth

If your child yelps from pain after a sip of orange juice, he might be suffering from a canker sore. These tiny round craters on your child's mouth, tongue or gums just wait for something acidic like orange juice to come along and sting them into action. The official name for canker sores—*aphthous ulcers*—means "fire sores." And if your child is one of the unlucky ones who is prone to getting them, it won't take you long to understand how this painful eruption got its name.

MEDICAL ALERT

When to See the Doctor

"Any sore in the mouth that lasts more than two weeks ought to be examined by a physician," says David N. F. Fairbanks, M.D., clinical professor of otolaryngology at George Washington University School of Medicine in Washington, D.C., and a spokesperson for the American Academy of Otolaryngology/Head and Neck Surgery.

A physician may prescribe a chewable antibiotic to cut down on any oral bacteria that could be prolonging the healing process, says Dr. Fairbanks. Or he may numb and cauterize the sore. If he chooses this particular option, he'll also probably apply silver nitrate, which will cause a dense scab to form over the sore's top. The scab will allow the sore to heal and also protect it from the digestive action of saliva.

"Most of the pain comes from mouth acids and digestive enzymes," says David N. F. Fairbanks, M.D., clinical professor of otolaryngology at George Washington University School of Medicine in Washington, D.C., and a spokesperson for the American Academy of Otolaryngology/Head and Neck Surgery. "The sore is a break in the surface that allows those acids to seep underneath the surface and literally eat away at the gum."

Canker sores usually appear one at a time, settling inside the lips or cheeks—especially where the gums meet the inside edge of the lips. They're usually caused or aggravated by certain foods, stress or some superficial irritation like nibbling on the inside of lips and cheeks. Fortunately, they only take up residence for a week or so and then disappear. While they're on their way out, however, the following tips may help your kid feel better.

Neutralize that acid. "Have your child chew chewable Tums, Rolaids, Maalox Plus or Pepto-Bismol to cut down on the acid in his mouth when he has a canker sore," suggests Dr. Fairbanks. "As many as one Tums or Rolaids every three to four hours is safe for a child."

Douse the fire with water. "Have your child rinse his mouth three or four times a day with lukewarm water to clean the area and make it feel better," says Paul Rehder, M.D., a pediatric dermatologist in private practice in Oxnard, California.

Coat it. Apply a protective gel such as Zilactin, after first drying the sore with a cotton swab, suggests Dr. Fairbanks. Use as often as the package directs.

Numb it. "Get your child anesthetic lozenges to suck on," says Dr. Fairbanks. He recommends lozenges containing benzocaine, such as Chloraseptic, available at most pharmacies. A cold Popsicle or a cool bowl of Jell-O can also do the trick.

Tackle the inflammation. "Acetaminophen [Children's Tylenol], an anti-inflammatory, helps reduce the discomfort for some children suffering from canker sores," says Dr. Fairbanks. Check the package directions for the correct dosage for your child's age and weight. If your child is under age two, consult a physician.

Avoid nuts that irritate. If your child seems prone to canker sores, you should have him avoid nuts and peanut butter, suggests Dr. Fairbanks. (Walnuts and pecans are especially pain-provoking—and so is coconut.)

Cancel the candy bars. Sweets and chocolate frequently induce canker sores. "Therefore, for some kids, eating an Almond Joy, Snickers or virtually any chocolate-nut candy bar will result in misery the next day. Such bars frequently contain sugar, chocolate, coconut *and* nuts," says Dr. Fairbanks.

Axe the acids. Highly acidic foods or juices can be real yowl-raisers, says Dr. Fairbanks. These foods include pineapple, grapes, plums, tomatoes and all forms of citrus fruit.

Supply something chewy. If your child is in the habit of biting the insides of his cheeks and getting canker sores,

WHEN TROUBLE COMES IN BUNCHES

If a child gets a whole group of canker sores on the back of his throat, it's a condition called herpangina, according to David N. F. Fairbanks, M.D., clinical professor of otolaryngology at George Washington University School of Medicine in Washington, D.C., and a spokesperson for the American Academy of Otolaryngology/Head and Neck Surgery. Those clusters of sores, caused by a virus, can continue spreading from the tonsil up onto the soft area of the palate and beyond, advises Dr. Fairbanks.

"This whole crop of sores, which won't appear anywhere else in the mouth, hurts like mad," he says.

Fortunately, once a child has had herpangina, she can't get it again. Treat it the same as you would regular canker sores, says Dr. Fairbanks, and in five to seven days the whole crop will disappear.

you might want to suggest that he chew some sugarless gum when he gets stressed or hungry, says Dr. Fairbanks. "Anything that scratches the inside of the mouth will trigger a canker sore in someone who's susceptible."

Brush the old-fashioned way. "Avoid electric or rotary toothbrushes if your child tends to suffer from canker sores," warns Dr. Fairbanks. The vigorous brushing provided by mechanical devices may also scratch the gum and initiate the canker formation process, he says.

Ditch an old brush. An old brush can also contribute to sores, adds Timothy Durham, D.D.S., assistant professor of dentistry at the University of Nebraska Medical Center College of Dentistry in Omaha. "If your child's toothbrush frays, she can scratch the soft tissues of her gum." And with some kids, that's all a canker sore needs to get started.

CAVITIES

Learning to Live Without

Look, Ma, no cavities!" beams the cherubic-faced child in the television commercial. And that's exactly what every parent likes to hear.

A clean report—"No cavities!"—is quite possible these days, according to Luke Matranga, D.D.S., president of the Academy of General Dentistry and chairman of the Department of Comprehensive Dental Care at Creighton University Dental School in Omaha.

Of course, nothing can substitute for good dental care, and most dentists recommend visits every six months after the age of two. But along with the dentist's attention, excellent at-home habits can go a long way toward preventing cavities. Here's how.

Caring for Teeth

Skip baby's bedtime bottle. Lull your baby to sleep with a lullaby—or a bottle filled with clear water—instead of a bottle with milk or juice, says Dr. Matranga. When your baby falls asleep with milk or juice in his mouth, the sugars in those beverages can decay teeth when they combine with plaque, a "film" on the teeth that encourages bacterial growth. In fact, most cases of extensive infant tooth decay are known as "baby bottle syndrome," he says.

Clean your baby's gums. Good dental habits start early—even before teeth come in. "You should get your child used to mouth care by wiping her gums with a moist, soft cloth right after she eats," says William Kuttler, D.D.S., a dentist in Dubuque, Iowa, who has been treating children for more than 20 years.

Direct the brushing. Start brushing teeth as soon as they appear, using a round-tipped, soft-bristle baby's toothbrush *without* toothpaste, says Jed Best, D.D.S., a pediatric dentist and assistant clinical professor of pediatric dentistry at Columbia University School of Dentistry in New York City.

Continue to assist your child with brushing as long as he needs it, Dr. Best advises.

"A good rule of thumb is that if your child is dexterous enough to tie his own shoes, he can probably brush his own teeth," says Dr. Best. "Until then, you can let your child do the best he can, then go over any spots he's missed."

Let your child choose the toothbrush. When your child is old enough to do the brushing, she's more likely to enjoy it if she has a toothbrush she likes—one festooned with cartoon characters, for example. "As long as the toothbrush is appropriate for a child—with a small head and soft, round-tipped, nylon bristles—your child can select it on her own," says Dr. Matranga.

Find fluoridated toothpaste. After your child has six or seven teeth, it's time for her to start using toothpaste. "Choose one that is fluoridated, but not tartar control," advises Cynthia Fong, a registered dental hygienist and assistant clinical professor in the Department of General and Hospital Dentistry at the University of Medicine and Dentistry of New Jersey/New Jersey Dental School in Newark. Some tartar-control products can be abrasive, she explains, and tartar buildup isn't a common problem in children. Also, make sure your child knows which tube of toothpaste is exclusively hers. She'll feel more important knowing that toothpaste is hers alone.

Brush twice a day. Many people—children and adults alike—do only a perfunctory job of brushing. It takes time to remove plaque and debris from teeth, and once a day isn't enough. "Your child should brush his teeth for two to three minutes at least twice a day," says Dr. Best. One brushing should be just before bed, so food particles or plaque don't remain on your child's teeth overnight.

Introduce flossing early. As soon as your toddler has two back teeth that touch, it's time to start daily flossing. But you'll be in charge of this task for quite a while—likely until your child is seven or eight, says Dr. Best. "This takes even more manual dexterity than brushing," he explains.

AVOIDING DENTAL PHOBIA

You probably know what dental phobia is—that horrible gut-churning feeling that makes you want to bolt for the car the minute you step into the dentist's office, even if you're just there for a routine checkup.

If you don't want your child to develop this irrational fear of the dentist, you need to start early. First, don't let your child sense that you expect him to be afraid of the dentist or that you're uncomfortable there. Kids are experts at picking up your feelings. "Don't make a big deal out of going to the dentist," says Philip Weinstein, Ph.D., professor at the School of Dentistry and in the psychology department at the University of Washington in Seattle. "Keep it as matter-of-fact as going to the supermarket."

Also make sure you get your child to the dentist *before* any dental problems arise, says Dr. Weinstein. This way, that first visit can be a new and exciting experience, rather than a frightening and possibly painful one. The first visit should be sometime between the first and second birthday.

Many dentists specialize in treating children, and a pediatric dentist might be much more experienced in this area than your own dentist. A thoughtful dentist will explain to your child what he's doing and why and give her some measure of control over the procedure. "He will suggest that the child raise her hand, for example, if something is bothering her during treatment," says Dr. Weinstein. "He might give her a mirror to watch and ask her to 'help.'"

Sit to floss. The easiest way to floss your child's teeth is to sit *behind* her while she's standing or kneeling, with her head in your lap. "Now she's in a position similar to that in a dentist's chair," says Fong. This will let you reach your child's teeth more easily and see what you're doing.

Floss in front of the TV. Flossing doesn't *have* to be done in the bathroom. If your child gets impatient while you're flossing his teeth, change locations. "Most kids will balk less about flossing if you can get him to a place he likes," says Dr. Matranga. "So park yourself in front of the televi-

TEST THE TEETH-CLEANING ROUTINE

Okay, you've bought a fluoride toothpaste and a brightly colored toothbrush for your child, you've showed him how to brush and floss and you check the toothbrush every night to be sure it's wet.

Your job is done, right?

Wrong. Your child could be conscientiously brushing and flossing daily and *still* not be getting his teeth clean. To check, use special disclosing tablets you can get from your dentist, says John Brown, D.D.S., a dentist in private practice in Claremont, California, and past president of the Academy of General Dentistry.

Have your child chew the tablet after he brushes. If the brushing job hasn't been adequate and some plaque remains, those spots will be stained red temporarily. And you'll know that you (or your child) need to brush his teeth more thoroughly.

You should also control how much toothpaste your child squeezes out onto the toothbrush, says Cynthia Fong, a registered dental hygienist and assistant clinical professor in the Department of General and Hospital Dentistry at the University of Medicine and Dentistry of New Jersey/New Jersey Dental School in Newark. A pea-size amount is just right, she says.

"If you use too little toothpaste, your child doesn't get its full anti-cavity value, and if you use too much, your child will wind up swallowing a good deal of the toothpaste," warns Fong. She also suggests that you keep toothpaste out of the reach of children who might be tempted to eat it. Although it doesn't happen often, getting too much fluoride by swallowing or eating toothpaste can cause tooth mottling.

sion, place your child's head in your lap and do the flossing there."

Try a mechanical toothbrush or an irrigator. The buzz of a special mechanical appliance can make daily tooth care more appealing to some children—and can cut the time required as well. "Electric or battery-operated toothbrushes do an excellent job of cleaning the teeth, in about half the time of manual brushing," says Dr. Matranga. Oral irrigators that shoot a stream of water onto the teeth help get food particles out from between teeth. But parents shouldn't assume that oral irrigation is a substitute for brushing and flossing, he says.

Preventing Tooth Decay

Eat less often. There's a reason many dentists recommend limiting between-meal snacks. Whenever your child eats, the teeth are bathed in food particles and sugars that can cause decay. "The more often food comes in contact with teeth, the more chance there is for decay," explains Dr. Matranga. If your child brushes after each snack, the damage is limited.

Pick snack foods carefully. Some snacks are worse for teeth than others, notes Dr. Kuttler. Dentists say the *best* choices are cheese, air-popped popcorn and raw vegetables. Fresh fruit is also acceptable, according to Dr. Kuttler, but it's not a first choice because fruit contains natural sugars. Candy, high-carbohydrate snacks such as cookies and cakes, and dried fruit are poor choices because they leave a sticky residue on the teeth that encourages decay. "And the worst culprit is soda, because of its acid and sugar content," Dr. Kuttler says, and juice can also be harmful.

This doesn't mean you have to deny your child these foods or drinks, but your child should only eat or drink them when he can brush afterward, advises Dr. Kuttler.

Grasp at straws. If your child does drink soda or juice, she can minimize the potential tooth damage by drinking from a straw. The straw directs the beverage *past* the teeth, so they aren't "bathed" in sugars. "A straw limits the time the drink is in contact with the teeth," says Dr. Kuttler. "So less damage is done."

Rinse with water. After your child has had a snack or a meal, have him swish plain water in his mouth. "This re moves some of the loose food particles and sugar," says

Fong. Brushing is better, notes Fong, but when a toothbrush isn't available, swishing is better than nothing.

Supply sugarless gum. Gum is another option: Chewing on sugarless gum for about 20 minutes can help clean teeth, says John Brown, D.D.S., a dentist in private practice in Claremont, California, and past president of the Academy of General Dentistry. "Chewing gum stimulates saliva flow, and saliva helps clear debris and plaque-forming substances from the teeth," explains Dr. Brown.

Set a good example. If your child sees you brushing and flossing your teeth and choosing snacks that are healthy for your teeth, it's more likely that she will do the same. "Good tooth care is a learned behavior," says Dr. Kuttler. "If parents put a high value on their own dental health, their children are much more likely to want to do the same."

CHAPPED LIPS

Soothe That Kisser

I t's one thing to watch your child lick her lips in anticipation of eating a yummy ice cream cone. It's quite another to watch her lick her lips over and over—trying without success to ease the irritation that comes from chapped lips.

Fortunately, your child needn't suffer if you use these tips from our experts.

Slather on petroleum jelly. "Wet your child's chapped lips 10 to 20 times a day with cool water for about 30 seconds and then slather on a thick coating of Vaseline petroleum jelly," says Paul Rehder, M.D., a pediatric dermatologist in private practice in Oxnard, California. "The Vaseline doesn't taste that good, but even when habitual lip-lickers lick their lips, the saliva won't get through the Vaseline."

Keep a lip balm in your kid's pocket. Any readily available lip balm such as ChapStick is suitable for use by kids with chapped lips, says Rodney S. W. Basler, M.D., assistant professor of dermatology at the University of Nebraska Medical Center in Omaha. But it has to be reapplied every time your child eats or drinks anything. Otherwise it won't work.

Don't go for flavored lip balms. Ignore the pleas of your child for such exotic lip-balm flavors as Mucho Mocha or Torrid Tangelo, suggests Dr. Rehder. "Some kids like to eat the flavored kinds right off their lips, causing even worse chapping. Stick with the unflavored lip balms instead. They're more likely to stay where they're needed," he says.

Go for the sunscreen combo. "It's a good idea to protect your children's lips from cancer as well as from chapping," says Dr. Basler. Regularly apply a lip balm that contains sunscreen whenever your child goes outdoors.

Borrow from the bees. Carmex, an over-the-counter product that comes in a little tin and is made of beeswax and phenol, is better than any prescription medicine for chapped lips, says Dr. Basler. If regular lip balm isn't strong enough to help your child, Carmex might do the trick

Heal with hydrocortisone. For chapping that refuses to yield to either lip balm or Carmex, try an over-the-counter 1 percent hydrocortisone ointment, says Dr. Basler.

Encourage less licking. Chapping is caused by dehydration. So if your child's lips feel dry, she'll automatically lick them to restore moisture. Unfortunately, as soon as the moisture from licking evaporates, her lips will be drier than ever.

With older children, you should discuss what's causing their lips to be chapped, suggests Dr. Basler. They may not understand how evaporation causes the problem, but they can certainly understand how licking the lips can make them hurt even more. With a few reminders, your child can become aware of this habit—and stop herself from doing it.

CHAPPED SKIN

The Best of the Balms

Scratch, scratch, scratch, scratch.

"Kevin, stop that!" Kevin looks up at you with a frown. Telling him to stop scratching his dry, chapped little arms isn't much help. What do you expect him to do? his frown seems to ask.

Fortunately, there are several things *you* can do to soothe Kevin's chapped skin—and a dozen more things you can do to keep it from recurring.

First, it helps to understand that water is what keeps the outer skin layer soft. Chapped skin is a result of dehydration. It frequently runs in families and is most common during the late fall and winter months in northern states, although any child can get it anytime, no matter where he happens to be.

Fortunately, there are a number of things a parent can do. When some part of your child's skin is rough, red, itchy and scaly, try these expert remedies.

Treatment

Apply bath oil directly to the skin. "Skin hydrates from the inside out, so apply a good bath oil directly onto your child's skin after bathing," says Rodney S. W. Basler, M.D., assistant professor of dermatology at the University of Ne-

---

MEDICAL ALERT

When to See the Doctor

If your child is itchy over a wide area of his body, or if his skin is cracking, seek professional help, says Rodney S. W. Basler, M.D., assistant professor of dermatology at the University of Nebraska Medical Center in Omaha. Bacteria can invade the skin through such cracks and cause infections.

braska Medical Center in Omaha. The oil puts a barrier on the skin to keep moisture from evaporating into the ozone.

"Use a good bath oil like Alpha-Keri," says Dr. Basler. "Apply it to your child's skin while he's still damp, to lock in moisture." But he advises against baby oil, because that just sits *on* the skin rather than being dispersed *into* the skin. (Bath oils have ingredients that act as dispersants to make sure oil gets into the top skin layer.)

Smear it. "If your child drools in his sleep, the skin around his mouth may get chapped," says Dr. Basler. Use petroleum jelly or zinc oxide (which comes in an ointment) just in the mouth area to protect the skin from chapping. Apply it right after his bath and before bed.

Start the moisturizer habit. "Teach your child to use a light, unscented moisturizing lotion whenever she washes her hands," says Dr. Basler. "She can apply the moisturizer anywhere her skin tends to get dry," Keep a squirt bottle handy on the sink—right beside the soap.

Leave the desert. A room humidifier is a must, says Dr. Basler. Ask your pharmacist for advice on models, then buy the best you can afford and place it in the room where your child spends most of his home time. It will not only help relieve his dry, chapped skin, but will help prevent any recurrence as well.

Preventive Care

Play dirty. "Teach your child to take a five-minute shower or a short bath," suggests Jane S. Wada, M.D., a dermatologist in private practice in Montrose, California. "Twice a week or every other other night is enough for young kids. Older children who are more active can supplement their baths and showers with sponge baths to clean the essential areas."

Soft-soap it. "Don't let your child wash her face with a harsh soap that strips oil from her skin," says Dr. Basler.

"Cleansing bars like Dove are the best. Deodorant soaps are the worst."

Spot clean the pertinent parts. "If your tiny baby's skin is dry, don't use soap when bathing her," says Dr. Wada. With a newborn's skin, all you really need to do is spot-clean the folds—particularly around the knees, neck and diaper area.

Skip the powder. Avoid following a bath with either talc or powder, says Dr. Basler. Both can dry the skin.

Rinse well. "Be sure your kids rinse their mouths well if they're using a fluoride toothpaste," says Dr. Basler. Fluoride toothpaste is a known irritant to skin. If a smear of toothpaste dries on your child's chin, or he drools during sleep, the toothpaste residue may irritate the chin and cause chapping.

Banish bubbles. Avoid bubble baths if your child tends to chap easily, says Dr. Wada. "Bubbles irritate the skin."

Pat-a-cake. Always pat your child dry, and teach her to do the same, suggests Dr. Wada. Rubbing with a towel can chafe the skin and set the stage for chapping.

Dress your child in soft clothes. "Irritating clothing contributes to chapping, especially when it's made of coarse fibers like wool," says Dr. Basler. Be especially aware that denim has a tendency to chafe the skin, particularly when it gets wet.

Choose mild detergent. Some very strong detergent soaps—particularly those with additives—cause chapping, says Dr. Basler. After all, the word "detergent" means "to take out oil." Avoid using strong detergents on your child's clothing until the chapped areas have cleared up. Try Dreft or Ivory Snow instead. The detergent residues on your child's freshly laundered clothes are just as likely to take out oil as the detergent in your washer.

Toss out dryer sheets. The residue from dryer sheets impregnated with fabric softener can also cause chapped skin, says Dr. Basler. It stays on the clothes and may leach moisture out of your child's skin. Instead of using sheets, switch to a liquid softener, he suggests. Or try one that's combined with your detergent.

Go from pool to shower. Children can get chapped skin just from getting out of a swimming pool and toweling down, says Paul Rehder, M.D., a pediatric dermatologist in private practice in Oxnard, California. The towel roughs up the top layer of skin and dries it out.

Instead of toweling down when the swim session is over, either have your child take a cool shower or sprinkle cool water on his skin for two or three minutes, suggests the dermatologist. "Then apply a moisturizer like Vaseline to trap water in the skin."

CHICKENPOX

Tips for Minimal Misery

A t first your child just doesn't feel well. "Sorta tired," is all he can tell you. When you put him to bed, you notice one little bump on his tummy—maybe a bug bite, you think.

In the morning, that little bump has been joined by a flock of others, and some of them show tiny clear water blisters.

Say hello to the chickenpox.

It's a fairly harmless malady that can strike babies and children as well as adults. For a week or more, the discomfort is almost continual. First there may be mild fever, then blisters, itching and, finally, scabbing. In very rare cases, chickenpox can lead to more serious ailments.

For parents, this uncomfortable malady offers just one consolation: After your child has had it, chickenpox are usually gone for good. (Unless, that is, you have another

MEDICAL ALERT

When to See the Doctor

In rare cases, the chickenpox virus can cause encephalitis, and it has also been linked to Reye's syndrome. Both ailments are life-threatening brain inflammations, so give your pediatrician a call if you have *any* doubts about your child's symptoms, advises William Howatt, M.D., professor of pediatrics in the Department of Pediatrics and Communicable Diseases at the University of Michigan Medical School in Ann Arbor. And always contact your pediatrician when your chickenpox patient has:

- Fever after the sores have begun to scab over.
- High fever accompanied by severe headache, vomiting, disorientation or convulsions.
- Pain when the neck is stretched.

You should also contact the doctor if your child has more than a few sores that are excessively swollen, red or painful. These may be infected. Your doctor may want to prescribe antibiotics.

susceptible child in the house who hasn't been through it before.)

Here's how the experts suggest you keep your child with chickenpox as comfortable as possible.

Supply pain relief. If the fever or itching is making your child unbearably uncomfortable, you can give her acetaminophen (Children's Tylenol), says William Howatt, M.D., professor of pediatrics in the Department of Pediatrics and Communicable Diseases at the University of Michigan Medical Center in Ann Arbor. Check the package directions for the correct dosage for your child's age and weight. If your child is under age two, consult a physician. If the fever isn't making your child uncomfortable, however, don't try to lower it: "It's actually one of the body's disease-fighting mechanisms," explains Dr. Howatt.

And *never* give a child with chickenpox aspirin, because it has been linked with Reye's syndrome, a potentially life-threatening complication, says Dr. Howatt.

Dress your child lightly. "The cooler you can keep your child's skin in the first 48 to 72 hours, the less discomfort he'll have," says F. T. Fitzpatrick, M.D., a pediatrician in private practice in Doylestown, Pennsylvania. Avoid bundling your child up, and dress him lightly in cotton clothing or pajamas. Cotton is the best choice because it's the least irritating to the skin, he says.

Supply cooling relief. Another way to help lower your child's temperature is to bathe her skin with a cool cloth or put her in a cool bath, says J. Owen Hendley, M.D., professor of pediatrics and head of pediatric infectious diseases at the University of Virginia School of Medicine at Charlottesville. Be sure the water isn't so cold your child shivers, however.

Try an itch-relieving bath. A bath in colloidal oatmeal— oatmeal that's been ground to a fine powder—can help soothe the itch, says Kenneth R. Keefner, Ph.D., a pharmacist and associate professor of pharmacy in the School of Pharmacy and Allied Health Professions at Creighton University in Omaha. You can find this product at most pharmacies under the brand name Aveeno, and directions for use are on the box. But take special care that your child doesn't try to stand in the bath, because this product can make the bathtub quite slippery, says Dr. Keefner.

Or soothe with soda. Baking soda is a perfectly good substitute for colloidal oatmeal, according to Dr. Keefner. Stir about a half-cup of baking soda into a shallow bath or a full cup in a deep bath. Use a washcloth to spread the bath water over all affected areas of skin.

Cool the itchy spots. If your child has one or two spots that are particularly itchy, wring out a washcloth in cool water, lay it on the area for five minutes and repeat as needed. "Coolness on the site of the itch can counteract the itching," says Dr. Hendley. If the cloth is rough on one side, however, put the *smooth* side next to the skin to avoid irritation, he suggests.

Keep your child fresh and clean. Children with chickenpox should get a daily shower and shampoo to keep the sores clean and help prevent infection, says Dr. Fitzpatrick. Also, while it may be tempting to let your groggy child fall asleep in the same pajamas she's worn all day, she should have a clean pair for the night, he says. (If your child is still in diapers, they should be changed frequently.) Not only is the clean clothing comforting, but the change can reduce the risk of the sores getting infected.

Try to control the scratching. If your child is old enough to understand, explain that he should try not to scratch, because scratching can cause infection or scarring. But chances are your child can't *completely* ignore the raging itch all the time, so supply a cool, wet washcloth he can scratch gently with, suggests Dr. Hendley. "This will help keep him from ripping his skin open," he says.

Clip nails short. Trim your child's fingernails as soon as chickenpox strikes—and keep them trimmed short, says Dr. Fitzpatrick. Even after the worst is over, he recommends trimming the nails twice a week for several weeks afterward. Scratching with sharp nails can lead to a bacterial infection in the sores, and that can lead to permanent scarring.

Treat with an antibiotic. If a few of the pox show signs of infection such as redness around them or the presence of pus in open pox, apply an over-the-counter antibiotic ointment such as Neosporin or Polysporin, says Dr. Keefner. "But if more than a few of the sores are infected, contact your pediatrician," he cautions.

Control the itch with an antihistamine. "An oral over-the-counter antihistamine, like Benadryl Elixir, may help control the itching," says Dr. Hendley. "But even if it doesn't, at least it will make your child sleepy so he can get some of the rest he needs." Be sure to read package directions to make certain the product is recommended for your child's age. For the correct dosage, follow package directions or consult your physician. Some doctors don't advise Benadryl cream or spray because it could cause a reaction.

Or try calamine lotion with phenol. This type of calamine lotion works as a topical anesthetic and can help with the itching, says Edward DeSimone, Ph.D., a pharmacist and associate professor of pharmacy administrative and social sciences in the School of Pharmacy and Allied Health Professions at Creighton University. Just dab it on particularly itchy pox. Because this product can be absorbed through the skin, you want to apply it *just* to the pox— not smear it all over, says Dr. DeSimone. "Also, make sure that you don't exceed package directions, which specify that this lotion should not be used more than three or four times a day."

Avoid OTC topical hydrocortisone. These kinds of steroid creams and ointments are available in pharmacies and are ordinarily used to fight inflammation and itch, says Dr. Keefner. They will, however, inhibit the child's own immune system from fighting the virus in the area where it is applied and may even allow the pox virus to generate further, he says.

Keep your kids out of the sun. Children who have recently had chickenpox—as well as those who may be just about to come down with it—should be extra careful about sun exposure, says Dr. Fitzpatrick.

"Children who become sunburned during the incubation period of chickenpox, especially if they're close to the breakout time, will have a much worse case," he says. So if you know chickenpox is going around, keep your child off any sun-drenched playing fields or apply sunscreen with an SPF (sun protection factor) of 15 or higher.

Once the chickenpox is over, the skin remains particularly vulnerable to sunburn for about a year, says Dr. Fitzpatrick. So be especially careful with the child who has recently recovered. Again, be sure to apply sunscreen whenever he's going to be outdoors in direct sun.

CHOLESTEROL

Keep It under Control

Walk by an elementary school classroom and you'll see a bustle of activity—and a roomful of apparently healthy kids. It's tough to believe that some of these kids may already be on their way to developing heart disease—also known as coronary artery disease.

There's growing evidence that coronary artery disease begins in childhood. Studies have shown that as many as 25 children out of 100 have borderline high levels of blood cholesterol, the goo that helps make artery-clogging plaque. Often, the cause of high cholesterol in kids is a high-fat diet coupled with a lack of exercise.

Until age two, children do need a diet that's higher in fat than the recommended diet for adults. And doctors say you *shouldn't* give low-fat milk or foods to an infant. Once your child is two, however, it's time to start watching the diet.

You may choose to have your child's cholesterol level checked. But whether or not you know cholesterol levels, experts agree that childhood is the time to begin patterns that will last a lifetime and—studies show—prolong life. If you encourage a healthy diet and lifestyle for your children, you will help prevent high cholesterol and future heart disease. Here's how.

Turn off the television. Excessive TV watching is linked to high cholesterol in children, points out Saundra MacD. Hunter, Ph.D., research professor at Tulane University School of Public Health in New Orleans. Researchers in California who studied 1,100 children found that kids who watched television more than two hours a day were twice as likely as non-TV viewers to have high cholesterol levels.

To help limit viewing, give each child an allotment of a certain number of hours per week. Together, design a colorful chart where the child records her viewing. Or simply select specific programs the children can watch, and don't allow the television on at other times. You can also adopt this strategy for children who want to play video games for hours at a time.

Get the kids moving. "Ideally, kids should do some form of aerobic exercise at least three times a week," advises Peter Kwiterovich, Jr., M.D., professor of pediatrics and director of the Lipid Research Clinic at the Johns Hopkins University School of Medicine in Baltimore. To get the most benefit, children should exercise 20 minutes or longer—which shouldn't be at all difficult for active kids. "Any sport where the arms and legs are constantly in motion is good—bicycling, running, walking, swimming," he says.

Make low-fat dairy choices. Parents should limit the amount of fat in the diet of any child over the age of two, according to Matthew W. Gillman, M.D., assistant professor of medicine, pediatrics and public health at Boston University School of Medicine. You can help reduce your child's fat intake by limiting butter, margarine and high-fat dairy products such as whole milk, sour cream and ice cream. Whenever possible, use low-fat or nonfat substitutes. Many children like reduced-fat cottage cheese or yogurt, for instance.

Keep an eye on high-fat culprits. Instead of stocking up on chips and cheese curls, keep lower-fat pretzels, graham crackers or low-fat crackers in your cupboard, suggest Rebecca Pestle, R.D., a clinical nutritionist at Crawford Long Hospital of Emory University in Atlanta. For lunches avoid bologna, hamburgers and hot dogs that are usually high in fat. Your child will be better off with a lunch of low-fat cheese or fresh turkey or a chicken sandwich instead.

Switch gradually. Your family may rebel if you abruptly ditch whole milk, mayonnaise, ice cream, chips and fatty lunch meat and immediately switch to lower-fat products. Make changes gradually, suggests Pestle. "Go from whole milk to 2 percent, for example, then to 1 percent and finally to skim," she says. "Or use skim milk and add dry milk to it to give it a richer taste without adding fat." When you replace high-fat snacks and lunch meats with healthier choices, do it gradually rather than all at once.

Choose natural peanut butter. Peanut butter—like all foods made from plants—is cholesterol-free, but some types are healthier than others. The only fat in *natural* peanut butter—which contains only peanuts and sometimes salt—is peanut oil, which is a monounsaturated fat. Monounsaturated fats—when substituted for saturated fats—can help reduce the body's "bad" cholesterol, says Pestle. But most brands of peanut butter that are creamy or smooth contain hydrogenated vegetable oil, a saturated fat that can increase blood cholesterol levels.

Supply plenty of produce. Serve plenty of fruits and vegetables, suggests Dr. Gillman. Aim at five servings of these foods a day. They're not only low in fat, but are considered important disease fighters as well.

Take your children shopping with you—one at a time to prevent bedlam—and let them help select the produce. "Children are more likely to eat foods they've helped pick out," says Pestle.

Increase fiber intake. Fiber is another cholesterol-fighter. "Add oat bran and fruit to muffins or bread recipes," suggests Pestle.

Also look for legumes, such as beans and lentils, and whole grain wheat and rice. All are good sources of fiber. Even finicky kids can be tempted by interesting menus. Your child may turn up her nose at lentil soup, for example, but will likely enjoy a bowl of chili or baked beans.

Monitor your meat. Realize that you don't need to serve meat at every meal or even daily. Fish is an excellent low-fat protein source, as are beans, lentils and split peas when you combine them with grains or foods made with grains, such as rice or bread, says Pestle. Even a peanut butter sandwich served with a glass of skim milk packs a lot of protein.

Prepare meat the low-fat way. When preparing chicken, remove the skin and any visible fat, says Pestle. Your lowest-fat meat choices are turkey and chicken breasts. But you can choose other meats that are relatively low in fat.

ABOUT CHOLESTEROL SCREENING

At what age should cholesterol levels be checked? This is a controversial topic, points out Matthew W. Gillman, M.D., assistant professor of medicine, pediatrics and public health at Boston University School of Medicine, "Some experts recommend no screening whatsoever until adulthood." At the other extreme, the American Health Foundation recommends that every child have his blood cholesterol screened after age two.

A middle-of-the-road approach is to consider having cholesterol checked after age two if you are aware of a family history of early heart disease or if either parent has a cholesterol problem, suggests Peter Kwiterovich, Jr., M.D., professor of pediatrics and director of the Lipid Research Clinic at the Johns Hopkins University School of Medicine in Baltimore.

The American Academy of Pediatrics and the National Cholesterol Education Program Expert Panel (NCEP) recommend testing if any of the following risk factors are present.

- A grandparent, aunt, uncle or parent had a coronary artery bypass procedure or balloon angioplasty before age 55
- A grandparent, aunt, uncle or parent had a heart attack, stroke, angina or other cardiovascular disease before age 55
- Either parent has a cholesterol level above 240
- Your child has two or more risk factors for coronary heart disease, such as high blood pressure or obesity—or your child is exposed to cigarette smoke because someone in your household is a smoker

If you do have your child screened, realize that normal blood cholesterol levels are lower for children than adults. For children, the NCEP categorizes 170 milligrams per deciliter as acceptable, 170 to 199 as borderline and over 200 as definitely high. At borderline and high levels, your doctor will probably recommend further testing and perhaps a low-fat, low-cholesterol diet to ensure that it doesn't go any higher.

When selecting beef, buy the leanest cuts, such as sirloin, tenderloin, round and flank, she says. "Pork tenderloin and some hams are also very low in fat," she says. A good choice is fresh, unprocessed ham. Another tip to help you choose low-fat meat: Look for the word "loin" or "round."

And when preparing any meat, bake or broil it instead of frying to decrease the amount of fat, suggests Dr. Gillman. Also trim fat off any meat.

Check out school lunches. Many school lunches are notoriously high in fat and salt. Visit your child's school or look at the menus for a couple of weeks to determine whether your child's school offers low-fat choices, says Dr. Kwiterovich. "If your child's school lunches are too fatty, you should pack lunches," he says. Good lunch box selections are fruit or dried fruit; carrot and celery sticks; graham crackers, bagels or low-fat muffins; yogurt; popcorn or pretzels; low-fat cookies, such as vanilla wafers, fig bars or ginger snaps, and low-fat cheese, lean ham, natural peanut butter or chicken or turkey sandwiches.

Make changes a family affair. You can't expect your kids to exercise and eat-low fat fare when you're lounging on the sofa eating hamburgers and fries. "Children learn best by example," says Pestle. "If you set a good one, they're more likely to follow." And the foods you keep in the house should only be the ones your kids are allowed to eat, he adds.

Don't go overboard. Don't go nuts when it comes to cutting fat out of your family's diet. Not only can this backfire—your kids may get rebellious and sneak off to spend their allowance money on snacks at the corner convenience store—but you can actually reduce the fat and calories in a child's diet too much for optimal health, says Dr. Kwiterovich. "Moderation is the key," he says.

COLDS

The Fewer Caught, the Better

Some kids seem to have a cold brewing almost all the time, which is not surprising when you consider that approximately 200 viruses can cause the common cold. Most of these cold viruses are extremely hardy. They can survive for several hours on hands, clothing and hard surfaces as well as in the air, giving your child ample opportunity to pick up something infectious somewhere. Small wonder, then, that most kids average about six colds every year.

Spending seven days—more or less—soothing a child with a cold isn't most parents' idea of a good time. Before a typical cold runs its course, you'll have to deal with sniffles and sneezes, stuffiness and coughs, runny nose and scratchy throat, maybe even a low-grade fever. But it's reassuring to know that these symptoms seldom turn out to be serious.

"The vast majority of kids—even infants—do just fine with a cold," says Michael Macknin, M.D., head of the Section of General Pediatrics at the Cleveland Clinic Foundation in Ohio, clinical professor at Pennsylvania State University Medical School in Hershey and associate professor of pediatrics at Ohio State University Medical School in Columbus. "It's a very common ailment that rarely causes a problem," he says.

That doesn't mean that you should just ignore your child's cold, however. Although there is no cure for a cold virus (antibiotics only vanquish bacterial infections, such as those that cause strep throat or ear infection), you can give your child some relief from annoying symptoms. And you may be able to prevent some colds entirely. Here's what the experts suggest.

Boost immunity by breastfeeding your baby. "To prevent colds in infants—as best we can—it pays to breastfeed," notes Naomi Grobstein, M.D., a family physician in private practice in Montclair, New Jersey.

MEDICAL ALERT

When to See the Doctor

As long as your child has no fever and is eating and sleeping well despite her cold, there is no reason to go to the doctor, says Flavia Marino, M.D., a clinical instructor in pediatrics at New York University Medical Center, Tisch Hospital, and a pediatrician in New York City. "However, if the symptoms worsen, if there is a low-grade fever (100° to 101°) for a few days or if the fever shoots higher, it's time for a visit to the pediatrician. Your child may have a bacterial infection rather than a cold," says Dr. Marino.

If your child's runny nose and cough haven't improved after ten days, your child may have a sinus infection. "Sinusitis may follow a cold because the sinuses become inflamed and can't drain properly," says Michael Macknin, M.D., head of the Section of General Pediatrics at the Cleveland Clinic Foundation in Ohio, clinical professor at Pennsylvania State University Medical School in Hershey and associate professor of pediatrics at Ohio State University Medical School in Columbus.

Sinus infections are particularly common among pre-schoolers. "For a child under age 6 who's had a runny nose with or without a cough for ten days and isn't getting better, chances are close to 90 percent there's a sinus infection," Dr. Macknin says. For 6- to 12-year-olds, chances are 70 percent. Unlike a cold virus, a sinus infection should be treated with doctor-prescribed antibiotics, he adds.

"Breastfeeding can provide extra protection against those cold viruses to which the mother has already developed an immunity," she says.

Go easy on the acetaminophen for fever. "You don't have to treat a low-grade fever," says Dr. Grobstein. "Fever mobilizes the immune system and helps fight off infection." But if you choose to treat the fever because your child is intolerably uncomfortable, use acetaminophen—Children's Tylenol or any other brand, she suggests. Check the package directions for the correct dosage for your child's age and weight. If your child is under age two, consult a physician. "You should never give aspirin to your child with a virus," she adds, "because it has been linked to Reye's syndrome, a serious disease that affects the brain and liver."

Smooth something soothing on a sore nose. "Most children are not bothered by a runny nose, except when the skin around it becomes chapped and raw from frequent wiping," says Flavia Marino, M.D., a clinical instructor in pediatrics at New York University Medical Center, Tisch Hospital, and a pediatrician in New York City. To prevent that, she recommends applying a layer of petroleum jelly just beneath your child's nose as often as necessary.

Ask for hand washing. "Cold viruses are frequently transmitted through hand contact," says Dr. Macknin. "So simple hand washing is the best way to prevent the spread of infection." And be sure your child uses soap when she washes up, he says.

Put the squeeze on excess mucus. During the first few months of life, babies have a harder time than the rest of us if they're forced to breathe through the mouth, notes Dr. Marino. "Nasal blockage caused by a cold may make it difficult for an infant to nurse or drink from a bottle," she says. "But you can make breathing easier for your baby with the help of saline (saltwater) drops and a rubber suction bulb."

You can purchase saline solution (sold under brand names such as Ayr Saline Nasal Mist and Ocean) from a pharmacy. Or you can mix your own, dissolving ¼ teaspoon of salt in 1 cup of lukewarm water. "Put a couple drops into your child's nose and wait a few moments," says Dr. Marino. "Then squeeze the suction bulb and then insert the tip gently into one nostril. Slowly release the bulb to suction out mucus." After you dispose of the mucus in a tissue, repeat the procedure for the other nostril, he says. Be sure to sterilize the bulb afterward in boiling water.

Serve warm liquids. Offer your child plenty of warm drinks or soup, suggests Dr. Grobstein. "Warm liquids help relieve congestion, and they can also soothe a sore throat," she says.

Mix a mild gargle. Another way to soothe a sore throat is to have your child gargle with warm water in which some salt has been dissolved, says Dr. Marino. This can be repeated several times a day, she says.

Don't squelch a daytime cough. "Coughing is a protective mechanism that keeps bacteria and debris out of the lungs," says Dr. Marino. So leave the cough alone during the day. If coughing is keeping your child up at night, though, an over-the-counter cough suppressant may help him sleep, she says. "Check with your physician for the appropriate dosage," says Dr. Marino, "and schedule an office visit if the cough lingers for more than a few days or if fever persists."

Say okay to school. "Unless he has a fever or feels really lousy, there is no reason to make your child stay indoors or keep him home from school just because he has a cold," says Dr. Grobstein.

Ditch the decongestants and antihistamines. These over-the-counter cold medicines have never been proven effective for kids under the age of five, says Dr. Macknin. "They may work, but there's not a single article in the scientific literature for the last 40 years that support their use," he says.

Dr. Macknin concedes that decongestants, at least, may offer some symptomatic relief, but both types of remedies have side effects. "Decongestants may make a child hyperactive, and antihistamines may make him sleepy," he says. "And in some instances, kids may have other, more unusual or severe reactions."

The bottom line, Dr. Macknin says, is that cold medications won't make the cold go away faster. So unless your child feels truly miserable, don't use them.

Check for stress. Studies have shown there is a link between stress and illness. "When your child is very fatigued, worn out or under a lot a stress, she is more likely to become ill with a cold," Dr. Macknin says. If you discover that your child is facing a stressful situation, either at play or at school, consider what steps can be taken to relieve her concerns. Pressure at school, trouble with friends or too many activities may be contributing factors.

COLD SORES

Clearing Up a Pesky Problem

L ike many frustrated youngsters, Brad couldn't understand why *he*, of all people, kept getting one cold sore after another. "I don't even remember how young I was when I had my first one, but it was a real bummer having them recur as I was growing up," he says. "Every time I had an important exam or, as I got older, a big date, I could almost guarantee that I would get one."

Now as an adult, Brad Rodu, D.D.S., is a dentist whose passion is helping kids—including his own two children— avoid the cold sore anguish he suffered. It's a tough assignment because it's just about impossible to prevent exposure to the herpes simplex virus that causes cold sores (also known as fever blisters). "Herpes simplex is so prevalent that virtually all of us come in contact with at least one strain of the virus before our fifth birthday," says Dr. Rodu, professor and chairman of the Department of Oral Pathology in the School of Dentistry at the University of Alabama at Birmingham.

"A grandmother who has a cold sore, for example, transmits the virus to her grandson when she smothers him with kisses," he notes. And that is just one way the virus is typically spread. It also can be passed along by shaking hands or sharing common household items like towels or dining utensils.

MEDICAL ALERT

When to See the Doctor

Although cold sores are unsightly and uncomfortable, they rarely require a physician's care, says Brad Rodu, D.D.S., professor and chairman of the Department of Oral Pathology in the School of Dentistry at the University of Alabama at Birmingham.

You should notify your pediatrician, however, if your child has a cold sore and also complains of difficulty seeing. It could be a sign that the virus has spread to the eyes, he says.

You also should bring a cold sore to the attention of your doctor if:

- Your child is less than 12 months old.
- It is the first time your child has had an outbreak of cold sores.
- The outbreak causes numerous painful sores on the lips, cheeks and inside the mouth.
- If mouth sores last longer than one to two weeks.

Your doctor will likely prescribe an ointment containing acyclovir, an anti-viral medication used to treat severe herpes virus infections.

Once exposed, your child may get sick with a fever, fatigue and headache. Those symptoms subside after a week or two. After that, one of two things can happen, according to Dr. Rodu.

If your child is lucky, the virus will lie dormant in a nerve, perhaps for his entire lifetime, without causing any further trouble. On the other hand, one in ten children will develop a patch of itchy blisters on the lips, gums, fingers, nostrils or even the eyes anytime from weeks to years after exposure to the virus. These small blisters rupture to form one large blister that eventually breaks and oozes, forming a yellow-crusted cold sore. After about seven to ten days, the sore disappears. Fortunately, many kids who experience this will never have another outbreak. But some children do continue to get them, off and on, for years afterward.

Often, these recurring cold sores appear during stress or illness or after exposure to sunlight or a cold wind. Once a sore forms, little can be done to shorten its stay. But there are some ways to prevent them and to make your child more comfortable if he gets one.

Try a tannic terminator. Studies conducted by Dr. Rodu show that over-the-counter drops (such as Zilactin-L) that contain tannic acid can, if applied soon enough, prevent a cold sore from forming or at least reduce its size. The key is getting your child to tell you when he begins feeling a tingling sensation in his lip. That's an early warning sign that a cold sore may appear in the next 4 to 12 hours, Dr. Rodu says.

"I tell my patients if they feel a cold sore coming on to put drops on early and often," he says. "If you apply the medication at the first sign of tingling and reapply it every hour, it will keep the sore very small."

Press a tea bag into service. Like some over-the-counter drops, tea contains tannic acid, a plant-derived substance that's used in tanning and dyeing as well as medicine. Researchers suspect that tannic acid has anti-viral properties. The over-the-counter medications are more effective, but you may want to try putting a wet tea bag on the sore for a few minutes once every hour to provide temporary relief until you can get to a drugstore.

Chill out the tingly spot. "If you put ice on your child's lip as soon as he tells you about the tingling, you'll slow the metabolic rate in the skin tissue where the herpes virus is growing. That could prevent a cold sore or at least result in a less severe outbreak," says Michael A. Siegel, D.D.S., associate professor of oral medicine and diagnostic sciences at the University of Maryland School of Dentistry in Baltimore. He suggests putting an ice cube on the affected spot for five to ten minutes, repeating about once every hour when possible.

Lubricate the site. Moisturizing ointments such as petroleum jelly help soothe the pain and prevent cracked and bleeding skin, Dr. Rodu says. Apply them as needed.

Send nourishment through a straw. "When a kid has a sore on his mouth, he tends to stop eating and drinking. That can lead to dehydration," Dr. Siegel says. "To insure that he gets an adequate amount of fluids and essential vitamins and minerals, give him things like sports drinks or liquid diet supplements that are essentially meals in a can. He can drink those through a straw so they don't come into contact with his sore lips." If your child is under four years old, however, be sure to check with you pediatrician before giving him a liquid-diet drink.

Keep those little hands busy. Urge your child not to touch the sore. He can not only spread the virus to other children that way but also, by touching the cold sore, he might cause a bacterial infection to develop at that site. "Kids naturally want to touch or pick at the sore, but you really need to make an effort to help them understand that doing so will only make the sore worse," says Ronald C. Hansen, M.D., professor of pediatrics and dermatology at the University of Arizona College of Medicine in Tucson.

Tell your child to ask you for more medication if the sore is bothersome, says Dr. Hansen. But also try to keep him occupied with distracting activities such as coloring or playing with building blocks.

Wash away the virus's chance to spread. If your child does touch the sore, make sure he washes his hands with soap and hot water immediately, says Dr. Siegel. Otherwise, he might spread the virus to others or to other parts of his body, such as the eyes or nose. In addition, wash all of his glassware, plates and eating utensils thoroughly in hot water or in a dishwasher to prevent exposing the next person who uses those items to the virus.

Go back to good-health basics. To help prevent new cold sores, make sure your child eats a balanced diet, gets regular exercise and plenty of sleep at night. "The healthier your child is, the less likely he is to get a cold sore," Dr. Rodu says.

Block out the sun. Fun in the sun can trigger a cold sore outbreak. To prevent it, make sure your child wears a lip balm that contains a sunscreen with a sun protection factor (SPF) of at least 15, Dr. Hansen advises. Reapply it every hour as necessary.

Bundle up against wintry blasts. Cold, windy weather is another infamous spark for cold sores. If your child is prone to developing sores, he should wear a ski mask or cover his face with a scarf when the wind howls and temperatures plunge, says Dr. Rodu.

Know when to stay at arm's length. If *you* get a cold sore, avoid direct contact with your child, including kissing, until it subsides. "Like the common cold, the cold sore virus is easily transmissible to someone else," Dr. Siegel explains. "Just because your child may have been previously exposed to the virus doesn't necessarily protect him from developing a fever blister."

COLIC

Calming the Chronic Crier

Your baby cries to communicate—to say that he is hungry, wet, cold, lonely, sick or bored. And if he's like most babies, he will also have fussy spells when he cries a lot for no apparent reason.

These periods of irritable crying usually fall into a pattern. Between the ages of two and six weeks, a child may cry for two to four hours a day. He may cry the most in the early evening. These fussy periods, as they become increasingly predictable, may seem endless to you, but keep in mind that they're a normal stage of development, and they won't last forever. By the time your baby is three months old, the crying should start to diminish to one to two hours a day.

If your baby has repeated episodes of crying that last for several hours at a time, be sure to consult your pediatrician. He may tell you that your baby has colic.

· A colicky baby may cry in a rhythmic pattern that often reaches a screaming level. He may clench his hands, flex his elbows and draw his legs tight against his abdomen. His face may look worried or tense, his belly seems tight and he has lots of gas. Sometimes he has a forceful expulsion of gas or a bowel movement right before or right after the bout of colic.

As many as one in five babies develops colic, yet it remains something of a medical mystery. Colic has been blamed on many things, including a hypersensitive nervous system, an immature gastrointestinal tract, food allergy and improper feeding technique. Although there is no consensus about the cause and treatment of this ailment, one thing is certain: Colic typically strikes otherwise healthy babies at age of 2 to 3 weeks and is usually over by the time the baby is 12 to 16 weeks old. And awful as it is to live through, it will not harm your baby in the long run, either physically or psychologically.

There is no surefire cure for colic except time, patience and perseverance, but some parents have found temporary relief using the following methods.

Take a systematic approach. What helps one colicky baby will do nothing for another, so you'll have to experiment to see what works with your child, says Russell S. Asnes, M.D., clinical professor of pediatrics at the College of Physicians and Surgeons at Columbia University in New York City and a pediatrician in Tenafly, New Jersey. "Take a systematic approach to determine the cause of your baby's cries," urges Dr. Asnes. "Check if he is hungry, wet, cold, wants some extra sucking on a pacifier or wants to be held. If he is warm and dry and has been fed recently, he may want company, so talk to him and rock him. If he is bored, take him out for a walk or a car ride."

No matter which approach you try, change tactics if the

crying continues for more than five minutes, says Dr. Asnes. Eventually you should hit on something that will work for your baby.

Take a cue from your baby. If you find that the more you try to comfort your inconsolable child, the more he cries, your baby's colic may be triggered by an overloaded nervous system, notes Peter A. Gorski, M.D., division head of behavioral and developmental pediatrics and assistant professor of pediatrics and psychiatry at Northwestern University Medical School in Chicago.

"If your baby has already had as much stimulation as he can handle, even calming techniques such as rocking, singing and talking softly are too much to take in and only serve to intensify your baby's irritability," says Dr. Gorski. Crying is one way for a baby to "shut out the world," observes Dr. Gorski. So when your usual methods of calming your infant aren't working, let him cry for 10 to 15 minutes and see whether he'll calm down by himself before you try anything else. "Hold the baby passively in your arms, or swaddle him and lay him down to rest," he says. "You may even find that avoiding direct eye contact helps him calm down sooner. After the crying spell, your baby should look wide awake and be ready to interact or be resting calmly. If not, consult your pediatrician." There may be a hernia or some other physical problem that's causing the prolonged irritability.

Try a regular feeding schedule. "Studies show that excessively sensitive babies are often small for their age. Their length is normal but they are thin. These babies, who indicate sensory overload by having colicky episodes, often do better with an organized pattern of caretaking," says Barry M. Lester, Ph.D., professor of psychiatry and human behavior and professor of pediatrics at Brown University School of Medicine in Providence, Rhode Island. "For some reason, organizing these babies' environment helps them organize their responses. Structure really helps," says Dr. Lester.

Help your baby gain control. "If your baby seems to be crying most of the time, take action to help him gain control over his nervous system," says Dr. Lester. "Whenever your baby is in a quiet, alert state, help him expand and lengthen this quiet time by introducing interesting toys and other objects, such as a safety mirror. Extending the calm periods helps the baby appreciate what it is to be in a quiet state and to enjoy the world. And it teaches him that he can learn to control his own irritability."

Be flexible. Feel free to try a lot of things for your colicky baby, says Dr. Lester. Turn him in a new position in the crib, seat him in an automatic swing, swaddle him or take him on an outing. "It may be hard, at first, to take a screaming child to a park or to the mall, but it might help him. Some colicky kids love that kind of stimulation and some don't. But you'll never know if it will help your own child unless you try it," he says.

Don't count on new formula. Many parents try switching to a soy formula in the hope that this will ease their baby's distress, but Dr. Gorski notes that it is very rare for colicky babies to be intolerant to milk. "A formula change usually gives that classic placebo effect. It may seem to work for a few days, but then it makes no difference," he says.

Check your feeding system. "Make sure that when you nurse or bottlefeed your baby, he is held in an upright rather than a horizontal position, and burp him well," says Dr. Asnes. "This helps prevent him from swallowing too much air, a source of discomfort. Also, if you use a bottle, check the size of the nipple hole. If it is too small, your child may be hungry—and frustrated that he can't get at the formula."

Try motion and music. Some colicky babies get temporary relief if they are swaddled and held next to your chest or carried in a front pack. Others may calm to the sound of music or the vacuum cleaner. "There are many ways to hold and soothe a baby, but there is no universal soothing method. Some techniques that work well for your baby will do nothing for another child," says Dr. Asnes.

Get support. "Don't let yourself become socially isolated. Parents of a colicky child need support." says Linda Gilkerson, Ph.D, senior consultant to the Infant Care Program at Evanston Hospital in Illinois and professor of infant studies at the Erikson Institute, which is affiliated with Loyola University in Chicago. Dr. Gilkerson advises that you turn to your pediatrician and family. "Also, make an effort to get in touch with other parents who have gone through it, since they are the ones who can truly empathize with your experience." Dr. Gilkerson suggests that you seek out a colic support group offered by a hospital, YMCA, church, synagogue or infant drop-in center.

Look for the real baby. "Try to see the child behind the tears. This little baby has a personality, and these tears are part of his personality for now, but they are not the whole baby. Focus on the other facets of his personality and realize the tears won't last forever," says Dr. Gilkerson.

Be good to yourself. Parents with a colicky child can become overwhelmed with feelings of rage, despair, guilt and inadequacy. "You have to figure out what will help you continue to have positive feelings about yourself and your baby, and do whatever you can to help yourself," says Dr. Gilkerson. At times, you may just have to hire an experienced babysitter, get out of the house and do something enjoyable.

CONSTIPATION

The Route to Regularity

Four-year-old Kara often goes three or four days without a bowel movement. That worries her mother, who is afraid Kara is constipated. But when she does go, Kara never has a problem moving her bowels. So even though her mother is worried, Kara has no complaints. Is she constipated—or not?

"Some parents think that unless a child has a bowel movement every day, there's something wrong," says Kevin Ferentz, M.D., assistant professor of family medicine at the University of Maryland School of Medicine and a family physician in Baltimore. "But regularity is a highly variable and personal thing. Even if a child has a bowel movement only twice a week, as long as there's no discomfort associated with it and the stool is relatively soft, then she's regular. She's not constipated."

In most children with true constipation, the cause is dietary, notes Dr. Ferentz. The digestive tract is designed to function best with a bulky, high-fiber diet—that means lots of whole grains, beans, fruits and vegetables. But for many kids, those aren't necessarily the foods of choice (at least, not *their* choice).

Other children, especially those being toilet trained, become constipated because of the changes they're going through, rather than their dietary habits. As part of their resistance to the training process, these kids become locked in what's been called the battle of the bowels with their parents. They literally refuse to go, and as a result their stools may become impacted.

Despite all the potential roadblocks to regularity, constipation in kids can easily be corrected and prevented. ("No child *ever* has to be constipated," says Dr. Ferentz.) Here's what you can do.

For Infants

Try a slick solution. Younger children and babies can be given glycerin suppositories. "These are very thin, bullet-shaped waxy substances that melt when they are inserted in the rectum," says Dr. Ferentz. "They relieve constipation in two ways: by stimulating the rectum and by 'greasing the skids' for smooth elimination. But use them only occasionally because regular use will make a child dependent and then they won't be able to have a bowel movement without them."

Glycerin suppositories for a child or infant can be pur-

MEDICAL ALERT

When to See the Doctor

Constipation can be a red flag for several serious physical or emotional conditions, cautions Marjorie Hogan, M.D., an instructor of pediatrics at the University of Minnesota and a pediatrician at the Hennepin County Medical Center in Minneapolis. When it occurs in infants, constipation *always* warrants a doctor's check, she says, because it can be a symptom of intestinal blockage.

Also, if your breastfed baby goes two or more days without a bowel movement, you should definitely contact your physician, according to Kevin Ferentz, M.D., assistant professor of family medicine at the University of Maryland School of Medicine and a family physician in Baltimore. For an older child, you should contact your physician if:

- Your child is in a lot of pain, his stomach is distended and he's not eating well. (This could be a blockage—or another intestinal problem.)
- There is blood in the child's stool.
- Your child seems to be withholding stools for emotional purposes, especially during toilet training.
- Your child has accidental bowel movements when he's not on the toilet. Withholding stools can, over time, lead to encopresis, a condition in which the child becomes so impacted that he loses sphincter control and some feces leaks out.

chased at any pharmacy, and directions for use are on the package.

Try using a thermometer. Once your infant's constipation is diagnosed by a physician, you can use a rectal thermometer approved for infant use to help her go. "Thoroughly lubricate the thermometer with petroleum jelly," suggests Dr. Ferentz. "Then stick it in the baby's rectum no farther than an inch-and-a-half and pull it out. Sometimes you'll get a 'present' along with the thermometer."

Try this sweet formula for relief. "For infants, a teaspoon of Karo syrup in a six- to eight-ounce bottle of formula, or ½ teaspoon in a four-ounce bottle, can soften a stool nicely," says Shirley Menard, R.N., a certified pediatric nurse practitioner and assistant professor at the University of Texas Health Science Center at San Antonio School of Nursing. The syrup draws water into the bowel and keeps stools soft, she says.

For Older Children

Give an over-the-counter laxative . . . but sparingly. If a child ten and over already has constipation, there are several over-the-counter medications that can provide relief temporarily. "For an older child, it's okay to use over-the-counter laxatives such as milk of magnesia or mineral oil," says Dr. Ferentz. "But only use them as advised by a physician. Mineral oil, in particular, shouldn't be used regularly because it interferes with the body's absorption of fat-soluble vitamins." Other laxatives, too, can cause problems if taken regularly. A child can become so dependent on them, she loses the natural urge to move her bowels.

Keep a daily food record. Write down everything your child eats and drinks each day, advises Marjorie Hogan, M.D., an instructor of pediatrics at the University of Minnesota and a pediatrician at the Hennepin County Medical Center in Minneapolis. This may allow you to pinpoint precisely what in your child's diet is causing bouts of constipation.

"If your child has been drinking a quart of milk a day, for example, you may have found the connection right there," says Dr. Hogan. Consuming too many dairy products can be constipating, she says. Other constipating foods frequently found in children's diets include applesauce, bananas and white rice.

Make some high-fiber muffins. "Dietary fiber helps keep stools soft," says Dr. Ferentz. "Unfortunately, in our society we take in way too few fiber-rich foods like fruits, vegetables, whole wheat breads and bran cereals."

WHEN A BABY GRUNTS AND GOES, ALL IS WELL

Three-week-old Jared seemed to put more effort into bowel movements than a power lifter going for a new world's record. He grunted and groaned and drew up his legs as though he were in pain. His mother, worried that her infant son was constipated, called the doctor.

"I don't think I've ever had a new mom who didn't call me to say that she thought her newborn was constipated because of all the grunting the baby was doing," says Kevin Ferentz, M.D., assistant professor of family medicine at the University of Maryland School of Medicine and a family physician in Baltimore. "Then when I ask if the stool is coming out soft, the typical response is, 'Yes, soft and watery.' When that's the answer, I know the child is not constipated."

"*All* new babies grunt," observes Dr. Ferentz. "It has nothing to do with difficulty passing the stool. Babies grunt because they don't have as much abdominal muscle strength as adults do, so they have to work at pushing the stool out. It's perfectly normal. They don't need any assistance."

You can introduce your child to fiber sources that are fun to eat. "For example, there's no reason why a child can't eat a bran muffin every day," he says. To make these muffins more appealing, add lots of raisins. "Most kids *love* raisins," notes Dr. Ferentz.

Serve snacks fit for a rabbit. When your child is hungry between meals, try giving him some raw vegetables, like carrots and celery. "Most kids like them because they're crunchy," says Dr. Ferentz. To make these snacks even more appealing, spruce them up with some add-ons. "A piece of celery spread with a bit of peanut butter is great for preventing constipation."

Disguise those "disgusting" vegetables. Maybe it's tough to get your child to eat cauliflower or broccoli—high-fiber vegetables that help the constipation situation. But you can camouflage those helpful veggies to make them more palatable, says Dr. Hogan. "Be creative. Try cutting them into different shapes. Tell him broccoli florets are little trees. If you have to, chop up vegetables and hide them in meat loaf where he can't find them."

Take advantage of fruit favoritism. Kids who won't eat vegetables usually will eat fruits. And many kinds of fruit are effective at getting things moving. "Offer lots of apples, pears and peaches," suggests Menard. "But hold back on bananas and applesauce, which tend to be constipating," she warns.

Offer liquids galore. "Make sure your child is drinking plenty of fluids, including fruit juices, because they too can help prevent constipation," says Menard. This is especially important if you're introducing more bran and other high-fiber foods into your child's diet. Liquids help bulk up fiber in the gut to form soft, easy-to-pass stools.

Don't start toilet training too soon. Kids who aren't ready to use the potty may withhold stools as a way to assert control over their own bodies, says Dr. Ferentz. "A two-year-old wants to be in control so desperately that if you tell him, 'You've got to go to the potty,' he'll actually try *not* to go—just to show you who's boss."

Instead of forcing the issue, wait and watch for signs of readiness on the child's part. "Most kids really don't express much interest in toilet training until they're close to three. That's when it's developmentally appropriate to begin," says Dr. Ferentz.

Turn over some control. Children engaged in a stool-withholding power struggle with parents may need to be given the freedom to make some decisions for themselves, says Dr. Ferentz.

"You may need to look at other control issues in the child's life—for example, what clothes he wears, or what kind of sandwich he eats for lunch. If you let him have more say in these matters, he'll feel like *you're* starting to let go—and that's important to him," Dr. Ferentz suggests. "The child may be able to relax and pass stools more freely."

COUGHING AT NIGHT

Hints for Sounder Sleep

On Monday your son's sleep was disturbed by a dry, hacking cough. Since then, the cough has been keeping him and everybody else up. Now it's Friday night, and even the dog is howling.

Of course, you are doing your best to ease those nasty nighttime symptoms. You've rubbed some strong-smelling ointment on his chest, dosed him with a multi-symptom cough-and-cold medicine and turned up the heat in his room. Now you're wondering if you should ask the doctor for some antibiotics. Unfortunately, according to the experts, none of those measures actually helps to stop the coughing.

"The most common reason for a child's nighttime coughing is a viral infection," says Blake E. Noyes, M.D., assistant professor of pediatrics in the Division of Pulmonology at Children's Hospital of Pittsburgh. "And that's the kind of illness that can't be treated with antibiotics."

Because coughing is an important mechanism for keeping the lungs clear, you don't want to stop it completely. "If your child has a viral illness, his natural defense mechanisms are temporarily impaired. The cough helps keep the lungs clear of bacteria and other irritants," says Dr. Noyes. "If you suppress the coughing completely, you are wiping away an important defense against a more serious bacterial infection such as pneumonia."

Although in many cases it's best to leave a nighttime cough alone, doctors say there are steps you can take, when necessary, to make your child more comfortable.

Offer lots of drink. The traditional recommendation, "Drink plenty of liquids," is still good advice when your child has a cough. "Fluids such as juice, water or clear broth are some of the best expectorants around," explains Robert C. Beckerman, M.D., professor of pediatrics and physiology and section chief of pediatric pulmonology at Tulane University School of Medicine in New Orleans. Flu-

MEDICAL ALERT

When to See the Doctor

It's important that your child be checked by a doctor to determine the cause of any severe or persistent cough, says Blake E. Noyes, M.D., assistant professor of pediatrics in the Division of Pulmonology at Children's Hospital of Pittsburgh. "Nighttime coughing may be due to a virus, a bacterial infection, asthma, something your child swallowed that is partially blocking the airway, irritating fumes or, in some cases, a more serious disease such as cystic fibrosis," he says.

You should consult a physician, advises Dr. Noyes, if your child:

- Coughs continually throughout the night.
- Coughs up phlegm.
- Has a fever.
- Has difficulty breathing.
- Has a cough that has lasted more than ten days.

---

ids can loosen up a dry, hard cough and help expel phlegm. And unlike cold medications, there are no side effects, Dr. Beckerman says.

"A hot drink, in particular, can be a soothing comfort when your child has a cough," says Dr. Noyes. But any type of drink will do. "When kids get stuffed up, they tend to breathe through the mouth, which dries out the throat and leads to a cough. Just keeping the mouth and throat moist may reduce the coughing," he says.

Turn down the thermostat. If your child's cough strikes during the winter months when the house is heated, you should turn the thermostat *down* at night, not up. "Hot, dry air will irritate a cough. But if you set the thermostat lower, the cooler air will preserve some humidity," says Naomi Grobstein, M.D., a family physician in private practice in Montclair, New Jersey.

Don't rush to vaporize. Although it seems sensible to add some humidity with a vaporizer, that's not always a good idea. "Vaporizers are hard to keep clean," notes Dr. Beckerman, "and they tend to be a breeding ground for mold and bacteria." If your child is allergic to mold or has asthma, a vaporizer could make the cough even worse, he says.

Skip the chest rub. "Petroleum products, which create a warm feeling on the chest, do nothing to ease a cough," says Dr. Beckerman. And if the child inhales or swallows a chest-rub product, it could possibly lead to a form of pneumonia, he cautions.

Try an antihistamine. If you know that your child's cough is caused by an allergy, an antihistamine at bedtime may help him get some sleep. "Allergic coughs may be helped by over-the-counter drugs such as Benadryl Elixir," says Dr. Beckerman. Be sure to read package directions to make certain the product is recommended for your child's age. For the correct dosage, follow package directions or consult your physician.

Choose the right cough medicine. "If your child has been up for a few nights with a bad cough, you can try a cough medicine containing dextromethorphan and guaifenesin, such as Robitussin-DM or Vicks Pediatric Formula 44e," says Dr. Grobstein. "Basically, any products with these two ingredients will do," she adds. This type of over-the-counter preparation will loosen up the mucus a bit and provide very mild cough relief. "Dextromethorphan is not 100 percent effective," she says, "but that's actually good, because you shouldn't try to suppress a cough entirely."

Caution: Don't give potent cough medication to a child who is under one year of age, says Dr. Beckerman. "The cough reflex is controlled in the brain stem, and if you give a very young child something to suppress it, you might also suppress breathing," he says.

CRADLE CAP

Coping with a Crusty Crown

That yellow, dry crust marring the perfect beauty of your infant's scalp may look unsightly. But cradle cap, a common skin inflammation that's most noticeable in infants (though children of all ages are susceptible), is usually not dangerous.

Surprisingly, a mild case of cradle cap isn't even irritating to your baby. But it is worth treating if it starts to spread or grow thicker. So if you see that telltale "cap" appearing like crust on the scalp, here are some easy ways to cope.

Leave it alone. If the cradle cap is mild and confined to the scalp, it can be safely left alone, says Karen Wiss, M.D., assistant professor of medicine and pediatrics and director of pediatric dermatology at the University of Massachusetts Medical Center in Worcester. "Cradle cap may look irritating, but for the most part, it is not bothersome to the baby," she says.

Slack off from shampooing. "Wash your baby's hair no more than every other day, using a gentle baby shampoo. Overwashing has a drying effect and can aggravate cradle cap," says Luisa Castiglia, M.D., a pediatrician in private practice in Mineola, New York.

Use a toothbrush. If you do want to do something about cradle cap, scalp brushing may help. "At the first sign of cradle cap, parents should use a drop of baby oil or cooking oil to loosen up the flakes on the baby's scalp and then lightly brush the scalp with a soft toothbrush. This loosens a lot of scale, which can then be removed by shampooing your baby's hair with regular baby shampoo," says Fran E. Adler, M.D., a pediatrician in private practice in Upper Montclair, New Jersey. This treatment is not a quick fix, but if you persist, you may see gradual improvement over time.

Switch shampoos. If the scale becomes very thick, it can

MEDICAL ALERT

When to See the Doctor

If you start to see a lot of yellow crusting, pus, redness or tenderness, your child may have developed an infection, says Karen Wiss, M.D., assistant professor of medicine and pediatrics and director of pediatric dermatology at the University of Massachusetts Medical Center in Worcester. "An infection can develop if your child is old enough to scratch his scalp and introduce bacteria into the skin. If this happens, it is easily treated with oral antibiotics prescribed by a doctor," says Dr. Wiss.

You should also alert your doctor if your child's cradle cap stubbornly resists home treatment. It may be a sign of a more serious problem, she says.

be annoying to your infant and may even become infected, notes Dr. Wiss. She suggests shampooing the baby's hair twice a week with an over-the-counter dandruff shampoo such as Sebulex. "Use a small amount of shampoo, and avoid getting it into the baby's eyes. It won't harm the eyes, but it will sting," says Dr. Wiss.

Dr. Adler adds that you'll get the most out of the dandruff shampoo treatment by keeping the lather on for five minutes before rinsing.

Try a special liquid. For very thick cradle cap, Dr. Wiss recommends loosening the scale by using Baker's P & S Liquid, a mild, mineral-oil-based solution available at drugstores. "Apply the P & S Liquid at night, comb through the scale with a fine-toothed comb and wash it out in the morning," she says.

"The baby's fontanelle [the soft spot on the skull] is a delicate area, but it won't be damaged by gentle combing and brushing," adds Dr. Castiglia.

Watch out for creeping. If cradle cap starts creeping down behind your baby's ears and onto the neck, it definitely needs treatment, notes Dr. Adler. If your doctor okays it, treat the affected areas with 0.5 percent or 1 percent hydrocortisone cream, which is available over-the-counter. If you apply the cream three times a day, it should clear up that crust immediately, she says. Be sure to consult your pediatrician, however, because this is strong medication, according to Dr. Adler.

CRANKINESS

Getting Away from the Whine Routine

When kids turn cranky, a lot of parents take it personally. "He's just doing it to get his way," is one interpretation of Johnny's pouts and whines. Some kids are *temperamentally* cranky, suggests William Sobesky, Ph.D., assistant clinical professor of psychiatry at the University of Colorado Health Sciences Center and research psychologist at Children's Hospital, both in Denver. "You don't need to think of it as intentional or take it personally. It's just the way the child is wired."

But other kids do use crankiness as a form of manipulation. They quickly learn that "Mommy hates it when I whine and cry at the mall, so she buys me a chocolate chip cookie." Here are a few tips to head off crankiness *before* it becomes a habit.

If there's a problem, take care of it. Perhaps the most common cause of crankiness is a physical need. "The child is tired or hungry or bored," says Dr. Sobesky. "Give her time for a nap or, if you're out, put her on your shoulder. Get her something to eat or distract her."

Don't respond to whining. "If your child uses whining to get your attention, say very simply, 'I don't understand you when you're whining,'" suggests Robert Mendelson, M.D., a pediatrician and clinical professor of pediatrics at

Oregon Health Sciences University in Portland. "Tell the child, 'When you're ready, come and tell me what's bothering you and then we'll talk about it.' As soon as the whining stops, say, 'I'm glad you're feeling better.' "

Pay attention to the good stuff. Kids who are using crankiness to get attention should get attention for other, more pleasant things they do. "The child who is picked up every time she smiles, coos and gurgles learns that when she wants attention all she has to do is smile, coo and gurgle," says Dr. Mendelson. "Don't reward negative behavior by giving her attention *only* when she's cranky. If you do, you'll just see more of that behavior."

Raise a do-it-yourselfer. Kids use crankiness and whining as a way of saying *"Do this for me!"*

"They whine because they can't tie shoes, their blocks fall down, they don't want to go to bed or they don't want to eat. Whining is a flag that is signaling, 'Please teach me some skills,' " says Edward Christophersen, Ph.D., clinical psychologist at Children's Mercy Hospital and professor of pediatrics at the University of Missouri–Kansas City School of Medicine.

Rather than leaping to their aid at the first whine, give them some time to figure out what to do on their own, suggests Dr. Christophersen. If they need some instruction, make your explanations brief and simple—and make it clear that you're confident they can do the task themselves. "The more you help," warns Dr. Christophersen, "the more dependent children become."

Explain the facts of life. With older children, explain that their crankiness is working against them, suggests Lottie Mendelson, R.N., a pediatric nurse practitioner in Portland, Oregon, and coauthor of *The Complete Book of Parenting*, with her husband, Robert. If you tell the child how annoying it is when she's constantly cranky, she'll be able to understand how crankiness affects other people.

CROUP

Chasing Off a Scary Cough

Your child has had the sniffles for a few days when suddenly he wakes up in the middle of the night with a strange cough that sounds like a seal barking. His voice is hoarse, and he's running a slight fever. He's also having trouble breathing.

After a panicky call to the doctor you learn that these are the symptoms of croup, a common viral infection of the vocal cords that strikes babies and preschoolers mainly during the fall and spring.

Though it's often thought of as a single ailment, croup is more accurately a symptom of many different viruses, says Marjorie Hogan, M.D., an instructor of pediatrics at the University of Minnesota and a pediatrician at the Hennepin County Medical Center in Minneapolis. "It can be very frightening—to both parents and children—because the swelling in the throat that causes the barking cough can also make breathing difficult," she says. Some children with croup also experience what is called stridor, a vibrating sound that occurs when they breathe in. It's especially noticeable when they cry.

In most cases, croup can be treated successfully at home with very simple measures. However, croup can sometimes be serious, and there are two life-threatening conditions that resemble it. So read "Medical Alert" on the opposite page before trying any of these home remedies.

Stay calm. The reason you need to stay calm is that you want your child to stay calm. "The symptoms of croup get worse when the child gets agitated," says Dr. Hogan. "As he's gasping for more breath, he breathes faster. If you can calm him, he'll breathe slower and more air can get in and out."

Turn on the hot water. If your child is having breathing difficulties, take him into the bathroom and turn on a hot shower to get the room really steamy, suggests Dr. Hogan.

MEDICAL ALERT

When to See the Doctor

"Most of the time croup is a benign disease that parents can readily deal with at home," says Marjorie Hogan, M.D., an instructor of pediatrics at the University of Minnesota and a pediatrician at the Hennepin County Medical Center in Minneapolis.

But a severe case can cause breathing problems that may require a visit to a hospital emergency room. "If the child's symptoms are really frightening you, call the doctor or go to the emergency room right away," says Dr. Hogan.

There are two other diseases that resemble croup, and both of them are life-threatening. One is epiglottitis, a sudden swelling of the cartilage flap at the top of the throat that can close a child's windpipe. The other is infectious tracheitis, an inflammation of the windpipe caused by a staph infection, which calls for antibiotics and often respiratory support. In both cases, says Loraine Stern, M.D., associate clinical professor of pediatrics at the University of California, Los Angeles, and author of When Do I Call the Doctor?, you may need to call local paramedics "if the emergency room is far away and the child is in real distress."

Here are some warning signs that indicate a medical emergency.

- Home remedies are not working
- High fever (103° to 105°)
- Crouplike symptoms that progress rapidly
- Unusual amount of drooling
- Inability to bend the neck forward
- The child is leaning forward and gasping for air
- Poor color (the child appears gray, blue or pale)
- Breathing becomes more and more labored, and the child's ribs are clearly visible at each breath
- Nostrils are flaring and the child is making a crowing sound with each breath
- The child cannot talk or cry
- The child looks frantic

If you suspect epiglottitis, it is imperative that you do *not* open the child's mouth to peer inside. "If you do that, the whole throat can close up and the child can go into respiratory arrest," says Dr. Hogan.

"The child will be able to breathe more easily in the steam. No one is really sure why this works, but it may decrease the inflammation so the swelling goes down."

Hit the cold air. One of the curious things about croup is what happens when panicky parents bundle their child into the car for the drive to the hospital. "Suddenly, the problem stops," says Dr. Hogan. "For some reason, cold air—like steamy air—can be really beneficial." So you may be able to help your child just by opening the window (if it's a cool night) or by taking him into an air-conditioned room.

Use a humidifier. "Turn your cool-mist vaporizer up full blast," says Shirley Menard, R.N., a certified pediatric nurse practitioner and assistant professor at the University of Texas Health Science Center at San Antonio School of Nursing. "You can either let the vaporizer douse the entire room or direct it toward the child." You need to get a lot of moisture into the air before this will be effective, she says.

Some experts recommend a warm-mist vaporizer, "but I always recommend the cool mist because if the child gets out of bed and falls on it, he won't burn himself," says Loraine Stern, M.D., associate clinical professor of pediatrics at the University of California, Los Angeles, and author of *When Do I Call the Doctor?* "Just be sure to use a vaporizer with a filter that's designed to filter out impurities, because those can aggravate breathing difficulties in an allergic child." Clean the vaporizer often, following the manufacturer's instructions.

Control the fever. "Children who have a fever tend to breathe faster to cool off their bodies, and that makes their breathing more difficult," says Dr. Stern. You can give your child acetaminophen (Children's Tylenol) to bring the fever down. Check the package directions for the correct dosage for your child's age and weight. If your child is under age two, consult a physician.

Give plenty of fluids. "We all lose some fluid from the

body with each breath. But for the child breathing harder and faster with croup, this can become a real problem," says Menard. "You can give the child frequent, small sips of an over-the-counter electrolyte replacement fluid such as Pedialyte—or even Gatorade." But any clear liquid—like broth or apple juice—will help restore fluids to the child's body.

Sleep with the child. Croup is scary. For your own peace of mind, it might be best to sleep in the same room as your child, says Dr. Stern. That way you'll be right there if he experiences breathing difficulties. For some reason croup tends to get worse at night. "It may be because the body produces less of the hormone cortisone at night. There's some evidence that cortisone can help a little bit with croup," says Dr. Stern. If you can't sleep in the same room as the child, use a monitoring device that will alert you if there's any problem.

CRYING

How to Still the Sobs

For most parents, a crying baby is no laughing matter. Many babies cry an hour or more each day, frustrating their parents who know that crying is a baby's only language yet are unable to translate it. When is it hunger? When is it pain? When do those plaintive wails that touch us to our very core mean, "Come and pick me up"?

What most parents learn in the first three months of a newborn's life is that comforting a crying baby is a matter of trial and error. Eventually, the signals will become clear, as parents get better at guessing what baby wants. But in these early few months, a lot of crying seems to be a general plea for comfort.

Should you *always* comfort a crying baby? In general, the experts say, a baby under 12 weeks may need frequent

---

MEDICAL ALERT

When to See the Doctor

Even though crying is normal in infants, there are times when prolonged or insistent crying could be a signal to call your doctor, according to Edward Christophersen, Ph.D., clinical psychologist at Children's Mercy Hospital, professor of pediatrics at the University of Missouri–Kansas City School of Medicine and author of *Baby Owner's Manual: What to Expect and How to Survive the First Year*. Be sure to call your child's physician right away if:

- Your child's cry is high-pitched and painful rather than fussy.
- Your baby cries constantly for more than three hours.
- Diarrhea, vomiting, high fever or other signs of sickness accompany the crying.

---

holding and cuddling to help him settle down. After three months, babies should be given the opportunity to learn to comfort themselves, or crying may become a habit. Here are a few comforting techniques to try—but results are not guaranteed.

Check for physical causes. "Make certain nothing is hurting the child," says Dena Hofkosh, M.D., assistant professor of pediatrics at the University of Pittsburgh School of Medicine and coordinator of the Infant Development Program at Children's Hospital of Pittsburgh. Look for open diaper pins, scratchy clothing, a crib toy poking your baby in the tummy. Also, look for fever or other symptoms of illness, such as a rash. Did the baby burp after his last feeding? If not, he may be having gas pains.

Try a quick pick-me-up. Some babies cry just because they want to be held, and as long as the baby is under 12 weeks old, you shouldn't hesitate. "A lot of parents think they'll spoil babies if they pick them up when they cry, but that's just not the case," says Dr. Hofkosh. "A study done at McGill University found that babies who were held more cried less."

Give daily love pats. Touch your child briefly and gently 50 to 100 times a day even when he doesn't need it. Essentially what you are doing is providing unconditional love and rewarding noncrying behavior at the same time, says Edward Christophersen, Ph.D., clinical psychologist at Children's Mercy Hospital, professor of pediatrics at the University of Missouri–Kansas City School of Medicine, and author of *Baby Owner's Manual: What to Expect and How to Survive the First Year.*

Tune in to the Fussy Hour. Many babies have a predictable fussy period each day. Although it can occur at any hour, it often comes around dinnertime, when the whole family is home and meal preparations are under way. "Once you're convinced that's what it is, think of that crying period as an exercise time for your baby," says Robert Mendelson, M.D., a pediatrician and clinical professor of pediatrics at Oregon Health Sciences University in Portland. "It's the baby's way of jogging, burning off the excess energy he has." So you might just want to let these crying spells run their course.

Bring on the rhythm and music. "A lot of babies respond well to a recorded heartbeat," says Dr. Mendelson. There's something primal and soothing about the rhythmic thump-thump that was their piped-in sound track for nine months. Playing music can also help: Many crying babies are distracted by George Gershwin's "Rhapsody in Blue," Raffi's "Baby Beluga" or anything that happens to be on the radio. Your humming can be very soothing to a fussy child. Even a running vacuum cleaner or clothes dryer can calm him down.

Put them in motion. A walk around the house might soothe your infant. Your baby may also respond to gentle rocking, either in your arms or in a baby swing or cradle. "For very irritable babies, vertical rocking seems to work," she says. Hold the baby on your lap or shoulder and rock up and down gently, applying some pressure to the chest and belly. "Babies like frontal pressure, which is almost like being tucked into the womb again," says Dr. Hofkosh.

Take a ride. For some babies, a drive in the car is like a tranquilizer. When one of her daughters was a baby, Dr. Hofkosh recalls, "we drove around for an hour-and-a-half in a pouring rainstorm because I couldn't deal with the crying anymore. I figured it was better than sitting home and waiting it out."

Use a baby carrier. "Some babies love the close comfort of being held on your chest in a front pack," says Dr. Hofkosh. "Some parents like the backpack, but it may be better if the baby's front is in contact with Mommy or Daddy. It's also convenient. You can get things done with the baby sleeping there. I know I ate many meals with my daughters in a front pack."

Change positions . . . but not too much. Like the rest of us, babies can get bored or uncomfortable staying in the same position, says Lottie Mendelson, R.N., a pediatric nurse practitioner in Portland, Oregon, and coauthor of *The Complete Book of Parenting*, with her husband, Robert. Some babies like to be vertical on your shoulder, while others like to peer at the world from your lap. But don't switch too frequently, says Dr. Hofkosh. "Some babies take a longer time to adapt to a particular position so you need to avoid going quickly from one to the next." Give the baby time to figure out whether she feels okay in the new position, advises Mendelson.

Turn down the light and noise. Babies who are easily overstimulated—or those who have had a big day full of strange faces and voices and a lot of handling—may need a little time to decompress, particularly before bed, says Dr. Hofkosh. By turning down the lights and keeping voices low, you can help the overstimulated baby relax.

Don't plug cries with food. "It's very satisfying for parents who hear a baby cry to be able to do something about it, and feeding is the most primal nurturing activity we can do," says Dr. Hofkosh. But she advises against feeding as the first response to a baby's cry.

Babies do cry when they're hungry, but that's far from the only reason, notes Dr. Hofkosh. A baby who cries when she's bored will probably stop crying if you nurse or give her a bottle, but you will miss the opportunity to learn what her cries *really* mean and you'll be training her to think of eating as something you do when you're bored.

As a rule of thumb, says Dr. Hofkosh, most breastfed babies feed every 90 minutes to 2 hours and bottle-fed babies can often wait 2 to 2½ hours between feedings. "If she cries sooner than that, it makes sense to try other things before offering food again," says Dr. Hofkosh.

Take a break. It's almost impossible for parents to remain calm when they have a crying baby on their hands. Every "wah" seems to be saying, "You're a bad parent." But you're not a bad parent if your child is crying, especially if you've done everything you can to console him," says Dr. Mendelson. "A truly fussy baby is often inconsolable, which can drive parents crazy."

Parents need to make sure they get regular breaks from a fussy baby, he suggests. Arrange to get an hour or two off daily—and possibly an entire afternoon off once a week—leaving the baby with a grandparent or trusted babysitter. And have an occasional evening out with your partner just to recharge.

Remember, this too shall pass. "Recognize that crying, especially in a challenging baby, is time-limited," says Dr. Hofkosh. "Tell yourself that you can help your baby be okay even though he's the kind who cries all the time. Remind yourself it isn't a personality trait that's going to last forever."

Give them some time. After a baby is 12 weeks old, you can begin to change your strategy. Rushing to comfort a crying baby or child at the first peep deprives her of a wonderful learning experience, says Dr. Christophersen. If you take care of her every need, she'll never learn how to calm herself, he warns. "The only way I know to reduce crying is by teaching self-quieting skills," he says. So wait a few minutes—how long is dictated by your tolerance for crying—to see if the baby can find a way to quiet herself. If she's not in true discomfort, a baby over the age of about 12 weeks will often distract herself by playing with her feet, sucking her thumb or examining her surroundings rather than screaming for you.

Put your baby to bed awake. Bedtime is often the best time to teach babies how to self-quiet, says Dr. Christophersen. Though there's a real temptation to nurse or rock babies to sleep, parents and babies eventually pay the price of sleepless nights (and cranky next days) because the baby comes to associate nursing or rocking with falling asleep. That may be fine at 8:00 P.M., but it's not such a pleasure at 3:00 A.M. when the baby begins crying for her "sleeping pill," in the form of a long rocking session.

"If a baby nurses before bedtime and gets drowsy, carry her, maybe bounce her around a little, talk to her, change her diaper, wipe her gums and put her to bed," says Dr. Christophersen. "She may go, 'Wah, wah wah,' and then she'll be gone. Best of all, she'll learn how to put herself to sleep. And if you know your baby can self-quiet, you won't feel like you're abandoning her."

Take your baby out of the crib before he cries. "A lot of parents use their babies as a snooze alarm," says Dr. Christophersen. "After 12 weeks, many babies who once woke up crying wake up babbling. But their parents don't pick them up until they cry. That teaches the child he *has to* cry before you'll pick him up. I'd much rather have parents teach children they get picked up for babbling and cooing, not for screaming."

CUTS, SCRAPES AND SCRATCHES

Remedies for Minor Wounds

Your son has taken a spill off his skateboard and comes home looking like an extra from a *Friday the 13th* movie. His right leg is bloodied from a scrape that stretches from thigh to calf. He has six or seven light scratches on his face and a nasty, deep-looking cut over his eye that is bleeding heavily.

Before you reach for your first-aid kit, you should know that cuts, scrapes and scratches are not all equal and may need different treatment. Cuts and scratches slice through the skin to a varying degree, while scrapes are caused by the skin rubbing against something abrasive such as gravel, wood or cement.

Serious wounds need the prompt attention of a doctor (see "Medical Alert" on page 140). But most minor cuts, scrapes and scratches can be taken care of at home. Here's how.

Cuts

Apply Pressure. Cuts can bleed a lot, which can be scary, but in almost every case, bleeding can be controlled with direct pressure, says Samuel Wentworth, M.D., a pediatrician in private practice in Danville, Indiana. "Take a clean cloth or gauze pad and apply pressure directly over the wound. If you don't have a cloth around, you can even use your hand alone. In either case, you may have to use a fair amount of pressure to get the bleeding to stop," says Dr. Wentworth.

If you can't stop the bleeding, get emergency medical care. Do not apply a tourniquet. "Tourniquets can cut off circulation to the limb and ultimately cause more problems than they solve," he says.

Cleanse and bandage. "Wash the cut thoroughly with

MEDICAL ALERT

When to See the Doctor

"If the cut seems very deep or gaping, or if there is a lot of bleeding, it should be seen by a doctor and sutured. If it is on the face or hand, you should ask for a plastic surgeon," says Ann DiMaio, M.D., director of the pediatric emergency room at the New York Hospital—Cornell Medical Center and assistant professor of pediatrics at Cornell University Medical College, both in New York City.

"If you think that a cut needs stitches, don't put off your doctor visit. If you wait more than eight hours, your doctor can't close the wound because bacteria may have entered, and closing the wound would invite infection. Also, if you wait and let a wound heal on its own, the scar that results will be a lot worse than one on a cut that has been sutured or stitched," says Dr. DiMaio.

If your child has received a major cut on the arm or hand, make sure he can move his hand, wrist and fingers. If he can't, a tendon may have been cut, warns Samuel Wentworth, M.D., a pediatrician in private practice in Danville, Indiana. Call a doctor immediately.

soap and water, cover it with antibacterial cream and, if the cut is minor, use a butterfly bandage to close the wound," says Fran E. Adler, M.D., a pediatrician in private practice in Upper Montclair, New Jersey. These butterfly-shaped bandages are sticky all over and keep the edges of the skin together so that the wound heals with a nice, straight scar.

Leave it alone. "Once a butterfly bandage is on, leave it in place for a couple of days. It usually takes 24 to 48 hours for the skin to knit together and heal, and you don't want to disturb the healing process by removing the bandage," says Dr. Wentworth.

Check your child's tetanus status. Make sure that tetanus shots are up-to-date. If the shots aren't up-to-date, see your doctor for a booster, says Dr. Adler.

Scrapes

Wash it. "The most important thing to do with a scrape is to wash it well with soap and water to remove all the little particles of dirt and grit. If these are not removed, they can result in permanent scars," says Ann DiMaio, M.D., director of the pediatric emergency room at the New York Hospital—Cornell Medical Center and assistant professor of pediatrics at Cornell University Medical College, both in New York City.

Soak it. If your child is really upset about having his scrape washed, run a bath and let him soak in the tub for a while. (Warn him, though, that he may feel some mild stinging initially.) "Most kids don't mind taking a nice soapy bath, and once your child has soaked, he'll be used to the feeling of the water on the wound. At that point, it won't be so bad when you take a washcloth and soap and really wash the area," says Dr. Adler.

Brush it. "Dirt can become very embedded in the scrape, and you may need to use a soft nailbrush to clean out the wound," says Dr. Wentworth. He admits that your child probably won't be happy about the procedure and that if the scrape is extensive, you may want to take your child

---

MEDICAL ALERT

When to See the Doctor

If a scrape is weeping clear fluid, it's okay, but if it contains blood or pus or there is redness that is traveling away from the wound, the scrape has become infected and needs to be treated with a course of oral antibiotics, says Samuel Wentworth, M.D., a pediatrician in private practice in Danville, Indiana. See a doctor if you see any sign of infection.

Cuts and scratches can get infected too. Again, watch for swelling, pus or a traveling area of redness. And if you suspect infection, see your doctor.

to an emergency room, where a doctor can give a local anesthetic before cleaning the wound.

Pat it, dab it, cover it. Pat the area dry and apply a dab of antibiotic cream. "The scrape will heal best if you leave it uncovered, but kids love Band-Aids, and it won't hurt to use one if it makes them feel better," says Dr. Adler. She suggests that you remove the Band-Aid at night, though, after bath time. "The Band-Aid will peel off easily after a soak in the tub, and then the scrape should be left uncovered for the night," she says.

Protect it. "Although leaving a scrape uncovered promotes faster healing, if your child is going to play in the dirt, cover any open wound with a loose-fitting bandage. When your child gets home, remove the dressing and wash the wound," says Dr. DiMaio.

Watch for weeping. "If the scrape is weeping (oozing clear fluid), apply an over-the-counter antibiotic cream according to the directions on the label. Some antibiotic creams need to be applied twice a day, while others need three or four applications," says Dr. Wentworth. He recommends washing the area before each application and covering it afterward with a nonstick bandage, such as Telfa, which prevents the scab from binding the bandage to the wound.

Scratches

Clean it out. Wash the scratch well with soap and water, advises Dr. Adler, and leave it uncovered. "A scratch may bleed and hurt, but it won't be deep enough to need stitches or a butterfly bandage. We don't worry about scratches unless they are deep, dirty or numerous."

Consider the source. If your child has been scratched by an animal or by a dirty implement such as a nail, it is a good idea to check on your child's tetanus status. It's unusual to develop tetanus from a scratch. But it can't hurt to be cautious, says Dr. Wentworth.

DANDRUFF

Putting the Hex on Telltale Specks

Having dandruff is not something to be ashamed of," asserts Guy S. Webster, M.D., Ph.D., assistant professor of dermatology at Thomas Jefferson University in Philadelphia. And if your child is dandruff-prone, you might have to remind him that the doctor says not to worry.

When telltale specks of dusty white appear on the shirt collar and shoulders of school-age children, they may come in for quite a ribbing from the other kids. So it's good if parents can offer an explanation and reassurance along with some helpful treatments.

Dandruff is simply an overenthusiastic turnover of skin cells on the scalp. Everybody's scalp sheds, but if a child has dandruff, the skin sheds too quickly and too much. The child may complain that his scalp feels itchy, and you're likely to find some white flakes.

MEDICAL ALERT

When to See the Doctor

Consult a doctor if your child's dandruff doesn't respond to two weeks of home treatment. And you shouldn't delay seeing the doctor if the child complains that his scalp is painful or extremely itchy, says Guy S. Webster, M.D., Ph.D., assistant professor of dermatology at Thomas Jefferson University in Philadelphia. He also recommends taking your child to the doctor if you detect hair loss, notice that the scalp seems inflamed or see some scaliness and inflammation on other parts of the body.

Other scalp conditions that resemble dandruff in some ways are cradle cap (usually in infants), ringworm, seborrheic dermatitis and psoriasis. These conditions usually aren't serious, but it takes a doctor to diagnose and treat them, according to Dr. Webster.

Though dandruff is not as common in children as it is in adults, kids do get it. If you see a scalp problem that *looks* like dandruff, go ahead and try some home treatment to see if it clears up, recommends Karen Wiss, M.D., assistant professor of medicine and pediatrics and director of pediatric dermatology at the University of Massachusetts Medical Center in Worcester. But she cautions, "If the dandruff doesn't respond within two weeks, your child's symptoms may be related to other conditions that need a doctor's diagnosis and treatment."

Here are the dandruff-fighting home treatments our experts suggest.

Buy a good dandruff shampoo. "A good dandruff-fighting shampoo is important because it reduces the scaling on the scalp and allows medication to penetrate where it is needed," says Alvin L. Adler, M.D., a dermatologist and attending physician and clinical instructor in dermatology at the New York Hospital—Cornell Medical Center and Beth Israel Medical Center, both in New York City. To ensure that you are buying an effective product, spend a moment in the drugstore reading some labels. Look for a dandruff shampoo that lists tar or salicylic acid among the ingredients, says Dr. Adler.

Shampoo often. Your child should start out using the shampoo at least twice a week, says Dr. Adler. Many doctors suggest that if the dandruff doesn't go away, the child should shampoo twice a week with dandruff shampoo and also shampoo frequently with the regular kind. And if the child still has dandruff, use the dandruff shampoo even more frequently than twice a week.

For the child who is reluctant, make a game of lathering up. And make the bath-and-shampoo part of your child's schedule, so it becomes routine.

If the dandruff doesn't resolve with shampoo alone, a topical steroid medication may be needed, Dr. Adler says. Check with your pediatrician or a dermatologist.

Use nongreasy hair fixatives. If you have an older child who has just started to use styling products, make sure that you buy nonoily gels or mousses. "Greasy or oily condition-ers and styling products will just make dandruff worse," Dr. Adler says.

Keep an eye out for recurring flare-ups. "Dandruff is easy to control but not to cure," says Dr. Adler. After your child's dandruff is under control, you can switch back to regular shampoo, but be alert for signs of itchiness or flak-ing. "Count on it—there will be another flare-up," Dr. Adler reminds parents. Keep dandruff shampoo in the cabi-net and get your child to use it at the first signs that dandruff is back.

Look out for stress. "No one knows why some people get dandruff and others don't, but stress can provoke it," says Dr. Adler. If your child gets frequent dandruff flare-ups, check out the possibility that she may be under too much pressure. You can help her reduce stress by talking about school and everyday problems and allowing more free time without planned activities.

DAWDLING

Methods to Get Things Moving

Lisa is 3 and her mother, Katherine, is 33, but at 7:30 every morning, it's Mom who comes closest to having a tantrum. If you've ever tried to get a small child moving in a hurry, you'll empathize with Katherine's strug-gle.

Frustration isn't a strong enough word to describe what you feel when your preschooler takes a half-hour to find her shoes or your 7-year-old can't do his homework because it takes him forever to round up a pencil and paper or your 11-year-old makes the whole car pool wait, morning after morning, no matter how many times you've said, "Today you're leaving *on time*."

Yet grown-up tantrums, pleading and nagging aren't the answer, agree the experts. There's usually a message behind the dawdler's molasses-like movements. Figure it out and you're halfway there. Here are some suggestions for coping.

Recognize that it may be normal. "Dawdling is a normal part of development in young children," points out Cynthia Whitham, a licensed clinical social worker and staff therapist at the University of California, Los Angeles, Parent Training Clinic and author of *Win the Whining War and Other Skirmishes*. "So sometimes you may just have to relax and accept it. The child's behavior will probably get better as she matures." But even older children may need a couple of reminders or an incentive, she notes.

Teach some clock-watching. "Preschoolers don't have

IS YOUR CHILD TRYING TO TELL YOU SOMETHING?

If your school-age child is dawdling all the time, it may seem as though he's purposely trying to irritate you. That may be *precisely* what's happening, says William Womack, M.D., associate professor in the Department of Child Psychiatry at the University of Washington School of Medicine and codirector of the Stress Management Clinic of Children's Hospital and Medical Center, both in Seattle. "You need to think about the meaning of the dawdling behavior. Does your child dislike the activity that's being postponed? He could be trying to say to you, 'The rest of my life is unpleasant so I'm going to make you pay by holding back now.'"

"We make lots of decisions *for* our children," notes Dr. Womack, "and as a result, they may feel helpless. If there are frequent tests of will between you and your child, take a look at whether he is able to make decisions in other areas of his life. If he has decided that a particular elective activity is not his cup of tea, it might be best to allow him to drop it rather than force him to continue when he insists on dawdling."

much concept of time, so urging them to get ready because you have to be someplace 'on time' means very little to them," says William Womack, M.D., associate professor in the Department of Child Psychiatry at the University of Washington School of Medicine and codirector of the Stress Management Clinic of Children's Hospital and Medical Center, both in Seattle. "Once kids learn how to tell time in first or second grade, it's easier to get them to do things on time." Teaching your child to read the clock—then checking the time together—helps to make her more aware of *when* you have to get things done.

Only interrupt when you must. "No one on the planet likes to be interrupted, yet all day long we're interrupting children's play to get them to do things we want them to do," notes Whitham. When a child resists being interrupted, we mistakenly call it dawdling. Rather than interrupt suddenly, give your child a "warning" announcement, so she knows there's a change-of-activity coming up. For example, you might say, "In five minutes it will be time to turn off the TV and come to dinner."

Praise the child who shows stick-to-it-iveness. Whitham suggests parents say, "Good job!" when a child does something quickly. Praise anything the child does that is efficient and the opposite of dawdling. By the time a child is nine or ten, he understands the concept of being organized, so you can begin praising him for that. Some children respond well when you say, "Good planning!"

Use the star system. "Buy some colored stars and a calendar that contains large boxes," suggests Robert R. Butterworth, Ph.D., a Los Angeles-based clinical psychologist specializing in treating children and adolescents. Then use those stars as awards for prompt behavior, he suggests. "If your child regularly dawdles over homework, for instance, explain that from now on, for every day he does his homework promptly, he gets a star on the calendar." Agree that once he gets a certain number, he'll get a reward, suggests Dr. Butterworth.

Put on a happy face. For preschoolers who can't read

yet, draw or cut out pictures of the tasks the child needs to do, suggests Whitham. Then place "happy face" stickers on a chart next to tasks that have been completed. "The positive approach works best," she notes.

Give positive attention. A child who drags his feet may actually be getting more attention from his parents for dawdling than he would for being efficient, according to Dr. Butterworth. "Attention can be either negative or positive," he says. "Children don't look at the type of attention they get, but rather at its intensity." In other words, if you say, 'Oh, you came on time,' that's only a three on the attention scale (even though it's positive). But if you yell, 'I'm tired of you always being late,' that's an eight on the attention scale (even though it's negative). "That's why it's so important to give *lots* of positive attention," says Dr. Butterworth.

Make it clear. "Find out if your child is having trouble understanding what he's supposed to do," says Dr. Butterworth. "Make your expectations crystal clear." With an older child, you can sit down and actually write out a schedule of the week. "That way, both you and the child know exactly when things need to be accomplished," he says.

Avoid labels. "It's easy for kids to be labeled slowpoke or lazy," reminds Whitham. They also "get labeled" when you make statements like, "You're *never* ready on time" or "You're *always* late." These labels can become self-fulfilling, points out Whitham. Instead, treat your child as if you expect him to get things done and to be places on time.

Give one command at a time. Preschoolers can only respond to one command at a time, says Whitham. "Don't surround your requests by a huge paragraph. Make a short, clear statement ending in a period, such as 'Go get your shoes. Then come back to me, and I'll tell you the next thing.' "

Make eye contact. Some children become "immune" to

WHEN A COUNSELOR CAN HELP

It's time to get professional counseling, says William Womack, M.D., associate professor in the Department of Child Psychiatry at the University of Washington School of Medicine and codirector of the Stress Management Clinic of Children's Hospital and Medical Center, both in Seattle, if you're experiencing this worst case scenario: Your child is stubborn, resistant and opposed to doing just about anything, and everybody in the family is yelling and screaming at everybody else. A professional can provide therapy to help get the family back on track.

Another get-help situation is when the child is unable to do things which are really in her best interest. Such dawdling can be a way of postponing tasks that are scary or seen as too difficult. It may be that your child's schoolwork is too challenging, or that she is anxious about attending a dancing or sports activity.

Also, if dawdling is a consistent problem and the tips here don't seem to help, you should consider taking your child to the pediatrician for a medical checkup. "If your child doesn't come when he's called, you want to be sure his hearing is okay and that he is processing information correctly," says Cynthia Whitham, a licensed clinical social worker and staff therapist at the University of California, Los Angeles, Parent Training Clinic and author of *Win the Whining War and Other Skirmishes.* "There's a slight possibility he could have a receptive language disorder or other form of learning disability."

long-distance commands shouted at them by a far-away parent. Whitham suggests first calling your child to come to you—or going over to your child—rather than yelling a command across the house. Then look directly into her eyes when making your request.

Pace yourself. Whitham suggests that parents look at the pacing of their own lives. "Are you overworked? Are you a Type-A personality? Are you the one who's always rushing? If so, consider your child's dawdling as a sign that *you* need to slow down," she says.

Discuss the upcoming events. Ask a school-age child, "What's your plan? You have that TV program you enjoy watching and you have this homework assignment. How do you plan to fit everything in?" According to Whitham, this helps the child take responsibility, and she'll be more motivated to get a task done so she can move on to things she enjoys.

Get ready . . . get set . . . get out the stopwatch. "Little children get a big kick out of being timed or racing with you," says Whitham. When you need your child to get moving quickly, say, "I'll time you," or "Let's see how fast you can go." Use a stopwatch or the second hand of a watch. Be sure to praise success with comments like, "Wow, ten seconds—was that fast!" As a last resort, use timing in this way: "I'm going to count to three, and I want you to run and get your shoes."

DIAPER RASH

Soothing Baby's Ruddy Buns

C loth . . . or disposable? It's the first, critical decision that parents make about their newborn's immediate future.

But whichever diaper you choose, the goal is the same— to keep your baby's bottom as dry as possible through those incontinent first years of life. Succeed in that, and your infant has a pretty good chance of avoiding that ruby-red bane of babies' buns—diaper rash.

Diaper rash is what happens when a baby's sensitive skin is kept in contact with urine- or fecal-soaked diapers for any length of time. The moisture breaks down the skin's natural protective oils, and a red, irritated, bumpy rash appears. The makeup of the diaper is irrelevant: Doctors say diaper rash can happen whether your baby wears cloth *or* disposable diapers.

MEDICAL ALERT

When to See the Doctor

Diaper rash usually goes away after two or three days of care, but if it doesn't, contact your doctor. Your child may have more than just a routine diaper rash.

"If the rash is becoming beefy red, involves the creases of the groin and has round pink spots radiating from the red area, your child may have a yeast infection," says pediatrician Lynn Sugarman, M.D., a pediatrician with Tenafly Pediatrics in Tenafly, New Jersey, and an associate in clinical pediatrics at Babies Hospital, Columbia Presbyterian Medical Center in New York City. Yeast infections are often a side effect of taking antibiotics, but they may occur for other reasons, too. "A yeast infection is not serious and can be easily treated with an anti-fungal medication such as Lotrimin or Mycostatin cream, after seeking advice from a physician," says Dr. Sugarman.

"Also, see your physician at the first sign of anything that looks like a pimple or blister in the diaper area," suggests Dr. Sugarman. "Your child may have a staph infection. This is particularly important if your baby is a newborn, but no matter how old your child may be, he'll need antibiotics to take care of this bacterial infection."

Fortunately, diaper rash is rarely serious. But just try telling that to your uncomfortable infant who's wiggling, kicking and complaining with a preverbal vigor that keeps you hopping. You're sure to lose some sleep before it's over—but luckily, prompt action and a few preventive steps can usually take care of that rash. Here's where to start.

Change frequently.   "Paper or cloth diapers work equally well as long as you change them whenever they're wet or soiled," says Sam Solis, M.D., chairman of the Department of Pediatrics at Children's Hospital in New Orleans, assistant professor of pediatrics at Tulane University School of Medicine and a pediatrician in Metairie, Louisiana. At home, that's easy enough to do. But be sure to carry enough diapers when you're traveling as well.

Abolish plastic pants. If your baby is in cloth diapers, don't cover them with plastic pants except when you absolutely have to. "Plastic pants keep the moisture in, which is just what you don't want," says Dr. Solis. "Moisture can cause or worsen diaper rash." He recommends thick cloth diaper covers as a better alternative, since they allow the skin to breathe.

Go natural. If you change your tot frequently enough, she might not need any powder at all. But if you do need a baby powder, use plain cornstarch, recommends Daniel Bronfin, M.D., staff pediatrician at the Ochsner Clinic and assistant clinical professor of pediatrics at Tulane University School of Medicine. "A lot of people, particularly grandparents, enjoy applying powders and baby lotion after a diaper change, but these won't prevent diaper rash," says Dr. Bronfin. "In fact, because these products usually contain perfume and additives, they may even *cause* a rash."

Wipe out wipes. In an ideal world, a baby's bottom would be cleaned with mild soap and water and rinsed well with every diaper change. But most parents use wipes that may contain alcohol, perfume and soap that remain on the skin, notes Lynn Sugarman, M.D., a pediatrician with Tenafly Pediatrics in Tenafly, New Jersey, and an associate in clinical pediatrics at Babies Hospital, Columbia Presbyterian Medical Center in New York City. "Wipes can be irritating to the skin, especially when your baby has a diaper rash. At the first sign of a rash, switch to soap and water," says Dr. Sugarman.

Use a spray bottle. Dr. Bronfin recommends removing stool with warm water mixed with a drop or two of baby oil. "Use a spray bottle to spray the mixture on the diaper area, then wipe it off with a clean cloth," he suggests. This method will be less irritating to your baby.

Air it out. The diaper rash will heal faster if you let air get to the area. "Try to let your baby go without a diaper for 10 to 15 minutes after each diaper change," suggests Dr. Solis.

Try a sitz bath. When a rash is really uncomfortable, a sitz bath helps restore moisture to the skin and speeds healing, says Dr. Solis. "Two or three times a day, fill the tub with a few inches of warm water and let your child sit in the tub and play with his toys. You only have to do it for five to ten minutes each time, but it really makes a difference," he says.

Create a barrier. Protect irritated skin from further contact with waste by applying a thick layer of an over-the-counter barrier cream such as Balmex ointment or A and D Ointment, suggests Dr. Sugarman.

Snip some elastic. If your child is outfitted in disposable diapers, there's some custom tailoring you can do to get the air circulating a bit better, according to Dr. Bronfin. Put the diapers on as loosely as possible, rather than snug at the waist and snip some of the elastic from the bands around the leg openings, he suggests. And make sure you choose a diaper size that is roomy enough to allow for some air space.

DIARRHEA

When a Minor Has a Major Mess

An occasional "accident" on the way to the potty is one thing. But when your child has diarrhea, the accident looks more like an awful disaster. Frequent passage of unformed or watery stools is more than just messy—it's also potentially dangerous.

"Diarrhea depletes the body of fluid, and if that fluid is not replaced, the body will draw from its stores. When that happens, the child runs the risk of dehydration," says Shirley Menard, R.N., a certified pediatric nurse practitioner and assistant professor at the University of Texas Health Science Center at San Antonio School of Nursing.

Diarrhea can be the result of dietary factors, such as too much fruit juice or fiber. With babies, just the introduction of a new food may be enough to cause diarrhea. But it's often caused by viruses.

Whether or not it's caused by a virus, the diarrhea most parents see is usually the acute form. Although it doesn't last long, acute diarrhea is the most dangerous because it's often accompanied by fever, which increases the likelihood of dehydration. Some children, however, develop a mysterious bout of what is called chronic nonspecific diarrhea that has no known cause and is usually harmless. At the onset of any diarrhea, however, it really takes a doctor to tell the difference.

Diarrhea is one of those childhood ailments that usually responds well to care at home. But because it can have life-threatening side effects, or can be the symptom of a more serious illness, you'll want to give the doctor a call before trying any of these suggested remedies.

Drink, drink, drink. This is the most important piece of advice health professionals have to offer. For a child with diarrhea, drinking lots of liquids is the only thing that will prevent dehydration. Ice pops, crushed ice with or without flavoring or even a cold wet washcloth to suck on can be helpful.

Menard recommends, in addition, clear liquids such as Kool-Aid, tea, ginger ale and oral rehydration solutions (sold in drugstores). For older kids, Gatorade is also fine, according to Menard.

Babies up to 20 pounds who have diarrhea and are feverish or vomiting should be getting about 3 ounces of liquid per pound per day to avoid dehydration; children over 20 pounds should get 1 to 1½ ounces of fluid per pound daily.

When your child's hungry, resume feeding. Some experts still recommend the so-called BRAT diet once your child wants to eat again. BRAT stands for bananas, rice, applesauce and toast. "Those are all foods that bind the bowels," says Loraine Stern, M.D., associate clinical profes-

MEDICAL ALERT

When to See the Doctor

"Parents should always call their child's doctor immediately at the first sign of diarrhea," says Marjorie Hogan, M.D., an instructor of pediatrics at the University of Minnesota and a pediatrician at the Hennepin County Medical Center in Minneapolis. She warns that diarrhea can be a symptom of many other ailments that can only be diagnosed by a doctor.

With infants especially, there's a real danger of dehydration. According to Dr. Hogan, parents should be alert to these warning signs.

- No urination (no wet diapers) for some time
- Crying without tears
- Loss of skin elasticity
- Dry mouth
- Sunken fontanelle (the soft spot at the top of an infant's head)
- Lethargy or listlessness
- Diarrhea accompanied by vomiting (which may increase the likelihood of dehydration)

And you should get in touch with the doctor again if your child's diarrhea persists longer than three weeks, if stools contain blood or if there is severe abdominal pain or vomiting.

Children who are between the ages of about six months and three years and have diarrhea are also at risk of developing a condition called intussusception. "The bowel telescopes in on itself as a result of the violent force exerted by the bowel muscles," explains Shirley Menard, R.N., a certified pediatric nurse practitioner and assistant professor at the University of Texas Health Science Center at San Antonio School of Nursing. "If your child suddenly has severe pain and dark stools, which look like currant jelly, it's a medical emergency," she says. Call your doctor or the emergency room at once.

sor of pediatrics at the University of California, Los Angeles, and author of *When Do I Call the Doctor?* But according to Dr. Stern, newer research suggests the BRAT diet may prolong the viral infection that causes the diarrhea.

Instead of the restricted BRAT diet, most experts recommend offering the child with diarrhea a choice of all foods—except for milk—and allowing him to eat whatever appeals to him.

But *don't* offer milk or milk products. "A lot of children have trouble digesting milk when they're sick," says Marjorie Hogan, M.D., an instructor of pediatrics at the University of Minnesota and a pediatrician at the Hennepin County Medical Center in Minneapolis. "That's because illness frequently causes superficial damage to the intestines that disrupts normal production of lactase, the enzyme that helps digest the lactose in milk."

DON'T BE ALARMED BY THE COLOR

"Stools come in all sorts of cockamamy colors," says Loraine Stern, M.D., associate clinical professor of pediatrics at the University of California, Los Angeles, and author of *When Do I Call the Doctor?* A child's oddly colored bowel movement can be frightening to a parent, but usually there's a perfectly logical explanation and no cause for alarm.

Red stools, for example, can result from something as minor as a tiny burst blood vessel caused by straining or as ridiculous as too much Kool-Aid. "Sometimes laxatives can give stools a reddish color. So can beets and food dyes in cereal," says Dr. Stern.

Licorice, iron medication, spinach and Pepto-Bismol can make stools look black, says Dr. Stern. Sandy, gritty stools can be caused by pears. And even bananas can cause unusual looking stools.

But Dr. Stern also warns that red stools—or stools with flecks of red—can signify internal bleeding, which is quite serious. So if there's no ready explanation for the color, call the doctor.

If your baby is on a cow's milk formula, switch over to a soy or hypo-allergenic formula that doesn't contain lactose. You can find these nonmilk formulas in most pharmacies. If your baby is breastfeeding, though, you need to continue breastfeeding "as much as you can" to keep up his strength, says Dr. Stern.

Read baby formula labels carefully. If you've been mixing baby formulas incorrectly, you may have inadvertently caused your baby's diarrhea, says Dr. Hogan. Review the labels and make sure your measurements are exact.

Cut back on fruit juice. In babies, especially, too much fruit juice can cause diarrhea or make it worse. Some experts recommend serving only two or three small portions a day, says William B. Ruderman, M.D., Chairman of the Department of Gastroenterology at the Cleveland Clinic—Florida in Fort Lauderdale. For children under one, the serving sizes should be no larger than one-third cup of vitamin C-rich juice (like orange juice). If your baby wants more, dilute it with water.

Cut back on fruit, too. Children under one who have diarrhea problems should eat no more than 1/4 to 1/3 cup of soft fruit at each serving—and no more than three servings a day, says Dr. Ruderman. Be alert, too, for fruit that's in prepared or packaged food—such as figs in Fig Newtons.

Fatten up the diet. There is some evidence that a low-fat diet can promote a certain kind of chronic diarrhea in children, explains Dr. Ruderman. Experts suggest adding margarine to vegetables, and serving fish, poultry and meats that have moderate amounts of fat. In addition, children under the age of two should normally drink whole, rather than low-fat, milk.

Avoid artificial sweeteners. Foods that contain artificial sweeteners such as sorbitol and saccharin may promote diarrhea, according to Dr. Ruderman. Read labels, and avoid food products with these additives whenever possible.

Watch those bottoms. A child with diarrhea may suffer

from a painful irritation of the anus. That's because the enzymes that help us digest food are also present in stool, and those enzymes irritate the anal area, says Dr. Stern. "When you have diarrhea, stools go through very quickly and frequently these enzymes also start to 'digest' the skin."

If irritation develops, wash the child's bottom with running water and some soap to get the enzymes off. "Don't just use wipes," says Dr. Stern. "Rinse their bottoms well and dry them off well, too."

Don't use drugstore remedies ... *unless* **you call the doctor.** Over-the-counter anti-diarrhea products are available for children, but that doesn't mean they're recommended by physicians. In fact, not all pediatricians and family physicians are in agreement over whether they should be used at all. "My feeling is they should be used only for a day, if there are no other complications," says Dr. Stern. "They just slow the diarrhea down a little bit so the child is more comfortable, but they don't cure anything." Before you use any anti-diarrhea medication, Dr. Stern recommends that you consult with your pediatrician.

DIZZINESS

Steps to Stop the Spinning

Your five-year-old didn't eat much lunch, and he's been running around all afternoon. But when he comes inside, he seems a bit unsteady. It's not until he says, "I'm dizzy," that you realize what the problem is.

Since dizziness can be caused by anything from missed lunch or a virus to epilepsy or a head injury, it frequently requires a doctor's care. In some cases, however, a little common sense can put stability back into your child's world.

Time for a bookmark. Reading in a car often triggers

dizziness. It's caused by a conflict between messages from the inner ear and messages from the eyes.

The solution? "Ask your child to stop reading and look ahead at something stable on the horizon," says Helen Cohen, Ed.D., assistant professor of otorhinolaryngology at Baylor College of Medicine in Houston. The dizziness will pass.

Lie down. If your child feels dizzy, tell him to lie down, slowly and gradually, says Sidney N. Busis, M.D., clinical professor of otolaryngology at the University of Pittsburgh School of Medicine. And suggest that he avoid sudden changes in position until the dizziness passes.

Watch the light. "When your child's dizzy, keep a light on at night," adds Dr. Busis. If he wakes up feeling dizzy, he can look around the lit room to get his bearings. And if your child needs to get up during the night, a light will show him what he can grab to help keep his balance.

Cool it. If your child gets dizzy after he's been soaking in the tub, have him drink something cool and lie down, says Edwin Monsell, M.D., Ph.D., head of the Division of Otology and Neurotology (the study of ear problems and diseases) at Henry Ford Hospital in Detroit. Anyone will feel dizzy if they soak in a hot tub and then suddenly stand up, he explains. That's because blood rushes to our skin to try to cool the body when we're soaking. When we stand up, it takes time for normal blood flow to resume—and meanwhile we may get dizzy.

With kids, this body reaction is very pronounced. Since children are so small, their bodies can get seriously overheated in hot water. That's one reason whirlpools, hot tubs and saunas aren't recommended for young children.

Keep up the drinks and eats. Make sure your child drinks a glass of water at regular intervals throughout the day, particularly in the summer, says Dr. Monsell. Dehydration can cause dizziness because blood volume is low.

If your child hasn't eaten in a while, this can also cause dizziness—but start him on a bland drink such as apple

MEDICAL ALERT

When to See the Doctor

While dizziness in children is most commonly caused by a virus, it can also be a sign of serious illness. Don't hesitate to take your child to a doctor if she experiences recurring episodes of dizziness or if one episode of dizziness lasts for more than half an hour. You should also get her to the doctor as soon as possible if she feels dizzy after a fall. And call for emergency assistance immediately if she loses consciousness after complaining of dizziness.

"If your child has fallen down and banged her head—even if the dizziness only lasts a few moments—I'd take her to a doctor to rule out a concussion or any other serious damage," says Helen Cohen, Ed.D., assistant professor of otorhinolaryngology at Baylor College of Medicine in Houston.

You should also check with a doctor if your child complains of ringing, pain or "stuffiness" anywhere in the head—particularly the ears. "Kids get ear infections easily," says Sidney N. Busis, M.D., clinical professor of otolaryngology at the University of Pittsburgh School of Medicine. And a bacterial ear infection can permanently affect your child's hearing if it's not promptly treated with antibiotics.

Dizziness may also be caused by an inner ear problem called nystagmus, which should be checked out by a doctor, according to Dr. Busis. The usual sign of nystagmus is a rhythmic movement of the eye characterized by slow movement in one direction, followed by quick movement in the opposite direction.

If your child's dizziness *is* caused by nystagmus, the problem can be alleviated with special exercises, according to Dr. Busis.

juice or a sports drink before serving food, adds Dr. Monsell. Steer clear of foods and beverages that contain caffeine, since that stimulant can be a prime cause of dizziness.

Check the medicine cabinet. Sometimes a medication

WHEN THEY DON'T KNOW THEY'RE DIZZY

Sometimes a child won't tell you she's dizzy because she doesn't know that *dizzy* is the name of what she feels.

But you can identify her problem by watching for a few simple clues. "A very young child may be feeling dizzy when she stops moving and puts her head against the bars of the crib. She's trying to stabilize things," says Helen Cohen, Ed.D., assistant professor of otorhinolaryngology at Baylor College of Medicine in Houston.

"A slightly older child who likes to read may suddenly put down her book and look around in confusion," Dr. Cohen notes. If you notice your child does this frequently, be sure to ask how she feels. From her description, you can usually tell whether she's dizzy or not.

your child is taking may cause dizziness as a side effect. Ask your doctor or pharmacist about a possible connection, suggests Andrea Beylen, a physical therapist at the Rehabilitation Department of Sequoia Hospital in Redwood City, California. If there is a connection, your doctor may be able to recommend a substitution.

Thumbs up for spinning around. Dizziness is to be expected if your child has been spinning around or rolling down a hill. If your child experiences dizziness, you can help her overcome the problem by doing a focusing exercise. "Tell her to sit still, stick out her arm and stare at her thumb," says Dr. Cohen. That should help the dizziness subside.

EAR INFECTIONS

Countering Chronic Flare-Ups

I f your child gets through her toddler years without an ear infection, her guardian angel must be working overtime.

"A middle ear infection, also known as otitis media, is one of the most frequently diagnosed childhood illnesses," says Michael Macknin, M.D., head of the Section of General Pediatrics at the Cleveland Clinic Foundation in Ohio, clinical professor at Pennsylvania State University Medical School in Hershey and associate professor of pediatrics at Ohio State University Medical School in Columbus. The root of the problem lies in the eustachian tubes, narrow passageways that connect the back of the nose and throat to the middle ear. When a eustachian tube functions properly, it allows air into the middle ear while keeping out bacteria and debris from the nose and mouth. It also permits any fluid that may collect to drain out.

Babies and young children, however, have very tiny eustachian tubes that tend to get swollen and blocked each time a cold, sinus infection or allergy attack comes along. A swollen eustachian tube can't do its job, says Dr. Macknin, and that makes your child more susceptible to middle ear infection.

When your child comes down with a middle ear infection, you'll probably know it—at around 2:00 in the morning when she awakens, crying and feverish. Ear infections are usually, but not always, painful and may be accompanied by irritability and some temporary hearing loss, notes Dr. Macknin. A full course of doctor-prescribed antibiotics should kill the bacteria, but fluid may remain in the middle ear, providing a warm, moist breeding ground for future infections.

If your child is taking antibiotics, follow your doctor's orders exactly. If you stop giving the medication prematurely because your child is feeling better, the bacteria might not be entirely wiped out. The survivors could multiply and bounce back, causing another infection, says Dr. Macknin.

Although your child should outgrow the tendency to get ear infections, lots of kids suffer with them throughout their preschool years. While you can't prevent ear infections completely, doctors say there are a number of ways you can reduce your child's chances of getting an infection. And even if your child gets one, you can make him more comfortable. Here are some suggestions.

MEDICAL ALERT

When to See the Doctor

If your child is still sick or in pain after three days of taking prescribed antibiotics for an ear infection, you should return to your doctor, says Charles D. Bluestone, M.D., professor of otolaryngology at the University of Pittsburgh School of Medicine and director of the Department of Pediatric Otolaryngology and the Otitis Media Research Center at the Children's Hospital of Pittsburgh. Your child may have a strain of bacteria that is resistant to the antibiotic she is currently taking, and she may need a stronger medicine to wipe out the infection.

"If your child is in acute pain, your pediatrician or otolaryngologist (a doctor who specializes in diseases of the ear, nose and throat) may perform a myringotomy," says Dr. Bluestone. "In this simple office procedure, a small nick in the affected eardrum relieves fluid buildup and pressure. This usually brings immediate relief from pain."

Treatment

Use a painkiller for short-term relief. Prescription antibiotics should provide pain relief within 12 to 24 hours. But while you wait for that relief to kick in, your child can take acetaminophen (Children's Tylenol) if he needs it, says Charles D. Bluestone, M.D., professor of otolaryngology at the University of Pittsburgh School of Medicine and director of the Department of Pediatric Otolaryngology and the Otitis Media Research Center at the Children's Hospital of Pittsburgh. Check the package directions for the correct dosage for your child's age and weight. If your child is under age two, consult a physician.

Don't rely on over-the-counter ear drops that contain a local anesthetic to relieve the pain. "None of them have been shown to be effective in controlled trials," Dr. Bluestone says.

Try some "warm-up exercises." Children with ear pain

may find warmth soothing. "I sometimes recommend that parents put two or three drops of warm mineral oil into their child's ear," says Gerald Zahtz, M.D., assistant professor of otolaryngology at Albert Einstein College of Medicine in New York City and physician at the Long Island Jewish Medical Center in New Hyde Park, New York. "But it's critical that the drops be the correct temperature. If they are too warm or too cold, you may induce dizziness. So aim for body temperature."

Hold the mineral oil bottle in your hand for about 15 minutes before you put in the drops. Or fill a large bowl with hot water and keep the bottle in the water for about 5 minutes. Test the oil against your skin before putting it in the ear.

Caution: Never use drops if the ear is draining, Dr. Zahtz advises.

Use a warm-water bottle. Dr. Zahtz recommends holding a hot-water bottle against the ear, but it should be filled

---

WHEN EAR INFECTIONS WON'T QUIT

Most ear infections clear up nicely with the help of an antibiotic, but your child may not be so lucky. If he has three ear infections within a six-month period, or two before he is six months old, additional measures may be needed, says Michael Macknin, M.D., head of the Section of General Pediatrics at the Cleveland Clinic Foundation in Ohio, clinical professor at Pennsylvania State University Medical School at Hershey and associate professor of pediatrics at Ohio State University Medical School in Columbus. Your doctor may prescribe prophylactic medication, antibiotics taken daily at a low, maintenance-level dosage to help prevent infections from recurring.

While your child is on prophylactic antibiotics, his ears will need to be checked by the doctor every month or two. If, during this time, your child is still getting infections, or if there is persistent fluid in the ear, your doctor may suggest other treatment, says Dr. Macknin.

with warm, *not* hot, water, he says. Also, wrap the bottle in a towel before placing it against the ear.

Preventive Care

Don't smoke around your child. Studies show that the children of smokers have more colds and ear infections than children of nonsmokers. "If you smoke, the best thing you can do for your child is to quit. But if you don't quit, at least smoke outside. Don't smoke around your child," Dr. Macknin says.

Breastfeed your baby. Breastfeeding provides a protective benefit, because anitbodies passed along in the breast milk may decrease your baby's chance of getting an infection, notes Dr. Bluestone. There also seems to be something in mother's milk that helps prevent bacteria from sticking to the mucous membrane of the throat, making it less likely that germs will travel up the eustachian tube into the ear, he says. "If you want to help prevent ear infections, you should breastfeed your baby for at least the first six months," Dr. Bluestone advises.

Feed baby in an upright position. When you bottlefeed or nurse your baby, keep his body in an upright position, especially if he tends to regurgitate a bit of his meal. "If your baby is in a horizontal position while feeding, regurgitated milk can pass into the eustachian tube, and possibly cause an infection," says Dr. Zahtz. This is less likely to happen if you hold your baby at an angle of 45 degrees or more while feeding, he says.

Consider a babysitter instead of day care. Babies under one year old are especially vulnerable to the many viruses in a day-care environment, according to Dr. Bluestone. As a result, they end up with more ear infections than children who are cared for at home, he says. If possible, consider delaying day care until your child is past this critical age.

Ask the doctor about milk allergy. In rare cases, recurrent ear infections may be due to milk allergy, says Dr. Zahtz. "If a child with chronic infections is less than a year old, I try taking him off all milk products for four weeks to see what develops." Don't make any diet changes without talking to your doctor first, though, advises Dr. Zahtz, or you could seriously compromise your child's health.

Watch for early signs of sinus infection. If your child has a cold, and the nasal mucus starts to thicken and become colored, consult a doctor. Thick yellow or green mucus may indicate a sinus infection that needs to be treated with antibiotics, says Dr. Zahtz. If the problem is treated early, there is a good chance that it won't lead to an ear infection, he says.

EARLOBE INFECTIONS

Help for a Piercing Problem

Your daughter has been lobbying hard for earrings. After all, she is the only one of her friends whose ears are not adorned with door knockers, shoulder dusters or hoops large enough to do the hula in. You wince at the idea of dangling so much metal from her ears—and what about the possibility of infection?

Fashion statements aside, earlobe infections do happen from time to time. "Whenever you insert an earring into the ear, you are inviting bacteria that live on the skin to hitch a ride on the earring and cause an infection within the earlobe," says Sam Solis, M.D., chairman of the Department of Pediatrics at Children's Hospital in New Orleans, assistant professor of pediatrics at Tulane University School of Medicine and a pediatrician in Metairie, Louisiana. "If the skin around the earring is red, swollen, scabbed, crusty or oozing, you've got an infection there," says Dr. Solis.

The first way to avoid infection is to have ears pierced by the right person in the right way. Find a dermatologist who pierces ears with an ear-piercing "gun," a device that pierces the earlobe with a sterilized earring, suggests Alvin

MEDICAL ALERT

When to See the Doctor

"If an earlobe infection does not go away on its own after a few days, you should definitely see your doctor," says Katherine Karlsrud, M.D., a clinical instructor in pediatrics at Cornell University Medical College in Ithaca, New York, and a pediatrician in New York City. It is unlikely that an earlobe infection will develop into something serious, but if an infection is ignored, it can turn into cellulitis, a creeping infection underneath the skin.

Cellulitis starts with a little bit of redness just where the earring is inserted. After that, it can spread over the entire earlobe, up the scalp, behind the neck and into the ear canal, according to Dr. Karlsrud. Cellulitis needs to be treated with antibiotics.

L. Adler, M.D., a dermatologist and attending physician and clinical instructor in dermatology at the New York Hospital—Cornell Medical Center and Beth Israel Medical Center, both in New York City. "Because a physician uses sterile equipment and techniques, the risk of infection is reduced," says Dr. Adler.

After that, here's what experts recommend to prevent infection or to nip it in the bud.

Keep ears clean. Treat newly pierced ears to a hydrogen peroxide wash twice a day, and follow up with an application of antibiotic ointment. Keep up this regimen for the first two to three days after piercing, then keep the area clean with plain soap and water, says Dr. Adler.

Go for the gold. Have your child wear earrings made of a pure metal such as silver or gold, says Katherine Karlsrud, M.D., a clinical instructor in pediatrics at Cornell University Medical College in Ithaca, New York, and a pediatrician in New York City. "Many people are sensitive to nickel, which is a metal commonly found in inexpensive earrings," says Dr. Karlsrud. The allergic reaction to that metal may lead to an infection.

Dr. Adler suggests that 24-karat gold earrings are worth the money when it comes to infection protection. "Ten- or 14-carat gold contains a certain amount of nickel, but 24-carat is the purest you can find in jewelry," he says.

Remove 'em. Remove the earrings at the first sign of infection. Your child may want to keep them in, but it's not a good practice. "The body has a real hard time fighting off an ear infection while the earring is in place," says Dr. Solis. "Take out the earrings, keep the area clean with soap and water, and the redness and swelling should go down by itself within a few days."

Get tougher. "At the first sign of infection, go back to applying hydrogen peroxide followed by antibiotic ointment twice daily," says Dr. Adler.

EATING PROBLEMS

How to Handle the Picky Eater

I 'm not hungry," four-year-old Andrew says sweetly, sitting at the dining room table, his untouched meal before him. His mother takes a deep breath, and the little vein in her neck begins to throb. Another dinner-time battle has begun.

Andrew has figured out how to drive his mother crazy: He eats only one brand of canned spaghetti for lunch, refuses dinner and whines for snacks up until bedtime.

Eating is one area where kids can begin to control their parents. Mom and Dad—worried that their slender, picky eater isn't getting enough nourishment—resort to threatening, bribing, cajoling or catering to their child to try to get him to eat.

Once an eating problem develops, it takes patience and

time to deal with it. Here are some hints from the experts to help you over the hurdle.

Assess your expectations. If your child eats small portions, don't worry. Some children don't need large amounts of food, says Alvin N. Eden, M.D., associate clinical professor of pediatrics at the New York Hospital—Cornell Medical Center, chairman of the Department of Pediatrics at Wyckoff Heights Medical Center, both in New York City, and author of *Positive Parenting* and *Dr. Eden's Healthy Kids*. Also realize that children can vary a lot in their day-to-day intake. They may be ravenous one day and pick at their food the next.

Serve small portions. "Put less food on your child's plate than you think he'll eat," says Quentin Van Meter, M.D., a pediatrician and associate professor of clinical pediatrics at Emory University School of Medicine in Atlanta. "Piles of food on a plate can turn off a child's appetite."

The appropriate portion size for kids is surprisingly small—and you can always serve seconds if the child wants more, points out Dr. Eden.

Snacks are fine—but keep them small. Your child may be turning up her nose at her nutritious dinner because her tummy is full of the chips she had after school. Don't deprive her of the after-school snack—but these snacks have to be small if you expect your child to eat a full dinner, says Barton D. Schmitt, M.D., professor of pediatrics at the University of Colorado School of Medicine, director of consultative services at the Ambulatory Care Center at Children's Hospital of Denver and author of *Your Child's Health*.

Limit the drinks, too. Many parents underestimate how filling juice and milk can be, says Dr. Van Meter. He recommends limiting juice to 6 ounces a day and milk to 16 ounces.

"The fats and sugars in these fluids can curb the appetite just enough to keep your child active and happy, but he won't be getting a balanced meal," he says. Soda is even

MEDICAL ALERT

When to See the Doctor

When a child is thin, it's often because he's quite active or just naturally slender.

But there are a few symptoms that should alert you that something may be wrong, says Barton D. Schmitt, M.D., professor of pediatrics at the University of Colorado School of Medicine, director of consultative services at the Ambulatory Care Center at Children's Hospital of Denver and author of *Your Child's Health*. Some illnesses, such as infestation with roundworms, can cause unnatural thinness. And preteens—girls especially—can develop a serious eating disorder called anorexia nervosa.

Call your child's physician if you notice that your child:

- Is losing weight.
- Has not gained any weight in six months.
- Has associated symptoms of illness, such as diarrhea or fever.
- Has lost weight suddenly.
- Gags on or vomits some foods.
- Has thinning hair.
- Develops fine, babylike hair on the body.

worse, because it fills up the child without supplying any essential nutrients.

Consider mini-meals. Some busy, active children function better on small meals throughout the day, says Corinne Montandon, Dr.P.H., R.D., assistant professor of nutrition at Baylor College of Medicine and the Children's Nutrition Research Center, both in Houston. Toddlers, in particular, may need nutritious small meals about two to three hours apart. This doesn't mean that Mom has to prepare meals on demand, however. Keep a supply of healthy snack foods on hand. "Give your child some cheese and fruit, or graham crackers and a small glass of milk," suggests Dr. Montandon. Then don't expect your child to eat a big meal at dinner.

Plan ahead. "Children who must wait too long between meals get so hungry that they get cranky," says Dr. Montandon, "and cranky kids do not eat well." If you know that your child gets famished because you can't get dinner on the table before 7:00 P.M., furnish a nourishing mini-meal earlier, or cook dinner ahead of time so you can serve it earlier.

Involve your child. Decide together what you are going to serve, advises Dr. Montandon. Offer nutritious choices and then let your child pick. "Children who are given the chance to make food decisions are more likely to eat what they choose," she says.

Let your child feed herself. When a child is pushing her food around the plate, it's tempting to pick up the spoon and try to tease her into eating, says Dr. Schmitt. Don't do it. "Once your child is old enough to use a spoon by herself (usually 15 to 16 months of age), never again pick it up for her," he says. "If your child is hungry, she will feed herself."

Refrain from forcing. Just about the worst thing you can do is force your child to eat, agree experts. This will frustrate you, make your child resentful and create a power struggle that no one will win—and it won't solve the problem, says Dr. Schmitt. "How much a child chooses to eat is governed by the appetite center in the brain," he explains. "If you try to control how much your child eats, he will rebel. Trust the appetite center."

Keep mealtimes pleasant. This is what you should concentrate on, rather than what your child does or doesn't eat, says Dr. Schmitt. "Draw your children into the conversation, and don't make mealtimes a time for criticism or arguments," he advises.

Forget about forcing your child to stay at the table with his food after the rest of the family has left. "This only develops unpleasant associations with mealtimes," says Dr. Schmitt.

Insist on politeness. Let your child know that he is ex-

DON'T WORRY—IT'S NORMAL

Suddenly it seems that your child is devouring an enormous amount of food at each meal, and you're worried that he's overeating.

But your child may simply be going through a growth spurt, explains Alvin N. Eden, M.D., associate clinical professor of pediatrics at the New York Hospital–Cornell Medical Center, chairman of the Department of Pediatrics at Wyckoff Heights Medical Center, both in New York City, and author of *Positive Parenting* and *Dr. Eden's Healthy Kids*. While in a growth phase, children may consume large quantities of food to keep up with the calories being burned. Just be sure that your child is eating a variety of foods and isn't loading up mostly on sweets or fatty foods.

If you're concerned, check with your pediatrician. Your child's pediatrician plots your child's weight and height on a special chart. If the child's growth deviates markedly from his usual patterns, that will signal that something is wrong.

Otherwise, relax—and keep plenty of healthy foods on hand for your hungry, growing child.

pected to be at the table on time, sit with the family while they eat and refrain from making faces and rude comments about the food, suggests Dr. Eden.

Never nag—or praise. Keep eating as matter-of-fact as possible, says Dr. Schmitt. Don't fuss at your problem eater for not finishing her food or praise her when she does. You want your child to eat to satisfy her appetite, not to please you. And never discuss how much or how little your child eats when you're in her presence.

Don't cook on demand. Never get up and make special meals for a picky eater, says Dr. Eden. Serve a well-balanced meal and let your child eat what she wants from what you have served.

Eliminate "gag" foods. Some kids have a natural aversion to foods that they associate with being sick. If a child happened to become ill after a certain food, that food may turn his stomach. Rather than force him to eat those foods, parents should avoid serving them, advises Dr. Schmitt. "Those foods should be put in a special category and simply eliminated from the menu," he says.

Avoid the dessert dilemma. This is a classic Catch-22. If everyone digs into a rich gooey cake for dessert but the noncater isn't allowed any, you're reinforcing the idea that "good" food is a reward for eating "bad" food. If you do give cake to the problem eater, you're letting her fill up on empty calories, explains Dr. Van Meter.

Your best bet is to serve nutritious desserts that are considered part of the meal: fruit, gelatin with fruit or yogurt, he suggests.

Ease your mind with vitamins. If you're worried about your child's intake of certain nutrients, ask your pediatrician about giving your child a daily vitamin and mineral supplement, says Dr. Van Meter. The supplement may not be necessary, but it can put your mind at ease.

ECZEMA

Strategies to Stop the Itching

This is one ailment that can *really* make a parent feel helpless. Your child is itching and scratching, and it's impossible to convince her to stop. Yet there seems to be no reason for this itchy ailment that can cause children to scratch themselves raw.

Eczema, also called atopic dermatitis, is usually associated with dry skin. It starts with a pink or red area that becomes itchy. After your child scratches, the skin gets rough and scaly or—in infants—may ooze and form a crust.

Eczema is common in babies between the ages of 2 months and 18 months, but it can occur at any age. In fact, about 10 percent of us have an outbreak of eczema at some

MEDICAL ALERT

When to See the Doctor

A doctor should always diagnose eczema, but once it's diagnosed you can treat most flare-ups at home. In some cases, however, the itchiness of eczema causes scratching and irritation so severe that open sores may appear on your child's skin. And that's where problems can develop.

"These open areas can become infected," says Karen Houpt, M.D., assistant professor of dermatology at the University of Texas Southwestern Medical Center in Dallas. "These require immediate medical attention, not only to heal the infection but also to bring the eczema flare-up back under control."

Signs of infection include pus or red streaks leading away from the scratch.

Also alert the doctor if your child has many open, scratched areas, and particularly, if any of them are bloody or have yellow crusts, says Dr. Houpt.

point in our lives, according to Hugh Sampson, M.D., a pediatric allergy/immunology specialist, professor of pediatrics and director of the Pediatric Clinical Research Unit at the Johns Hopkins University School of Medicine in Baltimore.

There's definitely a link between dermatitis and allergies. Many children with eczema come from families whose members suffer from hay fever, asthma and seasonal runny noses—and your child is more likely to have eczema if you or your spouse has had it. Also, everyday exposures to soaps, perfumes, dry air, heat or stress can trigger outbreaks of eczema. Generally, it waxes and wanes, though it often disappears completely as children grow up.

If your doctor has diagnosed your child as having eczema, he'll help you look for the factors that are triggering outbreaks so you can reduce your child's exposure. Because causes can differ, you may need to experiment to find what works best for your child. But here are what some of the experts recommend.

Limit bathing. Daily bathing isn't necessary, and it tends to make already dry skin even drier, says William Epstein, M.D., professor of dermatology at the University of California, San Francisco, School of Medicine. "Instead, you can sponge bathe the parts of the body that really need it—the hands, face, neck, armpits and (for babies) the diaper area." When you do bathe your child in the tub, make it quick—don't allow time for splashing or playing. "Get your child in and out quickly," says Bill Halmi, M.D., clinical assistant professor of dermatology at the Thomas Jefferson University Hospital in Philadelphia.

Try a soap substitute. If you use a soap substitute such as Neutrogena Rainbath shower and bath gel, your child can bathe daily, says Robert Rietschel, M.D., chairman of the Department of Dermatology at the Ochsner Clinic and clinical associate professor of dermatology at Louisiana State University and Tulane University School of Medicine, all in New Orleans. "It does an excellent job of keeping the skin relatively free of bacteria," he explains, "which in turn helps cut down on secondary infections."

Another good soap-free cleanser is Cetaphil, says Karen Houpt, M.D., assistant professor of dermatology at the University of Texas Southwestern Medical Center in Dallas. Don't expect it to lather up like regular soap, however.

Choose unscented products. A moisturizer or soap can contain fragrances that will trigger a flare-up of eczema. "Look for products that state that they're fragrance-free, such as the soaps Neutrogena and unscented Dove, and moisturizers like Neutrogena Norwegian Formula and Eucerin," says Dr. Houpt.

Keep it warm. Water should be warm enough to keep your child comfortable, but no warmer. "Hot water is more drying than warm water and tends to remove the oils from the skin," says Dr. Halmi.

Wash gently. Try to wash affected areas with water only or water and soap substitute. "But if you need to use a washcloth, be very gentle," says Dr. Houpt. "The tendency is to take soap and washcloth and really scrub the rash down, but nothing could be worse." Scrubbing and soap irritate the skin and dry it further.

Apply moisturizer liberally. Right after bathtime, while your child's skin is still wet from the bath, is the perfect time to apply moisturizers. "Mixing the oil with the water on the body will help hold some of the moisture in," says Dr. Epstein.

Dr. Rietschel recommends a cream such as Eucerin Creme rather than a lotion: "Creams are heavy enough to seal the skin and keep the moisture in," he says. Plain petroleum jelly will work, too (although it produces a rather slippery child). "Be sure to apply any moisturizer all over the body, not just to the affected areas," says Dr. Halmi.

Add cool compresses. "After applying oils or moisturizers, top with a cool compress for particularly itchy areas," says Dr. Epstein. "It helps soothe the skin." A washcloth soaked in cold water makes a good compress.

Keep nails short. To help limit the damage a baby or child can inflict on an itchy outbreak, keep fingernails clipped short and keep the edges of nails rounded, says Dr. Epstein. Another way to decrease nighttime scratching fits is to put mittens or socks on your child's hands at bedtime.

Keep 'em cool. Avoid overdressing or bundling up your child unnecessarily at night, because getting too hot can make the rash worse, says Dr. Halmi.

Choose snug PJs. "Loose-fitting pajamas can actually cause more rubbing and irritation to the skin than close-fitting ones," says Dr. Halmi. So choose knit nightwear over floppy, button-down PJs.

Opt for cotton. Cotton clothing is the best choice for your child to wear against sensitive skin, says Dr. Halmi. Avoid wool, which can especially irritate eczema.

Double-rinse clothes. Because detergents can irritate skin, run your child's laundry through a double rinse cycle to help remove detergent residue, says Stephen M. Purcell, D.O., chairman of the Department of Dermatology at Philadelphia College of Osteropathic Medicine and assistant clinical professor at Hahnemann University School of Health Sciences. Also, avoid fabric-softening dryer sheets, because they put chemicals in the clothing that can irritate the skin.

Humidify the surroundings. Dry air can contribute to itchiness, and most homes with central heating are too dry in winter. When the heat goes on, run a cold-air humidifier or place pans of water on or near heat outlets, suggests Nelson Lee Novick, M.D., a dermatologist and associate clinical professor of dermatology at Mount Sinai School of Medicine in New York City and author of *Super Skin*.

Reach for the hydrocortisone. "Hydrocortisone applied to the affected areas can help relieve the incessant itching of eczema," says Dr. Rietschel. Many hydrocortisone-containing over-the-counter products are available at pharmacies. Choose products in a 1 percent concentration and preferably ones that are ointment-based, rather than cream based.

"The ointment-based form tends to boost the potency of the cortisone because it seals it in and then drives it through the skin in slightly greater concentrations," says Dr. Rietschel. If you only have cream cortisone on hand, add a coating of petroleum jelly over the cream to produce the same effect.

Try an antihistamine. An over-the-counter antihistamine such as Benadryl may help quell the itch, says Dr. Houpt, but only give it before bedtime because it's likely to make your child sleepy. Be sure to read package directions to make certain the product is recommended for your child's age. For the correct dosage, follow package directions or consult your physician. Dr. Houpt advices against using an antihistamine product such as Benadryl Spray directly on the skin: The direct application may cause an allergic reaction.

Take stock of your child's diet. "There's a 20 to 30 percent chance that a food allergy may be causing your child's eczema," says Dr. Sampson. Children with eczema are most often allergic to eggs, milk, peanuts, wheat, soy, fish and tree nuts, although a child is usually allergic to only one or two of those foods. "If you notice a clear-cut pattern where a food consistently creates problems for your child, then it should be eliminated from his diet," he says.

Reduce stress levels. Stress can trigger eczema or make it worse, says Dr. Rietschel. Encourage your child to talk about problems, offer help with homework and cut down on your child's activities if the two of you decide there's just too much in the schedule. And try to keep calm about the rashes themselves, Dr. Rietschel says, so your own worries don't add to the child's stress.

FATIGUE

Tips to Recharge the Battery

M ommy, I'm tired!" Sure, you expect to hear that late in the afternoon, after your eight-year-old child has just spent the entire day playing with friends or racing around at a birthday party.

But what if your daughter says "I'm tired!" first thing in the morning or when she's on her way to the party? That's when her fatigue and droopiness are puzzling.

Toddlers don't complain of fatigue the same way as eight-year-olds, but they do get tired, too. The difference is that in toddlers, fatigue shows up as crankiness and whininess, says William Womack, M.D., associate professor in the Department of Child Psychiatry at the University of Washington School of Medicine and codirector of the Stress Management Clinic of Children's Hospital and Medical Center, both in Seattle.

Once you've ruled out possible physical causes of fa-

MEDICAL ALERT

When to See the Doctor

It's not normal for a child to be tired all the time, pediatricians agree. Fatigue can be a symptom of a variety of medical conditions, including infections, abscessed tooth, cold or flu, chronic nasal congestion, allergies, an underactive thyroid, anemia, parasites such as pinworms, or depression.

Here are a few symptoms that tell you it's time to check with a doctor.

- Fatigue that won't go away
- Sleeping much longer than usual or taking naps more often
- Problems sleeping
- Dark circles under the eyes
- Bad breath
- Persistent sadness and crying

Fatigue can also be caused by depression. "Childhood depression isn't unusual, but a lot of parents miss the signs," says William Womack, M.D., associate professor in the Department of Child Psychiatry at the University of Washington School of Medicine and codirector of the Stress Management Clinic of Children's Hospital and Medical Center, both in Seattle.

Watch out for sleep problems. "If your child has symptoms for two or three months, combined with a lowered energy level, seek professional advice, preferably from a child psychiatrist," says Dr. Womack.

Finally, excessive tiredness could also be caused by chronic fatigue syndrome, an illness that more often affects adults, says David S. Bell, M.D., an instructor of pediatrics at Harvard Medical School and in the Department of Pediatrics at The Cambridge Hospital in Massachusetts. If all other causes have been ruled out, ask your doctor if your child could be suffering from this ailment.

tigue, try our experts' perk-up suggestions. The odds are, your child will be outrunning you again in no time.

Build up slowly. If your relatively sedentary child suddenly acquires a group of active new friends, takes up a new sport or joins a play group, he'll likely be fatigued at first, says Robert R. Butterworth, Ph.D., a clinical psychologist in Los Angeles who specializes in treating children and adolescents. Explain to your child that it will take a while to "get up to speed." Encourage him to take things easy and get extra rest until he's used to the new activity.

Slow things down. Older children may be fatigued simply because they're doing too many things, says Dr. Womack. If your child participates in an after-school activity almost every day, plus sports or Scouts on weekends, you may need to cut out an activity or two.

Add in chill-out time. If your child is at school or day care all day, that can add up to a long, tiring day, says Frances Willson, Ph.D., a clinical psychologist in Sherman Oaks, California, and chairman of the Health Psychology Committee of the Los Angeles County Psychological Association.

If you can, arrange for your child to occasionally spend time with just a friend and a parent or sitter after school instead of always being in a large group. And some children, no matter what their age, benefit from a nap during the day. If none of these options are possible, give your child half an hour to an hour of quiet time when she gets home. Serve her a snack at the kitchen table while you prepare dinner, or have her rest quietly in her room with a book.

Go for more variety. On the other hand, a child without many activities or friends may not be fatigued at all—just bored by the same day-in, day-out routine. Try to add one activity that really appeals to your child, says Dr. Willson: "If your child likes getting attention, for example, you can motivate her by enrolling her in a performing arts class," she says.

You could break the routine by asking your child to

help you make dinner, going to the library together, having a different friend over to play once a week or playing board games in the evenings instead of turning on the television.

Set a bedtime hour. Children need a set bedtime to ensure they get enough rest, says Dr. Womack. To avoid disrupting sleep patterns, weekend bedtimes shouldn't be more than an hour different from the weekday bedtime.

On the average, 2- to 6-year-olds need 12 hours of sleep, plus a nap. Between 6 and 9 years of age, most children need 11 hours of sleep, and by age 12, about 10 hours. Children vary, however—some will need more, some less.

Supply a good breakfast and lunch. A child who dashes off to school without breakfast or with just a sweet roll is likely going to poop out during the day, says Dr. Butterworth. And the youngster who skips lunch will likely experience an afternoon slump.

If there's no time to cook breakfast, serve nonsugared breakfast cereals, toast, fruit, yogurt or whole-grain muffins. If your child won't eat school lunches, pack his lunch the night before, or have him do it.

Serve healthy snacks. Giving your child soda, juice, candy or cookies for snacks may provide quick energy, but his energy level will plummet afterward, says Donna Oberg, R.D., a registered dietitian and public health nutritionist for the Seattle–King County Department of Public Health in Kent, Washington. "His blood sugar will go below what it had been before he ate that 'quick energy' source," she says.

Better choices are fruit, vegetables, unbuttered popcorn or low-fat crackers. Some older children like chilled baby carrots and broccoli florets, she adds.

Supply plenty of vitamins. "I see children all the time who are deficient in nutrients such as vitamin B_6 and zinc," says Ray C. Wunderlich, Jr., M.D., who practices nutritional medicine in St. Petersburg, Florida. The best way to get these nutrients is with a balanced diet that includes at least five servings of fruits and vegetables daily. If you also include whole grains and two servings of meat, fish or other protein-rich foods, you'll be providing your child with all the nutrients she needs. (Beef, poultry, whole-grain products and brewers yeast are good sources of both zinc and vitamin B_6.)

If you're considering supplements, however, first discuss your child's diet with your doctor.

Watch out for dieters. Many youngsters, particularly girls, begin to diet at an early age, and the lack of calories can make a child feel exhausted, says Dr. Butterworth. If your child is just skipping desserts or she's choosing salads instead of french fries, you probably don't have to worry. But you should explain to your child that she needs plenty of nutrients and point out good food choices. If your child seems overly concerned about her weight or persists in dieting, arrange a visit to her doctor.

Look for an allergy connection. Allergies to certain foods can make a child tired. "Try keeping a food diary to determine whether certain foods seem to lead to more tiredness," Dr. Wunderlich suggests. Write down what your child eats, what time he eats it and how he felt throughout the day. If one food seems to trigger tiredness, try cutting out that food. Foods that are consumed in large amounts and most frequently are apt to be the food offenders.

Get problems out in the open. If you suspect that your child's malaise is the result of a fight with his best friend, problems at school or traumatic events in the family, encourage him to talk it out, says Dr. Willson.

Read-aloud stories can help a young child deal with some of the unpleasant things that may be going on in her life. For example, stories that deal with making friends, starting at a new school or dealing with loss can be very helpful, says Dr. Willson.

Set a good example. Is your child echoing your "I'm so tired" or "I'm pooped out"? Some fatigue can be learned. "If a child has a tired mother, a tired father or tired grandparents, he can pick up on that and mimic those symptoms

and behaviors," Dr. Wunderlich says. Try getting some
extra rest, if possible. And even if you are tired much of
the time, try not to complain about it in front of your child.

FEARS

Tactics to Take the Scare Out

The bogeyman. Monsters under the bed. Animal attacks. Being kidnapped. AIDS. At one time or another, your child may be beset by fears such as these.

"As a parent, you should understand that all these fears
are normal, but how you react to them can determine
whether fears go away, stay around or get worse," says
Sheila Ribordy, Ph.D., a clinical psychologist and director
of clinical training in the Department of Psychology at De
Paul University in Chicago.

Children may have different fears at different developmental stages. It's not unusual for a child who's been sleeping calmly in a dark room to suddenly, at age five, begin
begging for a night-light to keep monsters at bay. "Common fears among younger children are of imaginary things,
like the bogeyman," says Dr. Ribordy. "In spite of our
protestations that there aren't any monsters and ghosts,
until they're well into school age, children have a capacity
to believe there are.

"Older children, on the other hand, often become afraid
of things they hear about on TV: environmental contamination, AIDS, kidnappings, abuse. These messages are overwhelming to them emotionally," says Dr. Ribordy.

While at times it may seem like a scary world even to
adults, it is possible to make it a little less scary for children
by following these suggestions.

Help them use their imagination. It's imagination that
makes kids picture monsters lurking in the dark or believe
that a real, live animal or bug will suddenly attack them.

But they can also use their imaginations to beat those fears, says Thomas Olkowski, Ph.D., a clinical psychologist in private practice in Denver.

"Have a child imagine something she's afraid of, such as a dark room or a dog, and then visualize herself entering the dark room or approaching the dog without anything awful happening. She should practice a number of times until she finally feels comfortable," Dr. Olkowski suggests.

This can also work with older children whose fears might be based on more realistic concerns such as going to a dance, transferring to a new school or performing in the class play. Imagining themselves going through the steps is something like a rehearsal, he says, and gives them confidence when the real thing comes along.

Get real. After the child has practiced approaching his worst fears in his imagination, help him do it in real life, but in small steps, says Dr. Olkowski. "Set up situations in which the child feels absolutely in control. If the child is afraid of animals, for example, go to a pet shop, but just look through the window at first."

Read all about it. Nothing is better than information to help banish fears, both real and imaginary. "If a child is afraid of spiders and insects, for instance, he can read about them in a book," says Dr. Olkowski. Dr. Ribordy gave one young boy who was terrified of lightning a therapeutic homework assignment: "I sent him to the library to research lightning, as part of a science project. Learning about the phenomenon of lightning has desensitized him. Now he thinks about it in a different way. It's not an ominous, scary thing."

Offer reassurance. Kids need to be told that they have little to fear from what they fear. This is especially true for older children, says Dr. Ribordy. "They have very real fears about illness and death. They think, 'What would happen if I lost my Mom? What if I get AIDS?' "

When a child expresses such fears, you can respond by explaining just how low the probability is of any of those things actually happening to him, she says. "It also helps to assure your child that it's your job, not hers, to worry about such things," according to Dr. Ribordy.

Arm that child with a flashlight. Bedtime may be the time when your child's fears manifest themselves. That's when the hideous creatures of the night supposedly come to terrorize small, defenseless children in their beds. So you need to make your child less defenseless, says Dr. Ribordy.

She recommends giving a child her own flashlight. "To a child who is afraid of the dark, this symbolizes control," she observes. Even if the child doesn't use it, she knows the flashlight is always next to her bed and she can switch it on any time.

Fight monsters with a little magic. Sometimes it helps if you can empower the child in a special way. Barbara Howard, M.D., assistant clinical professor of pediatrics at Duke University Medical Center in Durham, North Carolina, advocates "monster spray"—a spray bottle containing a harmless substance, like water—for the parent to use at bedtime as a preventive measure to keep any imaginary creatures at bay. "You can use it once or as often as needed to reassure the child," says Dr. Howard.

"I've been criticized for suggesting this, because if you're preparing to 'exorcise' the monsters, doesn't that mean you're saying there actually are monsters? Logically speaking, you shouldn't do it," she says. "But, in fact, it works, because the child thinks the parent is all-powerful and accepts the spray as a potent weapon."

Deputize teddy. "Ask the child to pick out a teddy bear or other stuffed animal he feels good about to be his protector," suggests says Dr. Olkowski. "This also gives the child a sense of control over the things he fears, whether they're real or not."

Monitor TV viewing. "Be *very* careful about what your children are watching," says Dr. Howard. "There are a lot of scary things on TV." Sitcoms may be fine—but you certainly don't want a fearful child to watch shows that involve bloodshed, intimidation or violence.

Use relaxation exercises. Taking deep breaths or imagining a quiet, safe place can help a child relax and feel less fearful, says Dr. Howard. "Children are actually better at using these methods than adults. Have your child lie still and imagine herself drifting on a cloud or lying on the beach—something that would be relaxing and fun."

Set limits. Often, says Dr. Howard, those monsters kids are afraid of are *themselves*. "Nighttime fears especially are symbolic of things going on in their lives. If children's behavior is out of control during the day, they may feel they need protection from monsters at night," she says. "What they need is better structure in their lives and more discipline, by which I mean protection from their own aggression. If they're allowed to hit or to run rampant over their parents, who are supposed to be all-powerful, they're likely to have nighttime fears." By taking back control, you can help put those fears at rest.

Tell special bedtime stories. Since most kids are afraid of things they can't control, you should tell bedtime stories about characters who accomplished difficult tasks or overcame their fears, says Dr. Howard. "Tell stories of how someone mastered things he was afraid of or did something he didn't think he could do. You can tell stories from your own childhood, or read from a book, such as *The Little Engine That Could*."

Have a plan. "Children are reassured by having a plan," says Dr. Ribordy. "For example, we went though a period with my son when he was afraid the house would catch on fire. So we went out and bought a fire escape ladder, and every day for a week we practiced how we would escape in case of fire. He found that very reassuring, and his fear completely went away."

FEVER

What to Do When Your Kid Has a Temp

Her pajamas are rumpled, her face flushed and the tendrils of hair on her forehead are damp from sweat.

When your child seems feverish, your first instinct is probably to try to cool her off. But a warm child may not necessarily be running a temperature, and even if she is, lowering the fever isn't always the best solution, says A. Gayden Robert, M.D., a pediatrician and head of general pediatrics at the Ochsner Clinic in New Orleans.

Any concerned parent will call the doctor as soon as fever starts to escalate—and with good reason. It's important to find out what's *causing* the fever. But that doesn't mean you have to bring the fever down right away.

"The fever is a symptom, not an illness," says Dr. Robert, noting that fever is often caused by a viral or bacterial infection, such as the measles or flu. "It's a defense mechanism that helps a child fight the infection."

Most doctors agree, however, that you may need to treat a fever so your child can rest more easily. If your child is crying or irritable from the fever, you'll definitely want to lower it enough to make him more comfortable, says Carol Kilmon, Ph.D., R.N., a certified pediatric nurse practitioner and assistant professor at the School of Nursing at the University of Texas Medical Branch in Galveston.

So here's how to deal with high temperature to bring your child back to the comfort zone.

Taking the Temperature

Time your reading. The body's temperature fluctuates throughout the day, points out Sanford Kimmel, M.D., pediatrician and associate professor of clinical family medicine at the Medical College of Ohio in Toledo. It's generally highest in the late afternoon or early evening, and lowest in the morning. It can also be affected by exercise or hot foods. To get the most accurate reading, you should take

MEDICAL ALERT

When to See the Doctor

Fever doesn't usually require medical care, but there are certain red flags that indicate the need to consult with a doctor, according to A. Gayden Robert, M.D., a pediatrician and head of general pediatrics at the Ochsner Clinic in New Orleans.

If you have any concerns about your child's fever, check with the doctor, of course, but *always* call if your feverish child:

- Is crying inconsolably.
- Remains irritable even after the fever drops. (If you're giving acetaminophen—Children's Tylenol—to make the fever drop, allow 30 to 45 minutes for the medication to take effect.)
- Is difficult to awaken.
- Is confused or delirious.
- Has just had a seizure or has had them in the past.
- Has a stiff neck.
- Is having difficulty breathing even though the nose is clear.
- Has persistent vomiting or has diarrhea.
- Has had the fever more than 72 hours.

your child's temperature 30 minutes after he has quieted down or 30 minutes after he's had a hot meal or drink, advises Dr. Kimmel.

Take the right approach. A baby's temperature is most accurately measured with a rectal thermometer, which is shorter and has a thicker bulb than an oral thermometer, says Dr. Kimmel. Grease it with petroleum jelly, then insert the thermometer slowly no farther than 1½ inches, and hold it gently in place for at least three minutes. To do this you can put the baby on the dressing table or in your lap in the diaper-changing position, and lift the baby's legs for easy access. Or you may prefer to lay the child stomach

A DIFFERENT KIND OF FEVER

Your child's fever has stayed high for three days now, but your pediatrician has told you not to worry. Suddenly on the fourth day, the fever drops and a rash appears on her trunk, neck, face, arms and legs.

Do give your doctor a call—but don't panic. This isn't the onset of a new disease. It's a sign that what caused your child's fever was a harmless disease called roseola, says Daniel Bronfin, M.D., a staff pediatrician at the Ochsner Clinic and assistant clinical professor of pediatrics at Tulane University School of Medicine in New Orleans.

"You can't always diagnose it before the rash appears, but when we see a playful child one or two days into a fever in the 103° to 104° range without symptoms, we suspect roseola," he says.

Roseola is caused by a virus and occurs most often in infants between the age of six months and two years. There's no medication required, and you should only try to bring down your child's temperature if he's uncomfortable, says Dr. Bronfin. Realize that you'll only be able to bring it down a few degrees, however.

Although it seems to make your child irritable, the rash isn't itchy or uncomfortable and doesn't require treatment. It will disappear in a few hours to a few days. When the rash appears, the child is no longer contagious.

down across the lap, spread the buttocks and then insert the thermometer.

Switch to oral. When a child is four or five, he'll usually be able to cooperate in holding an oral thermometer under his tongue for at least four minutes, says Dr. Kimmel. Digital thermometers are fast, accurate and a little safer than traditional glass mercury thermometers, but they are also more expensive. Regardless of the type of thermometer used, make sure your child sits quietly, since any activity will raise the temperature.

Assess the readout. Although 98.6° has long been considered the classic "normal" oral temperature, some people routinely have a higher temperature—so your child could have a slightly higher reading and still be perfectly normal. Your child has a fever if his temperature is more than 100.4° measured rectally, 99° under the arm or 100° measured orally, says Dr. Robert.

Lowering the Fever

Give acetaminophen. Pediatric acetaminophen (Children's Tylenol) will help bring the fever down, says Beth W. Hapke, M.D., a pediatrician in private practice in Fairfield, Connecticut. These products come in liquid form for infants and toddlers and chewable tablets for older children. Check the package directions for the correct dosage for your child's age and weight. If your child is under age two, consult a physician.

Doctors caution that you should *never* give your feverish child aspirin, however, as it has been linked to a serious brain and liver ailment called Reye's syndrome.

Try a sponge bath. Give your child a lukewarm sponge bath for 15 to 20 minutes, says Lynn Sugarman, M.D., a pediatrician with Tenafly Pediatrics in Tenafly, New Jersey, and an associate in clinical pediatrics at Babies Hospital, Columbia Presbyterian Medical Center in New York City.

Put your child into a tub with tepid water, and sponge the water over her arms, legs and body. "As the water evaporates, it cools the body, which helps bring down the fever," Dr. Sugarman explains. Don't use water so cold that the child shivers. Shivering will actually raise the body temperature, defeating the whole purpose of the sponge bath.

If you don't want to take your child out of bed to bathe her, you can just loosen her clothing and sponge her from a basin.

Leave the alcohol on the shelf. Parents once rubbed down feverish children with rubbing alcohol, but doctors today discourage this practice. "Besides causing shivering, alcohol can be absorbed through the skin and cause a toxic reaction in your child," says Dr. Robert. And breathing the fumes can irritate your child as well.

Supply lots of fluids. A child with a fever breathes faster than usual, which makes him lose extra fluid. If he has diarrhea, even more fluid is lost. "So make sure your child sips some liquid—whatever his stomach will tolerate," advises Dr. Kilmon. "Make the drink cool, not hot, and give frequent, small amounts rather than trying to get lots down at once."

Any beverage kids will drink is fine, as long as you steer clear of colas, tea or coffee (these are diuretics that

---

FEBRILE SEIZURE: A SCARY EXPERIENCE

If your child has ever had a febrile seizure, you won't soon forget it. It's triggered by a rapid rise in temperature—often from an infectious illness such as tonsillitis—which apparently causes a change in the brain's electrical patterns.

Febrile seizures occur in about 1 child in 25, and in some cases, the feverish child lapses into unconsciousness. Other seizures can mimic an epileptic seizure with arms and legs twitching and jerking uncontrollably. You should alert your doctor of every febrile seizure.

When the seizure begins, follow these guidelines, advises John Freeman, M.D., a pediatric neurologist and professor of pediatrics and neurology at the John Hopkins Hospital in Baltimore.

- Turn your child on his side and make sure he can breathe freely; this way saliva or vomit won't block the windpipe
- Move harmful objects out of the way
- Don't try to wedge your child's mouth open; he will not swallow his tongue
- If the seizure lasts only five to ten minutes, call your doctor as soon as it ends
- If the seizure lasts more than ten minutes or your child has trouble breathing, get him to a hospital where he can receive anti-seizure medication

encourage fluid loss). And you can add some variation by supplying soup, a Popsicle or gelatin.

For nursing infants, regular feedings will provide enough liquid. If your infant has had diarrhea more than 24 hours, ask your doctor about giving him Pedialyte, an oral electrolyte solution available at drugstores, suggests Dr. Kimmel.

Keep clothing light. A child in flannel PJs or bundled in a quilt will overheat quickly, making the fever worse. "Keep your child lightly dressed, and have her sleep under a thin blanket or sheet," advises Dr. Sugarman.

Make meals optional. If your feverish child doesn't want to eat, don't urge her, says Dr. Kimmel. On the other hand, if she asks for pizza, that's okay, too. "If your child is in the mood to eat a certain food, it's probably okay to give it to her," he says.

A child who has had a stomach virus or upset stomach, however, will likely prefer something simple such as toast or crackers with some jelly. Other "comfort foods" such as oatmeal and mashed potatoes as well as bananas and pudding are also good choices, says Dr. Kimmel. Avoid fruit juices, however, as these can contribute to diarrhea.

Don't expect normal. Neither acetaminophen nor sponge baths will bring your feverish child's temperature down to normal, says Daniel Bronfin, M.D., a staff pediatrician at the Ochsner Clinic and assistant clinical professor in pediatrics at Tulane University School of Medicine in New Orleans. "If the fever was 104°," he says, "you may be able to get it down to 101°."

Keep your child home. As long as your child has a fever, it's best to keep him home. "The rule of thumb here is that a child can return to school after his temperature has been normal for 24 hours," says Dr. Robert. "Although we don't know for sure, we believe if the fever is gone, then the infectious risk is, too."

FLATULENCE

How to Lessen the Gas

Getting rid of excess gas that forms in the stomach and intestines can be a source of embarrassment for adults. For kids, though, flatulence is more often a source of entertainment. We all remember the friend in elementary school who cracked up the class by making body noises.

In all likelihood, however, he was not a hit at the dinner table or when the boss came to visit. For passing gas can quickly become a social problem for kids as well as adults.

While you'll want to help your child manage and control any gassy outbursts, it's important to remember that flatulence is completely normal.

"Concerned parents come in to the doctor and say, 'My child is very gassy and always passing wind.' But that's not necessarily a bad thing. It may seem bad for the people around the child, but it is absolutely normal to be gassy." says Kevin Ferentz, M.D., assistant professor of family medicine at the University of Maryland School of Medicine and a family physician in Baltimore.

In fact, it's *not* passing gas that causes the most problems, because gas trapped inside the body can be quite painful, says Dr. Ferentz.

If your child is especially gassy, it may be related to what he's eating, or to the bacteria living in his gastrointestinal tract. "Everybody's gastrointestinal tract is a little bit different," he says. "We're colonized with different bacteria and some of them produce more gas than others."

Fortunately, the problem responds well to simple remedies.

Serve something hot to drink. Try giving your child a cup of hot tea or some other warm liquid, suggests Dr. Ferentz. "This definitely seems to help for gas pains, although there hasn't been a lot of high-powered scientific research to find out why it works," he says. "My own theory is that it's because the heat makes the gas expand.

This may actually make the problem worse for a short time. But ultimately the heat allows the gas to escape by helping it expand around the area where it's trapped."

If you have an infant who is troubled by gas, you can get the same effect by putting a cloth-wrapped hot-water bottle on the child's abdomen for no more than 10 to 15 minutes at a time, Dr. Ferentz says. And it is important that the bottle is not so hot that it might burn the child, he warns.

Seek out simethicone. "Use an over-the-counter anti-gas medication that contains simethicone," says Dr. Ferentz. "This ingredient is very effective because it breaks up gas into smaller bubbles which are much less uncomfortable and easier to pass." Be sure to read package directions—or check with your physician—for the correct dosage for your child.

Watch for broccoli backlash. "Foods that are high in fiber, like beans, broccoli and cabbage, cause more flatulence than other foods," says Dr. Ferentz. These foods typically aren't big favorites with kids. But they are part of a healthy diet. If they seem to trigger a gas crisis for your child, cut back temporarily or experiment with alternative items.

Use an enzyme to tame those beans. "There's an anti-gas product called Beano, which apparently does work," says George Sterne, M.D., clinical professor of pediatrics at Tulane University Medical School and a pediatrician in New Orleans. Available at health food stores and some supermarkets, Beano contains an enzyme that neutralizes the gas-producing effects of beans. Just sprinkle a few drops on your child's bean burrito and see what happens.

Work out gas with a workout. An active lifestyle comes naturally for most kids. But in case yours is a couch potato, encourage him to get up and move around more, especially after meals. Exercise helps the body eliminate gas, says Dr. Sterne.

Give baby a lift and a pat. Babies can have an especially tough time passing gas, which then becomes trapped and painful to them, says Dr. Sterne. "You can sometimes tell when a baby needs to pass gas, because he looks bloated—he has a sort of full-up look. If you simply move the baby around, change him to an upright position and pat him a little bit, it will help him release the gas. Raising or tilting the head of a crib so the baby's head is up can also help," he adds.

Establish gas-free zones. Don't expect any home remedy to eliminate gas problems completely. "Flatulence is a normal bodily function," says Jeffrey Fogel, M. D., a pediatrician in Fort Washington, Pennsylvania, and staff physician at Chestnut Hill Hospital in Philadelphia. "So you should tell your child that passing gas occasionally is okay to do. But he will just have to handle it in a socially acceptable manner. What's acceptable? In the bathroom, in his room, but not at the dinner table or in some other social situation."

And if you doubt that kids really *can* control passing gas, Dr. Fogel urges you to try this test: "Tell your kid, 'If you pass gas in public, you can't play with your video games'—or whatever else is his current favorite pastime. You'll find he'll get really good at stopping it."

FLU

Ways to Soothe the Symptoms

Compared to a cold, the flu can bring major league misery to your child. Influenza—the medical name for the flu—is caused by a virus, just like the common cold. And many of the symptoms are similar—cough, runny nose, sore throat and fever. But if your child has the flu, she'll be much, much sicker.

There are three different influenza viruses—types A, B and C—but whichever strain your child catches, she's in for a rough time. A fever will zap her on day one and may last for an entire week. Along with the upper respiratory symptoms, she'll have chills and shakes, a "wiped-out" feeling, muscle aches and pains and reddened eyes. Some kids, especially infants, also have vomiting or diarrhea.

Ear infection, sinusitis or pneumonia may follow in the wake of influenza, but these secondary infections can be treated with antibiotics. Unfortunately, the flu cannot be stopped this way. (Antibiotics are useless against viruses.) Prescription anti-viral medications such as amantadine have been found helpful in shortening the duration of Influenza A, but their use is limited. To be effective, they must be given within 20 hours after the flu symptoms appear.

In most cases, all you can do for your flu-stricken child is to try and make life a little more bearable. You won't be able to take away all her symptoms, but you can alleviate some of them. Here's how.

Treat the fever, but only if it's high. If your child is really miserable because of aches and fever, acetaminophen (Children's Tylenol) is the treatment of choice. Check the package directions for the correct dose for your child's age and weight. If your child is under age two, consult a physician. If your child's temperature is approximately 102° or lower, however, do nothing for the fever, advises Naomi Grobstein, M.D., a family physician in private practice in Montclair, New Jersey.

"Fever mobilizes the immune system. And the reaction it creates helps ensure that your child will lie down and take it easy for a while—which is just what she should be doing," Dr. Grobstein says.

Caution: Never give your child aspirin when she has the flu, says Dr. Grobstein. "Studies have linked taking aspirin to Reye's syndrome, a severe disease in children that affects the brain and liver."

Raise the humidity. A cool-mist vaporizer placed near your child's bed can help make nasal secretions more free-flowing so your child breathes more comfortably, says Jack H. Hutto, Jr., M.D., chief of pediatric infectious disease at

MEDICAL	ALERT

When to See the Doctor

You should call your pediatrician right away if your child appears ill with a high temperature and other signs of flu, says Michael Macknin, M.D., head of the Section of General Pediatrics at the Cleveland Clinic Foundation in Ohio, clinical professor at Pennsylvania State University Medical School in Hershey and associate professor of pediatrics at Ohio State University Medical School in Columbus. Be sure to notify the doctor if your child begins suffering from excessive vomiting or diarrhea, has difficulty in breathing, is delirious, has ear pain or is urinating infrequently, says Dr. Macknin.

The flu will make your child feel very sick, notes Dr. Macknin, but he should occasionally perk up for 15 to 20 minutes, perhaps after being given some acetaminophen (Children's Tylenol; check the package directions for the correct dose for your child's age and weight, or consult a physician). "If he stops having good times mixed with the bad, call your physician," Dr. Macknin says.

All Children's Hospital in St. Petersburg, Florida. "Your child will benefit from the extra humidity, but be sure to clean the vaporizer often, following the manufacturer's instructions. These machines tend to collect mold and bacteria, which can get sprayed into the air," Dr. Hutto says.

Quiet those coughs in the night. If your child's cough is harsh and bothersome, give a nonprescription cough syrup containing dextromethorphan, a cough suppressant, says Michael Macknin, M.D., head of the Section of General Pediatrics at the Cleveland Clinic Foundation in Ohio, clinical professor at Pennsylvania State University Medical School in Hershey and associate professor of pediatrics at Ohio State University Medical School in Columbus.

"Don't try to suppress the cough around the clock, though," he says. "A cough provides a useful function by helping to clear the lungs of bacteria and debris. So treat it only when it is preventing your child from getting some sleep." Dextromethorphan is contained in many brands of children's cough medicine, including Delsym, Robitussin-DM and Triaminic-DM.

Replenish lost fluids. Kids tend to lose a lot of fluid with a fever, and even more if there is vomiting. So you should push fluids by offering your child a choice of things to drink. "We adults tend to offer things that make *us* feel better. But what seems good to you may not appeal to your child," says Dr. Hutto. "Children's taste buds are more sensitive than ours. So when they are ill, they tend to want really bland things without a lot of flavor or odor."

Try flat soda or diluted rather than full-strength apple

COPING WITH CHILLS AND SWEATS

The flu is accompanied by bouts of high fever, so it is likely that your child will experience some chills as his temperature rises, and some sweats when the temperature returns to normal, says Michael Macknin, M.D., head of the Section of General Pediatrics at the Cleveland Clinic Foundation in Ohio, clinical professor at Pennsylvania State University Medical School in Hershey and associate professor of pediatrics at Ohio State University Medical School in Columbus.

Mild chills precede every fever, says Dr. Macknin, but when there's a very high fever coming on, the chills may be accompanied by violent shaking that can last a few minutes. "When your child has chills, his brain is telling his body to raise its temperature," Dr. Macknin explains. "To get to the higher temperature, the body has shaking chills—a kind of forced exercise that generates the heat necessary to drive the temperature to the point set by the brain."

When your child's fever goes down, he may be sweating heavily. (The evaporation of the sweat helps cool the body off.) The cycle of chills and sweats is a normal one and doesn't need to be treated, according to Dr. Macknin. "Don't smother your child with blankets when he has chills, because very shortly, he'll be feeling too hot from the fever. A light blanket is usually all that is necessary," he says.

juice, he suggests. "A hot drink such as hot lemonade with honey may be soothing to the throat, but most kids tend to prefer cool drinks," he says.

If your child is vomiting, keep in mind that the worst is usually over within 6 hours, and kids usually stop throwing up after 24 hours, says Dr. Grobstein. "Your child will feel awful for a while, but it is not likely that he'll get dehydrated in such a short time," she says.

As long as your child's stomach is upset, a teaspoon or so of liquid at a time may be all you can expect him to swallow, Dr. Grobstein says. If your child vomits that small amount of liquid, wait 20 minutes and try again.

Opt for a pop. "Along with water, offer sugary drinks such as juice or a Popsicle, which is basically sugar-water that's been frozen. A small amount of warm chicken soup is a good addition because it provides sodium—an important electrolyte—and is soothing to the throat besides," suggests Dr. Grobstein. Electrolytes are key minerals that help keep the body's electrical charge in balance. And, she notes, "unless your child is very young, or has other health considerations, you can keep the electrolyte balance normal just by offering this variety of liquids."

It's usually not necessary to give a child Pedialyte, an over-the-counter fluid often recommended when a child is vomiting a lot, says Dr. Grobstein. While this beverage is formulated to maintain electrolytes, most kids hate the taste, she adds.

Serve some light bites. Your child won't have much of an appetite, but it is important to keep his blood sugar level up so that he'll have less tiredness, vomiting, headache and fussiness, Dr. Hutto says. "Think in terms of small carbohydrate snacks: miniature marshmallows, crackers, dry toast, plain bread. The snacks should be fat-free so that they're easily digested," he says.

Soothe the sore throat. Dr. Macknin recommends easing throat pain with nonprescription Chloraseptic spray. Or have your child gargle with saltwater. Dissolve ½ teaspoon of salt in a cup of warm water. "You can also offer throat

---

WHO NEEDS THE FLU VACCINE?

The federal Centers for Disease Control and Prevention in Atlanta recommend that kids with chronic heart or lung disease, asthma, diabetes or other chronic diseases should be given the influenza vaccine every year. Check with your doctor to find out if your child should be vaccinated.

---

lozenges, which kids seem to enjoy because it's like eating candy," Dr. Macknin says.

Dr. Hutto warns that very young kids can choke on throat lozenges, but a lollipop makes an acceptable substitute.

Give extra TLC. When he's feeling bad, your child will appreciate having some special attention from you. "Sit down and play a quiet game together, read a book, sing or cuddle your child if he finds it comforting," Dr. Grobstein says.

"Make your child's bed as comfortable and as soft as possible," adds Dr. Hutto. Some kids also may appreciate a gentle massage to stroke away their aches and pains, he says.

Watch out for a relapse. "It's typical for a child with the flu to be sick for three to four days, seem better for a day or two, and then get sick for another few days," says Dr. Grobstein.

Be on your guard against misleading morning temperatures. "Body temperature tends to be lower in the morning. So a child who registers 99° after breakfast may have a fever of 102° in the afternoon," says Dr. Grobstein. Your child should maintain a normal temperature for 24 hours before you let him go back to school, she says.

FOOD ALLERGIES

Keeping an Eye on the Edibles

Your three-year-old breaks out in hives after eating scrambled eggs. Or your infant begins to wheeze after eating anything made with wheat.

Food sensitivity affects 2 to 5 percent of children in their first few years of life, says Hugh Sampson, M.D., a pediatric allergy/immunology specialist, professor of pediatrics and director of the Pediatric Clinical Research Unit at the Johns Hopkins University School of Medicine in Baltimore. Fortunately, many children outgrow some types of allergies by the age of three.

If you suspect a food allergy, an allergist or your doctor can help you pinpoint the problem food or foods and tell you what to do if your child accidentally eats the food. In rare cases, you'll need to keep prescribed medications on hand to control anaphylaxis, a severe and potentially fatal reaction.

Once your child's doctor has confirmed an allergy, you need to help your child avoid that food and instruct your child, family and caregivers how to recognize a reaction and what to do if it occurs. Here's how to help keep your child safe from the offending food and what to do if she does eat it.

Become a wise shopper. "Learn the technical and scientific names for foods your child is allergic to," says Dr. Sampson. Milk, for example, can be present in foods under many names such as caseinate or whey, and eggs could be listed as albumin or ovomucin. If you encounter names you're not familiar with on a label, look them up before you allow your child to eat the food, or call the manufacturer and ask about the ingredients. And read label ingredient information every time you buy a food product; manufacturers sometimes change ingredients without warning.

Beware of cross-contamination. If you're cooking an

MEDICAL ALERT

When to See the Doctor

For those with a severe food allergy, eating or drinking even a tiny amount of the allergen can cause a life-threatening reaction called anaphylaxis.

"Although it's not a common occurrence, parents need to be able to recognize this emergency in its earliest stages," says Hugh Sampson, M.D., a pediatric allergy/immunology specialist, professor of pediatrics and director of the Pediatric Clinical Research Unit at the Johns Hopkins University School of Medicine in Baltimore. "Some children will have early warning signs, such as itching of the lips or tongue, before the full-blown reaction begins—which can occur as little as 5 to 15 minutes later. The earlier a reaction is treated, the better."

Here's what to look for.

- Hives
- Swelling, especially of the lips and face
- Tight feeling in the chest
- Difficulty breathing, whether from swelling in the throat or an asthmatic reaction
- Nausea or vomiting
- Diarrhea
- Cramping

If these symptoms occur, immediately give your child his prescribed medications, which help slow the reaction, and go immediately to the nearest emergency room. "Even if it turns out to be a false alarm, it's better to find that out at the hospital," says Dr. Sampson.

---

allergy-free dish for one child, be sure you don't stir it with the same spoon you're using for other dishes that might contain an allergen, says Anne Muñoz-Furlong, founder and president of the Food Allergy Network, a nonprofit organization in Fairfax, Virginia, established to help families cope with food allergies.

Be especially careful to wash all cookware, dishes and

tableware thoroughly with soap and water and rinse them well to be sure no allergen remains. It's a good idea to put all your cooking materials in the dishwasher and run them through a regular cycle.

Involve your child. "Allergic children should know what foods they're allergic to and be taught to be aware of their own bodily symptoms," says Gilbert Friday, M.D., professor of pediatrics and chief of clinical services of the Asthma and Allergic Disease Center at the Children's Hospital of Pittsburgh.

Explain to your child that certain foods make her body react, and that she should avoid them. For a young child, it may help if the two of you cut pictures of offending foods out of magazines and mount them on a poster. Explain symptoms to your child, and tell her she should let you or another adult know immediately when she feels those symptoms.

Role-play situations. "Your child may worry about avoiding temptation or may experience peer pressure to eat forbidden foods," says Muñoz-Furlong. "Role-playing possible scenarios can help him learn how to handle whatever comes up."

For example, pretend you're a friend of your child's at a birthday party, cajoling your child to taste ice cream although he's allergic to milk. Have your child practice saying no and explaining that the food will make him sick.

Reinforce the positive. "Compliment your child every time she turns down an allergy-causing food," says Dr. Sampson. "This builds independence and self-esteem, which is important because as she gets older it will ultimately be her responsibility to monitor her own diet."

Alert caregivers. "Before the school year begins, schedule a meeting with your child's teachers, school administrator, counselor, nurse, cafeteria personnel and office staff," says Muñoz-Furlong. "Explain to this team what foods cause a reaction, what precautions should be taken and emergency procedures. Provide them with the name and phone numbers of three emergency contacts."

AN EGG BY ANY OTHER NAME

Your child is allergic to eggs, so you serve oatmeal in the mornings and avoid products that list *egg* in the ingredients. Easy, right?

Whoa. It's not that simple. Eggs may also be listed on a packaging label by a variety of names, such as albumin or even ovomucin, points out Anne Muñoz-Furlong, founder and president of the Food Allergy Network, a nonprofit organization in Fairfax, Virginia, established to help families cope with food allergies.

For common allergies, here is a partial list of some ingredient words and foods to avoid.

Eggs: albumin, mayonnaise, ovalbumin, ovomucin, ovomucoid, Simplesse. A shiny glaze on baked goods also may indicate the presence of eggs.

Milk: artificial butter flavor, butter, butterfat, buttermilk, casein, caseinates, cheese, cream, curds, dry milk solids, lactalbumin, lactose, milk derivative, milk protein or milk solids, rennet casein, sour cream, sour milk solids, whey, yogurt. There may be milk present if the label indicates caramel color or flavoring, high protein flour, margarine or natural flavoring.

Wheat: bran, enriched flour, farina, gluten, graham flour, high gluten flour, high protein flour, wheat bran, wheat germ, wheat gluten or wheat starch, whole wheat flour. Wheat may be present if the label indicates: gelatinized starch, modified food starch, modified starch, starch, vegetable gum or vegetable starch.

Tree nuts: almonds, brazil nuts, cashews, filbert, hazelnuts, gianduja, hickory nuts, macadamia nuts, marzipan, nut butters, nut oil, nut paste such as almond paste, pecans, pine nuts, pistachios, walnuts. Also avoid natural extracts such as almond extract or wintergreen extracts.

Peanuts: cold pressed peanut oil, mixed nuts, peanut butter or peanut flour. Peanuts may be present in chili, candy, Chinese and Thai dishes, egg rolls, marzipan or soups.

Soy: miso, soy flour, soy nuts, soy protein or soy sauce,

continued

continued

textured vegetable protein (TVP) or tofu. Soy may be present if the label indicates vegetable broth, gum or starch.

This list is updated as new products come out, so for the most complete information, contact the Food Allergy Network, 4744 Holly Avenue, Fairfax, Virginia 22030-5647.

If medication is needed to control allergic reactions, supply medical information forms from your doctor with the allergy information highlighted, suggests Dr. Sampson. If changes in allergy or medication occur, alert the school team.

And furnish the same information for any family members or babysitters who take care of your child.

Create a special alarm signal. "Have your child create a signal to let the teacher know that he's having a reaction," says Muñoz-Furlong. "Tell family, friends and school personnel what the signal is." This signal could be a code word or a gesture such as pointing to the throat.

Take special care when eating out. Allergens can be present in foods where you don't expect them. Make sure you know what ingredients are in prepared food, says Dr. Friday. "I had a patient who ate what he thought was chocolate pudding at the school cafeteria," he says. "It turned out that peanut butter was an ingredient in the pudding, and he was highly allergic to peanuts. He had a severe allergic reaction within minutes."

Unless you can review the school menu with school personnel ahead of time, pack your child's lunch, and explain clearly to your child why he can't swap lunches with friends.

Plan before parties. Before your child attends a party or school function where food will be served, talk to the host so you know what will be served and the host will be aware of your child's allergies, says Muñoz-Furlong. If your child is allergic to anything on the menu, send along special treats that your child *can* eat.

Avoid bakery items. "Baked goods are notorious for including possible problem foods such as nuts, eggs, milk and other ingredients," says Muñoz-Furlong. It's much safer to bake items yourself, either from scratch or using mixes with labels you've carefully scrutinized.

Beware of deli meats. If your child is allergic to milk, you'll probably want to skip deli meats. "The same machine is often used to cut cheese and meat products, and can cause meat to contain trace amounts of milk," says Dr. Sampson.

Give an OTC antihistamine. "Most kids get itchy hives if they eat a forbidden food," says Dr. Sampson. "Over-the-counter antihistamines such as Benadryl Elixir will help relieve the symptoms." Be sure to read package directions to make certain the product is recommended for your child's age. For the correct dosage, follow package directions or consult your physician. Some doctors don't advise Benadryl cream or spray because it could cause a reaction.

Don't, however, substitute an over-the-counter product for one that your physician has prescribed. If your child has reactions severe enough to have prescribed medications, it's crucial to use them.

Buy a medical emergency necklace. "If your child suffers from severe food allergies—the kind that can cause anaphylaxis—have her wear a medical emergency necklace and carry a personalized emergency-care card listing your doctor's name and number, medications used and foods that can cause reactions," says Dr. Sampson. Your doctor can help you order the necklace, or you can buy one at a jewelery or drugstore.

Keep medicines handy. If your child has a severe food allergy, your doctor probably will have recommended an antihistamine. Where there is risk of a very strong reaction, a doctor may prescribe epinephrine (Adrenalin), which is available in two forms for home use: Ana-Kit, a syringe, and EpiPen, a pen-shaped applicator. If an antihistamine or epinephrine is prescribed, be sure that your child carries the prescribed medications at all times, cautions Muñoz-Furlong.

Packing the medications should be part of the daily routine, like putting on shoes or socks. You may want to get your child a special fanny pack to carry the medications in. Put a checklist by the door, and have your child check off the items he's carrying before he leaves the house. You should also keep extra medications around the house and in your purse or briefcase.

FOOT ODOR

Fresh Solutions to Sole Pollutions

L ooking at the tiny toes of a newborn baby, it's hard to believe that they'll someday be smelly old feet. But by the time that same kid is running around in overused sneakers, you'll be awed by the fragrance those feet can produce.

Not a *big* problem, of course. But an odoriferous one— that every child seems to have sometimes.

"Frequently, children's feet will sweat more than adults' feet," says Rosario Labarbera, D.P.M., chief of podiatry at The General Hospital Center at Passaic and at Saint Mary's Hospital in Passaic, New Jersey, and board member of the New York College of Podiatric Medicine. Often that perspiration is foul-smelling—a condition doctors refer to as bromhidrosis. The odor is very similar to that of rotten cheese.

Bromhidrosis in kids is mainly caused by the presence of fetid bacteria on the foot, according to Morton Walker, D.P.M., formerly a podiatrist in private practice in Stamford, Connecticut, and author of *The Complete Foot Book*. If a whiff of your child's feet is enough to disturb the peaceful life of your family, listen to what doctors have to say about sweetening the air at floor level.

Let those tootsies breathe. Choose shoes made from materials that breathe, such as canvas or leather, suggests Dr. Labarbera. These are less likely to encourage moisture buildup, he says. Avoid shoes made of plastic or other synthetic, nonporous materials that trap odor inside.

Change shoes—often. "When children wear the same shoes every day, that doesn't give them a chance to dry out," says Dr. Labarbera. Moisture that builds up from activity frequently accumulates in the shoes. Wet shoes can cause the skin to break down and smell bad. Sometimes the skin on a child's feet will even turn whitish from this ongoing wetness, says Dr. Labarbera.

To counter this, have your child alternate shoes daily so that each pair gets a chance to dry thoroughly. "If your child's feet are extremely smelly, change shoes twice a day," suggests Marc A. Brenner, D.P.M., a podiatrist on the medical staff of the Long Island Jewish Hospital in New Hyde Park and North Shore University Hospital in Manhasset, both in New York.

Switch socks. Dry socks may be the only thing protecting your child from malodorous feet. So change his socks as often as two or three times a day, if necessary, says Dr. Brenner. But don't put on just any socks. "Pure cotton

---

MEDICAL ALERT

When to See the Doctor

If your child's foot odor is powerful and the tips here don't seem to help, there may be a fungus or other infection involved, says Marc A. Brenner, D.P.M., a podiatrist on the medical staff of the Long Island Jewish Hospital in New Hyde Park and North Shore University Hospital in Manhasset, both in New York. Take your child to a podiatrist. You may need a prescription antibiotic salve or antifungal liquid to start the healing process.

socks tend to hold wetness in," says Dr. Labarbera. He recommends breathable socks made of blends of cotton and synthetics, such as acrylic and orlon, that wick perspiration away from the feet.

Dry and powder after bathing. While it may not eliminate odor, basic good hygiene can help. Encourage your child to bathe his feet thoroughly every day, says Dr. Walker. Just as important, be sure he dries his feet completely after bathing, says Dr. Labarbera, and applies a foot powder to absorb any remaining moisture.

Smooth on a deodorizer. Dr. Brenner recommends an over-the-counter deodorant cream called Lavilin. "It's

---

SOAK AWAY TROUBLE

Nothing like a good long soak to freshen up stinky feet. Each of the following foot soaks can help stop bacteria from growing, according to Marc A. Brenner, D.P.M., a podiatrist on the medical staff of the Long Island Jewish Hospital in New Hyde Park and North Shore University Hospital in Manhasset, both in New York.

In each case, have your child soak his feet in the mixture for five to ten minutes. Soaking can be as frequent as twice a day or as seldom as twice a week, depending on the extent of the problem and your child's ability to stay put.

Epsom salts: Dilute two tablespoons in two quarts of warm water. (This not only cleans the feet but also makes them drier afterward, according to Dr. Brenner.)

Vinegar: Dilute two tablespoons in two quarts of cool water for an acidic footbath.

Domeboro Astringent Solution: This pharmacy product comes in tablets or powder packets. Just dissolve it in water, following directions on the package, for a refreshing soak. Dry thoroughly, especially between the toes.

Betadine Solution: Dilute a teaspoon of this over-the-counter antibacterial agent in two quarts of cool water.

made in Israel and you can buy it in health food stores. It's perfectly natural and harmless for kids," he says. Read the directions carefully before applying the cream.

Try dropping in inserts. Shoe inserts, especially brands that contain activated charcoal, absorb perspiration, notes Dr. Brenner, who has found them to help some youngsters with smelly "sneaker feet." Although these inserts usually come in only one size, you can trim them to fit your child's shoes.

Cool those tootsies. "Dip a cotton ball in some rubbing alcohol and dab it on the child's feet to help dry them and cool them off," says Dr. Labarbera. Don't use alcohol if the child has any breaks in the skin, though. That would burn, he warns. Instead, use an antiseptic like Betadine Solution, which soothes, dries and cools without burning.

Look for sources of stress. Mental tension is another common cause of foot odor, according to Dr. Walker. In fact, the odor of perspiration that results from stress is considered more offensive than the exercise-generated kind. If your child's feet have suddenly become smellier lately, talk with him about stresses at school, at home or in his friendships. If you can help him deal with tension caused by change and uncertainty, the smelly-foot condition might get better.

FOOT PAIN

Tips to Take Away the Ache

O h, those aching tootsies! When your feet hurt, it seems like *everything* hurts, and that's just as true for a child as for an adult. When your child has a pinched toe or a scrunched heel, you'll probably hear a lot of crankiness and complaining.

Foot pain can have many different causes and can arise at many different sites. So you'll need to talk to your child and find out exactly where the pain is. Too-tight shoes are an obvious irritant, but there can be other factors. Heel pain, for example, can be caused by a stiff Achilles tendon. Pain under the middle of the foot is often the result of an arch problem. Toe pain is sometimes the result of a bunion. And blisters can turn up just about anywhere, as a quick inspection of your child's feet is likely to reveal. (If that's the problem, see page 52 for additional advice.)

Once you've zeroed in on the source of the pain, the following expert suggestions can help keep your youngster high-stepping and happy.

Ice away heel pain. Some children are especially prone to heel pain between the ages of 8 and 12, according to Suzanne Tanner, M.D., a pediatrician and sports medicine physician at the University of Colorado Sports Medicine Center in Denver. "Often this is because the Achilles tendon joining the calf muscle to the heel bone is too tight," Dr. Tanner says.

To relieve the pain, she suggests putting ice on the heel for 10 to 20 minutes after activity. Just be sure to wrap the ice in a towel so it isn't directly against the skin. If that doesn't work, heel lifts may help. These are available in many sizes at most pharmacies and shoe stores. "And have your child cut down on the amount of running and jumping he's doing," she adds.

Beat soreness by stretching. Stretching exercises may also help guard against heel pain. Here's an exercise Dr. Tanner recommends: Have your child stand facing a wall about two feet away. With his hands on the wall, have him move forward at the hip, leaning toward the wall. "This exercise loosens the calf muscle and the Achilles tendon," she says.

Bear down on stiff shoes. If the backs of your child's shoes are very stiff, they can irritate the heel and cause pain, says Elizabeth H. Roberts, D.P.M., professor emeritus of anatomy at the New York College of Podiatric Medicine

MEDICAL ALERT

When to See the Doctor

If your child complains of foot pain, check the foot for swelling, deformity (anything that looks abnormal), redness, warmth to the touch compared to the other foot or loss of sensation, says Eli Glick, a physical therapist at PhyCare Physical Therapy in Bala Cynwyd and Flourtown, Pennsylvania. If you discover any of these symptoms, see a doctor.

Even without these warning signs, also take your child to a doctor if there's no reduction in pain or swelling after four to five days, Glick says. Persistent pain or swelling could be a sign of a sprain or fracture.

If your child has diabetes, do not treat his feet at home without getting medical advice, he suggests.

in New York City and author of *On Your Feet*. "Whenever you buy a new pair of shoes for your child, press the heel of your hand against the back of the shoe to soften it."

Support your local arches. Always buy shoes with built-in arch supports. "If your child has a medium or high arch, it's especially important that the shoe provide support," says Dr. Tanner. "Not having enough arch support in the shoe may stretch the arch, causing fatigue and pain."

Say no to sandals. Stay away from sandals. They don't support your child's arches, says Rosario Labarbera, D.P.M., chief of podiatry at The General Hospital Center at Passaic and at Saint Mary's Hospital in Passaic, New Jersey, and board member of the New York College of Podiatric Medicine. "Foot fatigue can result from wearing sandals for long periods, and that can cause discomfort," he says.

Get the jump on impact injuries. If your child has been jumping rope or playing other jumping games on the pavement, and pain results, have her change the activity or continue on a mat, suggests Eli Glick, a physical therapist at

HELP FOR INGROWN NAILS

Ingrown toenails can be painful. "As a temporary measure to alleviate the discomfort caused by the side of the nail cutting into the flesh, put a wisp of cotton between the flesh of the toe and the ingrown nail," says Elizabeth H. Roberts, D.P.M., professor emeritus of anatomy at the New York College of Podiatric Medicine in New York City and author of *On Your Feet*.

To perform this simple procedure, use a narrow but *not* sharp instrument. "If your child is restless, you might try using the edge of an emery board. Make sure it's clean," she adds.

If the problem persists, and particularly if you suspect an infection, you should have your child seen by a doctor or podiatrist. "The signs of an infection may be redness, some oozing of pus and/or pain," says Dr. Roberts.

To prevent ingrown toenails from happening in the first place, teach your children not to tear their nails. And make sure the nails are cut straight across. "If the nail is left extending just a tiny bit further than the nail groove, there's less chance of it growing inward," says Dr. Roberts. "Additionally, be sure the shoes have not become too small, causing pressure on the flesh against the nail.

PhyCare Physical Therapy in Bala Cynwyd and Flourtown, Pennsylvania. Be sure your child is wearing appropriate footwear, too. A general-purpose sneaker or cross-trainer that has good padding and support is best, says Glick. Check the shoes periodically for wear and replace them when needed.

Give bunions a good soaking. If your child's foot pain is in the big toe and there is thickening and swelling of the joint, it may indicate the beginning of a bunion. "There's often a hereditary tendency to develop bunions, though they don't often show up before age ten or so," says Morton Walker, D.P.M., formerly a podiatrist in private practice in Stamford, Connecticut, and author of *The Complete Foot Book*. For temporary bunion relief, Dr. Walker recommends having your child soak his feet twice a day for 15 minutes in a warm Epsom salts solution deep enough to cover both feet completely.

Try a toe tug-of-war. Dr. Walker suggests the following exercise to relieve beginning bunion pain: Take a small but thick rubber band and—with the feet side by side—hook it around the child's two big toes. Then have him hold a small can (the size of a small can of mushrooms) between his two feet, cradled in the hollow created by the arch structure. Ask your child to try to pull his heels toward each other against the resistance of the rubber band. Dr. Walker says this stretches the big toes and pulls them away from the other toes, taking pressure off the affected joint.

If the shoe fits, let your child wear it. Ill-fitting shoes are the cause of most foot pain in children, according to Dr. Roberts. "To get a good fit, be sure there's a quarter of an inch between the end of the longest toe and the front of the shoe," she says.

Children outgrow shoes very quickly. Dr. Roberts suggests buying new shoes for your children every couple of months when they're very young. As they grow older, expect to purchase new shoes every six months or so. "Even at the age of 12, a year is too long to be wearing the same shoes," she says.

Go for new shoes. "Avoid hand-me-down shoes, even if they're the correct size," says Dr. Roberts. "A shoe inevitably takes on the contour of the previous wearer's foot."

FORGETFULNESS

Measures That Add to Recall

Your 2-year-old can't find his blanket. Your 10-year-old can't find his shin guards. Your 12-year-old can't find the phone number of the boy who sits next to her in homeroom. ("You know, Mom, the cute one with the leather jacket.")

Is there any child left in the universe who remembers anything at all?

"Actually, most kids have pretty good memories," says Jeanne Murrone, Ph.D., a clinical psychologist who specializes in working with children and adolescents and staff psychologist at the New York Foundling Hospital, a foster care agency in New York City. So if a child seems to be forgetful on a regular basis, there's probably a good reason for it, she says. For example, she may be totally disorganized or reluctant to take responsibility for her own actions. Some kids who have parents that are overcontrolling may end up being forgetful. And other kids are forgetful because they have overly permissive parents, according to Dr. Murrone.

Of course, some children may simply be absentminded by nature. "These are the kids who are on their way to becoming absentminded professors, sculptors, painters or musicians," says Dr. Murrone. "They're the ones who simply don't see the world in a logical, linear, step-by-step way."

Most parents don't want to stifle original thinking or artistic creativity by forcing their children to jump through memory hoops. But since all kids—even twentieth-century

---

MEDICAL ALERT

When to See the Doctor

"If, in addition to being forgetful, your child seems confused, drowsy, unable to focus or momentarily 'not there,' check with your pediatrician," says Daniel Rosenn, M.D., director of children and adolescent outpatient services at McLean Hospital in Belmont, Massachusetts, and an instructor of psychiatry at Harvard Medical School in Boston. These may be signs of a physical problem such as hearing loss or epilepsy, he says.

Mozarts—do have to function in the real world, they still have to remember to brush their teeth, put their socks in the laundry and not leave their shoes in the middle of the floor.

Whether your child's memory lapses fall into the frequent or sporadic category, there are some steps you can take to enhance recall.

Structure your child's day. This does not mean turning your home into a boot camp or regularly posting the day's schedule on your child's bedroom door. What it does mean, according to Dr. Murrone, is providing meals at regular times, sending your child to bed at about the same time every night and insisting that homework and chores be done around the same time every afternoon and evening.

"All children thrive when they have structure and consistency," she says. When each day is basically well-scheduled, most kids will then be able to concentrate on the details of their lives—the keys, soccer shoes, bikes and hair ribbons—that are frequently misplaced and forgotten.

Use visual cues. "Very small children really don't have any idea that they even *need* to remember anything," says Sandra Calvert, Ph.D., associate professor of psychology at Georgetown University in Washington, D.C. "They just do things." But if you can place visual cues in their path to literally prompt them to say things, the chances of getting them to "remember" what you want are pretty good.

"If your child always forgets her backpack, for example, put it beside the front door so she'll see it as she runs out," says Dr. Calvert. "Always put it in exactly the same place—don't move it around." Eventually picking up her backpack as she goes out the door will become a firmly ingrained habit.

Hand out appreciative "warm fuzzies." Once a child remembers to pick up her backpack, her keys or whatever else it is that you've told her not to forget, says Dr. Calvert, praise her. Let your child know that you are pleased. A "You *remembered*!" with a quick hug and a big smile is far more likely to keep her memory on track in the future than 47 nagging reminders uttered to deaf ears.

"I'm a firm believer that if you love your kids and you ask them to do things appropriate to their age, they'll do whatever they can to please you," says Dr. Calvert. "They want your attention. If they can get it by remembering, they'll be more likely to remember."

Dr. Murrone agrees. "When children remember to put their dishes in the dishwasher, for instance, reward them with a word of praise. This is particularly effective with children who tend to forget things because they may not have yet learned to accept responsibility."

Drop the negative baggage. Kids are also more likely to remember something if you make your request—to take out the dog, feed the goldfish or hang up a coat—in a calm, positive voice, says Daniel Rosenn, M.D., director of children and adolescent outpatient services at McLean Hospital in Belmont, Massachusetts, and an instructor of psychiatry at Harvard Medical School in Boston.

"Kids remember things that make them feel good, and they forget things that make them feel bad," he explains. "If you're angry when you tell your child to go upstairs and make his bed, for example, he may not be able to process what you've said. In fact, he may honestly not even hear what you say."

"Instead, the child hears your anger. He hears, 'I don't like you,'" says Dr. Rosenn. And he may be so overwhelmed by the idea that his mom or dad doesn't like him, that whatever request was made in the midst of that horrifying message won't even make it past his eardrums.

When something's too important to forget, underscore it. "If you want your child to remember something serious, *be* serious," advises Dr. Rosenn. "Let's say you want him to remember where you've put the spare house key, for example. When you tell him, 'The key will be under the rock by the back door,' say it in a serious voice.

"But try not to generate any anxiety by adding something like 'If you forget where it is, you won't be able to

STRIKE A BALANCE IN YOUR PARENTING STYLE

Unfortunately, when forgetfulness in a child stems from a parent's own behavior, it may be a little harder to remedy, says Jeanne Murrone, Ph.D., a clinical psychologist and staff psychologist at the New York Foundling Hospital, a foster care agency in New York City, who specializes in working with children and adolescents.

"Overcontrolling, authoritarian parents don't give their children enough room to breathe," she says. "The Archie Bunker style of parenting pushes children to go wild and rebel. And one perfect way to rebel is to 'forget' everything parents ask them to do."

Going to the other extreme in parenting style can also contribute to forgetfulness, adds Dr. Murrone. "Permissive parents—parents who say 'Well, if everybody else is doing it, I guess you can, too'—may be so flexible that they create a constant state of chaos for the child. And chaos leads to forgetfulness."

One solution is to develop a parenting style that strikes a balance somewhere between these two extremes, says Dr. Murrone. "That style, an *authoritative* style, enables children to function well." They get the stability and structure that's frequently lacking in permissive parenting, but they also get some of the freedom and space that's lacking in authoritarian parenting.

"The result," she says, "is a child who tends to be more responsible, organized and less likely to forget."

get inside, and a kidnapper could come along and get you.' All a child will remember of *that* message is the kidnapper part."

Drill it into memory. Practice is also important, according to Dr. Rosenn. "Take your child outside and show him the rock and the key. Then practice some dry runs," he says. Have your child lift the rock, pick up the key, unlock the door, then replace the key under the rock. Remember to praise him when he's finished.

"That will attach good feelings to remembering where the key is," says Dr. Rosenn, "and it will lock the key's location firmly into his memory.

FROSTNIP

Bundling Up and Thawing Out

Y ou expect your child to be rosy-cheeked after playing outside in cold weather, but sometimes Jack Frost's nip is more serious than playful. When cheeks and fingertips turn bright pink, your child may just be a bit chilled. But overexposure to subfreezing temperatures and wet weather can lead directly to frostbite.

If your child has serious frostbite, you'll want her to get immediate medical attention, according to Susan Fuchs, M.D., assistant professor of pediatrics at the University of Pittsburgh School of Medicine and attending physician in the emergency department at the Children's Hospital of Pittsburgh. Frostbitten skin is actually frozen and must be carefully thawed to avoid permanent damage. (See page 221.) And because kids are different from adults in their surface-to-body ratio and metabolism, they are more likely than adults to get frostbitten skin, according to Dr. Fuchs.

But often, an alert parent can detect the early warning signs. And when you find that your child is getting numb fingers and cheeks, it's essential to bring her indoors and get her warmed up before mild frost*nip* turns into frost*bite*.

So next time you meet winter weather or a windchill factor that makes you shiver, here are some hints to help you protect your child.

Treatment

Know the signs. Frostnip, the beginnings of frostbite, most often nips the cheeks, the tip of the nose and ears and the fingers and toes, says Dr. Fuchs, leaving them white and somewhat numb.

When your children are playing outside in the cold, call them in at regular intervals to warm them up with a hot drink and check for sodden mittens or freezing noses and cheeks. "Children don't understand what numb skin means, and they may be unwilling to suspend play activities to warm up," says W. Steven Pray, Ph.D., a registered pharmacist and professor of pharmaceutics at Southwestern Oklahoma State University School of Pharmacy in Weatherford. This is where Mom or Dad steps in.

Take off the togs. "As soon as you get your child indoors, remove all her wet clothing," recommends Marcia Walhout, R.N., a clinical nurse specialist in the emergency department of Butterworth Hospital in Grand Rapids, Michigan, who has treated many hypothermia patients. Wet clothes draw heat from the body, she notes—and the sooner you can get them off, the quicker your child will warm up.

Warm up slowly. One of the best ways to warm chilled body parts is in warm water. "Fill a sink or tub with water just above body temperature—about 104° to 108°F," says Karen Houpt, M.D., assistant professor of dermatology at the University of Texas Southwestern Medical Center in Dallas. If the fingers or toes are chilled, ask your child to keep her hands or feet in the sink or tub until full feeling returns. This can take up to 15 to 20 minutes.

But don't let your child control the water temperature, because she may burn herself without knowing it. "Higher temperatures can cause severe burns, because numb hands won't feel the heat," says Dr. Fuchs.

Handle with care. If you suspect frostbite, you can change your child's clothing and get her dry—but *don't* rub your child's hands or feet to help warm them. "When the skin is frozen there are actually tiny ice crystals inside," explains Walhout. "Rubbing the skin may cause those ice crystals to damage the cells, like little razors," she says.

Preventive Care

Choose the right fabrics. If you live in a cold climate, you'll probably find it worth your while to invest in special

MEDICAL ALERT

When to See the Doctor

If your child is frostbitten, prompt treatment is crucial to avoid infection or possible loss of fingers or toes. You also need to be on the alert for hypothermia, a drop in body temperature caused by prolonged exposure to cold.

Frostbite. "If your child's skin appears white and waxy and feels numb and hard, like a wooden stump, take him to an emergency room as soon as you get him into dry clothes," says Karen Houpt, M.D., assistant professor of dermatology at the University of Texas Southwestern Medical Center in Dallas.

If the feet are frostbitten, carry your child, says W. Steven Pray, Ph.D., a registered pharmacist and professor of pharmaceutics at Southwestern Oklahoma State University School of Pharmacy in Weatherford. Walking on frostbitten feet can damage them, he says. Don't rub frostbitten skin, adds Dr. Pray—and never rub snow on frostbitten skin.

"Don't attempt to thaw a frostbitten area if there's any possibility that it may refreeze," says Dr. Pray. "If the tissues refreeze, the amount of skin damage increases."

Hypothermia. When the body's temperature drops below 95°, it's a medical emergency that should be treated promptly by a physician, says Marcia Walhout, R.N., a clinical nurse specialist in the emergency department of Butterworth Hospital in Grand Rapids, Michigan, who has treated many hypothermia patients.

How can you recognize it? "A child exhibiting any strange behavior after exposure to extreme cold for an extended period of time needs medical attention," says Susan Fuchs, M.D., assistant professor of pediatrics at the University of Pittsburgh School of Medicine and attending physician in the emergency department at the Children's Hospital of Pittsburgh. Signs to look for include confusion, disorientation, sleepiness, apathy or paleness.

"If you suspect hypothermia, remove any cold, wet clothing and replace with dry clothing or warm blankets," says Dr. Fuchs. Be sure the arms, legs and head are covered, and get your child to the emergency room of the nearest hospital as quickly as possible.

cold-weather gear for your children. Good choices include clothing made of polypropylene or other man-made fabrics that wick moisture away from the skin, water-resistant gloves or mittens, and wool or polypropylene socks, says Brian Delaney, who operates Whiteface Inn Cross-Country Ski Touring Center in Lake Placid, New York. Also choose snow boots with removable liners that can be dried out, suggests Delaney, who often takes his four young children on snowy outings.

Go for the layered look. "Clothes worn in layers help trap the warmth," says Dr. Fuchs. Start with long underwear, then add a turtleneck and sweater under a water-resistant jacket. Because of the insulating effect of the trapped layers of air, this will keep your child a lot warmer than a heavy coat on top of a shirt.

Cover up. Pay special attention to extremities, says Dr. Pray. Mittens will keep small fingers warmer than gloves, and feet will stay warmer with wool or polypropylene socks. To help prevent frostbite above the neck, put a hat and scarf or a neck gaiter on your child, or a balaclava, a knitted mask that covers the face except for the eyes and mouth.

Consider windchill. Don't assume that your outdoor thermometer tells the whole story. "It's not just temperature that determines how dangerous the cold is," says Walhout. "Whipping wind causes the body to lose heat quickly."

Try the buddy system. Assign each child a buddy and tell them to watch their buddy's ears, nose and cheeks for changes in color, says Dr. Fuchs. "Your child may not know when her lips lose color, but her friend might see it," she says. "And a buddy may just be able to step in when it's critical."

GAGGING

Hints for Smoother Swallowing

Close your eyes and pretend you are a baby. For the first six months of your life, you have been getting all your nourishment by sucking on a nipple—and you do it rather well. Sucking is something that you practiced in the womb, could do at birth and have been doing ever since. You are a natural, and life has been a pleasant procession of liquids expertly extracted—until today.

Today, your father has put you in an infant seat and is waving a silver spoon with great enthusiasm. On the spoon is a heaping mound of white goo—tremendously exciting stuff by the look on Dad's face. The goo comes closer, closer, closer, then plop! He shoves it in your mouth. "Acchh," you gag. How the heck are you supposed to suck down that stuff? You spit the goo on Dad's new tie, then clamp your jaws shut. For the moment, feeding time is definitely over.

Although Dad might be alarmed because you gagged on your first bite of solid food, a certain amount of gagging is par for the course when a baby starts to eat. "Eating solid food is a learned process," says Robert Wyllie, M.D.,

---

MEDICAL ALERT

When to See the Doctor

Although the gag reflex is a normal reaction in many situations, babies and children should not be gagging on a regular basis, according to Robert Wyllie, M.D., head of the Section of Pediatric Gastroenterology at the Cleveland Clinic Foundation in Ohio. "If your child gags repeatedly or starts to turn red in the face or bluish around the lips, see your doctor," advises Dr. Wyllie. In rare cases, gagging may indicate a problem that requires medical intervention.

head of the Section of Pediatric Gastroenterology at the Cleveland Clinic Foundation in Ohio.

"With the sucking reflex, babies bring their tongues to the front of the mouth and then up toward the palate. They may take 10 to 20 sucks, and then take a big swallow. With solids, though, the tongue needs to swing the food to the *back* of the mouth—almost the opposite motion," notes Dr. Wyllie.

Learning to swallow solid foods is not easy for a baby. And during the learning process, he may gag if food starts heading toward his airway rather than toward his stomach. You can help make mealtimes a gag-free experience, though, by adopting some new feeding tactics. Here are some tips from the experts.

Wait until your child is sitting up. "If your child is gagging a lot while eating, he may not have reached the stage in his development where he's ready for the experience," says Flavia Marino, M.D., a clinical instructor in pediatrics at New York University Medical Center, Tisch Hospital, and a pediatrician in New York City. "Your child should be at least four or five months old before you start feeding solids," Dr. Marino says.

The cue? Introduce solids when your child can sit up fairly well by himself, suggests Dr. Wyllie. "When your baby eats sitting up, gravity will help him get food from the mouth down the esophagus," he says.

Start the meal with liquids. "When your child is really hungry, breastfeed or give a bottle first to take the edge off her appetite," suggests Eileen Behan, R.D., a registered dietitian and consultant at Sea Coast Family Practice in Exeter, New Hampshire, and author of *Microwave Cooking for Your Baby and Child*. "If your baby is less ravenous, it will be easier for her to manage the complex task of eating solid foods," she says.

Reach for rice. Rice cereal is an ideal first food because kids are seldom allergic to it, and it can be made very diluted by mixing it with extra milk, says Dr. Wyllie. "Your baby will have less trouble eating the cereal if the texture is more like the liquid he is used to swallowing," he notes. Once your baby can swallow rice cereal, you can gradually work your way up to foods that are thicker and have a coarser consistency.

Keep the first meals small. "Early solid-food meals are for practice, not sustenance," notes Dr. Marino. "A baby who is learning to eat needs just a few teaspoons of food per day to practice on. The main nutrition should come from breast milk or formula.

Try a tiny dollop. "When your child opens her mouth, place a pea-size portion of food on the front of her tongue," says Behan. "A large dollop of food is harder to deal with, and if you drop it in toward the back of her mouth, your child is much more likely to gag on it."

Easy does it. Don't try to force the issue if your baby is having trouble with a new food. "If your child is gagging on a particular food such as potatoes or strained beef, I recommend omitting that food from the diet for a few days, then trying it again in slightly finer texture," suggests Dr. Marino.

Don't overfeed. If your child vomits or gags at every feeding, you may be giving him more than he can handle," says Dr. Wyllie. "In the first year of life, a baby can't control his food intake very well, so it is your job not to overfeed him." Look for cues that your baby is full, says Dr. Wyllie. He may start turning his head away or closing his lips when the spoon comes near his mouth.

GAS PAINS

How to Burst the Bubbles

Babies get it, toddlers get it, school-age kids and teenagers get it. And so do parents. Having gas is part of the human condition. You could call it a great equalizer.

MEDICAL ALERT

When to See the Doctor

Ordinary gas pains should dissipate without much fanfare, says Abraham Jelin, M.D., assistant chairman of the Department of Pediatrics and director of pediatric gastroenterology at the Brooklyn Hospital Center in New York City. However, a persistent stomachache, especially on the lower right side of the abdomen—which might indicate appendicitis—should be brought to your physician's attention. "If your child looks very ill; complains of acute, persistent or chronic pain; or has pain accompanied by fever, vomiting, diarrhea or weight loss, consult your physician," says Dr. Jelin.

Gas can be caused by swallowed air, gas-producing foods or certain disorders that interfere with the body's ability to absorb food. Whatever its source, air in the gastrointestinal tract must come out—either through burping or by passing gas.

All babies are somewhat gassy, since they tend to suck in air as they breastfeed or drink from a bottle. "Some babies handle gas without a problem. But others, who may have an immature or spastic gastrointestinal tract, feel uncomfortable as they digest their food," notes Michael J. Pettei, M.D., Ph.D., associate professor of pediatrics at Albert Einstein School of Medicine of Yeshiva University in New York City, and co-chief of the Division of Gastroenterology and Nutrition at Schneider Children's Hospital of the Long Island Jewish Medical Center in New Hyde Park, New York.

"A baby should soon grow out of the problem on his own, but during the first few months of life, he may be very uncomfortable. He may draw up his legs and cry inconsolably whenever he feels the gas pain," Dr. Pettei says. "Some people call this condition colic—though not all 'colicky' babies have gastrointestinal problems."

On occasion, older kids may have gas-related stomach pain that lasts for a couple of minutes. If the pain persists or is prolonged, you should consult your pediatrician, says Abraham Jelin, M.D., assistant chairman of the Department of Pediatrics and director of pediatric gastroenterology at Brooklyn Hospital Center in New York City.

Infants and older children may get relief with some of the following gas-reducing tips.

For Infants

Try a different bottle. There are many different baby bottle designs, and there are also different sizes and shapes of nipples. If gas is a problem, try switching bottles, nipples or both. "Some kids may swallow less air when they drink from the combination of nipple and bottle that's right for them. So experiment with a few different varieties," suggests Dr. Pettei.

Feed at a 45-degree angle. Babies should be held semi-upright, at a 45-degree angle, when being fed, says Dr. Jelin. "Your baby still swallows air in this position, but the air that is swallowed forms an air bubble at the top of the stomach," he explains. The advantage to this is twofold: You'll have an easier time burping your baby, and there's less likelihood air will get past the stomach to the intestinal tract where it will cause more discomfort, Dr. Jelin says.

Burp baby in a vertical position. Dr. Jelin recommends that you burp your baby by holding her in an upright position. Lift her so her belly rests against your chest with her head on your shoulder. In that position, gas stays above the liquid in the stomach and is easily burped out. "Avoid burping your baby in a horizontal position such as across your knees," says Dr. Jelin, "since that makes it easier for gas to pass from the stomach to the small intestine."

Take a burp break. A baby who is troubled by gas often benefits from being burped halfway through a feeding, says Dr. Pettei. When your baby takes a pause from the bottle or breast, lift her gently to the upright position and see if she'll burp.

Don't feed too much. Encouraging your baby to eat more than he wants can make gas problems worse. "Let the baby determine how much he wants to eat," Dr. Pettei advises, "since overfeeding will only make him more uncomfortable."

For Older Children

Slow down the pace at the table. Older kids may have gas pain if they race through their meal and swallow a lot of air, says Eileen Behan, R.D., a registered dietitian and consultant at Sea Coast Family Practice in Exeter, New Hampshire, and author of *Microwave Cooking for Your Baby and Child*. "Check out your own eating speed, too," suggests Behan. "Your child may have learned his wolfish mode of eating from you. In that case, it will do everyone good if you deliberately try to slow down and enjoy the meal."

Scrutinize the veggies. Certain foods are high in complex carbohydrates that are not completely digested in the small bowel. These tend to produce gas. "Cauliflower, brussels sprouts, cabbage and broccoli are regarded as common offenders because they do cause some people to have a lot of gas," Behan says.

"If one or all of these vegetables are gas-pain triggers for your child, he'll start to feel discomfort about two to four hours after eating," she says. Using this guideline, you and your child may be able to pinpoint the troublemaker, and cut back on portion size. "These vegetables are really very nutritious and good for you. So if your child enjoys them, try to cut back rather than cut them out," she suggests.

Soak the beans. To reduce gassiness from dried beans, soak them for several hours in a few changes of water before cooking, advises Behan. "Soaking and rinsing beans does not detract from their protein content," she adds.

Drop in with relief. A few drops of an enzyme product called Beano sprinkled on beans just before eating may also help prevent gas, suggests Behan. Beano is available at health food stores and pharmacies.

Avoid sorbitol. Sorbitol, an artificial sweetener found in many sugar-free foods, including some chewing gums and mints, can cause a lot of distension and gas, says Dr. Jelin. If gas pain is a problem for your child, try eliminating foods made with sorbitol from his diet.

Guard against air gulping. "Anything that causes a child to swallow air may contribute to gas," Dr. Jelin says. So your child may need to cut back on chewing gum, sucking on hard candies and drinking carbonated beverages (especially through a straw).

Check out the dairy connection. In older children, gas may also be caused by lactose intolerance, says Dr. Pettei. Children with this condition don't produce enough lactase, the enzyme needed to digest milk sugar (lactose).

If you think you've spotted a connection between dairy food and your child's symptoms, see your doctor. Lactose intolerance can be diagnosed with a simple breath test. If it's found to be the cause of your child's gas pain, your doctor may recommend limiting dairy products, taking supplemental enzymes or drinking a special kind of milk that contains lactase.

GROWING PAINS

What It Takes to Stop the Aches

Sometime between the ages of four and nine, your child may experience what are commonly called growing pains. These mysterious pains occur in the legs—often at night—and may last for anywhere from minutes to hours and then disappear. These episodes usually occur several times per week and may continue for a year or more.

You might be surprised to learn that growing pains have nothing to do with growth. "Actually, a better name for the condition is simply limb pains of childhood," says Bram H. Bernstein, M.D., professor of clinical pediatrics at the University of Southern California and head of rheumatology at Children's Hospital of Los Angeles.

But doctors still don't have all the answers about growing pains. "In some children the pains seem to be located in the muscles, while other children get pains in the bones," notes Dr. Bernstein.

In many cases growing pains may be nothing more than muscle soreness caused by overexertion of tight muscles. "It's similar to how you or I might feel tomorrow if we climbed a mountain today," says Dr. Bernstein. "A lot of these children are quite active. The tight muscles don't hurt when they're doing things, but do begin to hurt when they relax at night. In other patients, though, we really never know the cause."

One thing experts do know about growing pains: They're not muscle cramps. Those are something else altogether—a severe pain, usually in a calf muscle, caused by spasm. "With cramps, you can usually see the muscle spasm. That's not the case with growing pains," says Dr. Bernstein.

There are a few simple remedies for growing pains. "But it's hard to predict which ones will be effective in any given case," he says. "Once your doctor has ruled out anything serious, like arthritis, you may need to try a number of remedies to find out what works for your child."

Reassure with calming words. Pain is scary to children, even if the cause is simply muscle strain, Dr. Bernstein notes. "Explain to your child that the leg pains are probably caused by overexertion and that they will soon pass. "Reassurance is the most important thing. Kids need to know that what they're experiencing is not the result of any terrible disease."

Fight the pain with a pain medicine. "A mild analgesic such as acetaminophen [Children's Tylenol] may be all the child needs," says Dr. Bernstein. Check the package direc-

MEDICAL ALERT

When to See the Doctor

Leg pain in children can sometimes be a sign of a serious condition, such as rheumatoid arthritis, says Bram H. Bernstein, M.D., professor of clinical pediatrics at the University of Southern California and head of rheumatology at Children's Hospital of Los Angeles. He advises contacting a physician if any of these symptoms accompany the pain.

- Fever
- Swelling of joints or muscles
- Exceptional fatigue, loss of appetite and weight loss
- Limping
- Morning pains upon awakening

---

tions for the correct dosage for your child's age and weight, or check with your physician. If a mild medicine doesn't work, he says, ask your doctor about ibuprofen, an anti-inflammatory drug, which is only available for young children by prescription. "Ibuprofen seems to work better than acetaminophen in many cases, though it's not clear why," he says.

Try a hands-on approach. "Growing pains respond very well to 'mother's massage,'" says Russell Steele, M.D., professor and vice chairman of the Department of Pediatrics at Louisiana State University School of Medicine in New Orleans. "Gently massage the child's legs in the area where the pain is located until he starts to feel better."

Warm up the sore spots. Heat may be soothing, particularly if the child's pains are from muscle soreness, says Shirley Menard, R.N., a certified pediatric nurse practitioner and assistant professor at the University of Texas Health Science Center at San Antonio School of Nursing. "A warm bath or shower, or even a heating pad can often bring relief," she notes.

Twenty minutes in a warm bath or under a heating pad is often all that's needed, adds Dr. Bernstein. However, don't leave your child unattended with a heating pad for an extended period because he might get *too* warm.

"Go camping" in the bedroom. As a preventive measure to stop future pain episodes, it may be helpful to keep your child's legs warm at night while he's sleeping. "You don't want him to sleep all night under a heating pad or an electric blanket, because that could be dangerous," says Dr. Bernstein. "But small children can be safely bundled up in a sleeping bag. The sleeping bag will keep your child's legs warm, and he'll probably enjoy it."

HAIR TANGLES

Keeping Locks in Line

I n the bathroom, your child stands wrapped in her towel, her hair a mass of tangles. But just approach her with a comb and you'll hear, "No! No! *Don't touch my hair!*"

A hair tangle—that twisted, knotted mat that snags your comb and won't let go—may not be your child's most serious problem in life, but it sure does make your child yowl when you try to pass a comb through it.

Why do kids get so many tangles, you ask? They earn them. "Kids play in the wind, roll in the leaves, pull winter hats on and off their heads, swim in the pool, sleep with wet hair, turn, twist and chew on their hair, and all without stopping to use a comb," says Harley Marks, owner and manager of Kids Cuts in New York City.

Impossible though it may seem, it's not hard to keep a child tangle-free, but she may need some help from you. Kids up to the age of six or seven need a lot of help to keep their hair in line, but even older kids who prefer to manage their own hair can benefit from some expert advice. Follow

GUM, TAR, SAP AND OTHER
STICKY PROBLEMS

If your child comes home from the park with a big wad of gum or tree sap in her hair, your first line of defense is not the scissors. "I find that Aveda's Nourishing Clarifying Gel, which is available in salons, sometimes does the trick," says hair care expert Elena Ciervo, manager of Kidz Kuts, a salon in Livingston, New Jersey. "Leave the gel on the hair and gum for about five minutes; rinse and comb out bit by bit."

Children's hair stylist Lorraine Massey, owner of New York Master Practitioners of Hair (N.Y.M.P.H.) salon in New York City, finds that ice helps by making the sticky substance hard. "Once you've frozen the gum, you can crumble it out with your fingers," she says. Massey likes to apply vinegar after icing the gunk, and then gob on conditioner. "The acid in the vinegar helps dissolve the stickiness, and the conditioner helps you work the comb through it," she says.

You might also try working some mayonnaise through the area, says Massey. "The heavy greasiness might help the gum to slide out of the hair."

Harley Marks, owner and manager of Kids Cuts in New York City, likes to use her mother's remedy—smooth peanut butter. "Mush some peanut butter right into the gum, and the hair will start to separate," says Marks. "Continue to separate the hair with your fingers, then work out the gum with a comb." Marks says you might have to repeat the procedure a few times before you get all the gum out.

Whatever you try, work slowly and distract your child with music, a story or a favorite television show.

these tips, from three children's hair care professionals, and your child will be well on her way to a more manageable mane.

Water down shampoos. "All shampoos, even baby shampoos, should be watered down with spring water," says Lorraine Massey, owner of New York Master Practitioners of Hair (N.Y.M.P.H.), a salon in New York City. "Manufacturers claim that their shampoos are really mild, but many actually have very strong detergents in them, which dry the hair and make it more prone to tangles."

As an added benefit, diluting shampoo will make it easier to distribute through the hair, she adds.

Use a gentle touch. Parents may inadvertently create tangles by piling hair on their child's head and then giving it a vigorous, lathery shampoo, notes Massey. "You'll disturb the hair shafts less if you gently massage the shampoo into the scalp and then carefully work the shampoo down the hair," she says.

Condition that coif. Using a conditioner after shampooing is a lifesaver—or at least a hairsaver, says Elena Ciervo, manager of Kidz Kuts, a full-service haircutting salon for kids in Livingston, New Jersey. Use a conditioner that is rich in protein and contains oils such as carrot, citrus, rosemary or grape seed. "Conditioners add lubricants to the hair and make it easier to comb out," according to Ciervo.

Tackle tangles tubside. Massey recommends applying the conditioner while your child is in the tub and then combing the conditioner all the way through to the ends

---

BREW YOUR OWN

For a truly mild shampoo that won't contribute to tangles, try making your own shampoo with your child. It's a fun, easy project and everyone's hair will benefit, says hair care expert Lorraine Massey, owner of New York Master Practitioners of Hair (N.Y.M.P.H.) salon in New York City.

First, buy a four-ounce cake of castile soap from the health food store or pharmacy. She recommends that you "grate it fine and add it to one quart of spring water. Simmer the mixture on the stove until the soap is dissolved, and then add a few drops of your favorite essential oils such as chamomile, citrus, rosemary, eucalyptus or carrot seed." Bottle the shampoo in a plastic container.

of the hair. Finish the detangling treatment with a good rinse and then comb the hair again, she suggests.

Squeeze and pat. "Try to towel-dry the hair gently," says Marks. "Vigorous toweling leads to more tangles." She recommends that you gently squeeze the excess moisture out of your child's hair and then pat it dry.

Try a detangler. When a child has major tangles, a detangling cream can't be beat. "There are a lot of detangling products on the market, but I prefer Paul Mitchell's product, The Detangler," says Ciervo. "Made from botanical extracts, it's gentle and can be used after every shampoo, if need be. But it is only available in salons."

Consider the right comb. Work out tangles with a medium-toothed comb, recommends Massey. "Combing out tangles works best, but don't choose a comb that is too wide-toothed because you'll miss the tinier tangles," she says.

Work your way up. If you start at the roots and try to yank your way down, your child will never let you near her with a comb in your hand. Instead, Marks suggests that you clip the unknotted hair out of your way and patiently work away on the problem area. "Never yank, and always comb from the bottom of the tangle to the top," she says.

Don't let her sleep on snarls. "Every day I see hair that is brushed on the surface but not underneath, where it gets knotted and matted," says Ciervo. If your child gets tangles, they'll get worse if she sleeps on them. The solution? "Brush through her hair every night before bedtime. Get that brush or comb right down to the scalp and through every strand," Ciervo says.

Sleep in style. After your child's hair is combed, have her sleep in a braid or a loose pony tail with a fabric-covered elastic band at the top and at the bottom, says Marks. "Keep the elastic band loose and not too close to the scalp because tension can damage the hair." The best coverings are made of terry cloth because they won't tear or damage hair.

HANGNAILS

Fix-Ups for Fingertips

A hangnail isn't a nail at all—and it might not even be a problem. It's just a little flap of dried skin on the side of a nail.

But a kid's hangnail is just asking to get chewed on, torn off or covered with playground grime. And with that kind of abuse, a kid's hangnail is more than a nuisance—it's a potential source of infection.

"Teach your child the right way to treat a hangnail, and you'll nip a lot of tough problems in the bud," says Patience Williamson, R.N., a certified school nurse at the Rand Family School in Montclair, New Jersey. Here's how.

Cream those cuticles. Hangnails are often the result of dry skin. "It helps to keep hands well-moisturized," says Williamson. She recommends that your child apply some hand cream around the cuticles after each bath.

Teach gentle care. Ask your child not to push the cuticle back or to pick at dry skin at the edge of the nail. "The cuticle is a natural protective barrier for the nail, and if your child cuts it or forcibly pushes it back, she may *cause* a hangnail, or introduce bacteria that may trigger an infection," says Scott A. Norton, M.D., staff dermatologist at Tripler Army Medical Center in Honolulu.

MEDICAL ALERT

When to See the Doctor

If your child has a swollen, red area at the base or side of his nail that is exceedingly tender or oozes pus when you press on it, see a doctor immediately, advises Scott A. Norton, M.D., staff dermatologist at Tripler Army Medical Center in Honolulu. "This bacterial infection, called a paronychia, may need to be drained or treated with antibiotics," he says.

Ask your child to wash it and wait. If your young child can recognize a hangnail, she should let you take care of it, suggests Williamson. "A child should wash and dry the affected area very carefully, cover the hangnail with a Band-Aid and then get an adult's assistance," she says. "But don't advise your child to try to fix the hangnail with a nail clipper or scissors. She can do far more damage than good," Williamson says.

Snip off the problem. "A hangnail should be removed with a clean nail clipper that has been rinsed with alcohol to prevent the spread of bacteria," says Dr. Norton. By trimming the far end of the hangnail promptly, you'll be removing any temptation for your child to pull or chew on the dead skin. "If you pull on a hangnail, you'll just tear some of the live skin," he says.

Fight infection with warm water. Examine the area around the hangnail every day for signs of infection. "If the skin around the hangnail looks as if it is getting red or tender, apply warm compresses to the area or soak the finger in warm water," says Dr. Norton. This treatment should be repeated three or four times a day for one or two days to increase the blood flow. Increased circulation brings antibodies to the area, which help fight infection, Dr. Norton explains.

Anoint it with ointment. Apply a dab of over-the-counter antibiotic ointment such as Aquaphor Antibiotic Ointment or Polysporin Ointment to the infected area three times a day and cover it with a Band-Aid, says Richard Garcia, M.D., a pediatrician and vice chairman of the Department of Pediatrics and Adolescent Medicine at the Cleveland Clinic Foundation in Ohio. Continue doing this until the infection clears and the hangnail can be loosened and trimmed without trauma. "Be sure that the antibiotic ointment you select does not have neomycin in it, because that often causes an allergic reaction," cautions Dr. Garcia.

Protect the site. To prevent sore spots from developing, encourage your child to practice good hygiene, says Dr. Garcia. "Stress the importance of keeping fingers out of the nose and mouth, washing hands frequently and cutting nails straight across so that the skin beside the nail is not traumatized," he says.

Discourage nail-biting. Nail-biting is at the root of many a hangnail, so encourage your child to break the habit. "Unfortunately, that's easier said than done," notes Dr. Garcia. "And nagging often makes the problem worse."

HAY FEVER AND ALLERGIES

Getting the Better of Allergy Onslaughts

Your child has an itchy nose that's running like a faucet. She has no fever, but she's sneezing, producing several ka-choos in a row. Her eyes are teary, red and swollen. All in all, she's just plain miserable.

"Hay fever," you think, and you may be right (although children under five aren't usually allergic to pollen). But what if it's the dead of winter with nary a blossom in sight?

Instead of reacting to pollen, your child may be allergic to something that floats around in the air year-round: dust mites, mold or animal dander. When a child is allergic to something she inhales, her body overreacts by releasing chemicals such as histamine that cause unpleasant side effects—congestion, itching, dripping and sneezing.

So what can you do? Most allergy specialists agree that allergy prevention begins in the home. "We put our major emphasis on avoiding contact with the allergen, which is a cheap and effective form of allergy treatment," says Peter LoGalbo, M.D., assistant professor of pediatrics at the Albert Einstein College of Medicine of Yeshiva University in New York City and director of the Asthma and Allergy Center, Schneider Children's Hospital of the Long Island Jewish Medical Center in New Hyde Park, New York.

The first step is to go to the allergist's office, where your child can be tested to find out what allergens are causing

MEDICAL ALERT

When to See the Doctor

If keeping your child away from whatever causes the allergy isn't adequate to quell symptoms, your physician will recommend other measures. "The second line of defense is medication, which can be effective but may have side effects. Finally, we turn to allergy shots if the first two fail," says Peter LoGalbo, M.D., assistant professor of pediatrics at the Albert Einstein College of Medicine of Yeshiva University in New York City and director of the Asthma and Allergy Center, Schneider Children's Hospital of the Long Island Jewish Medical Center in New Hyde Park, New York.

You may be able to treat your child with over-the-counter products, but you must ask your physician about the amount and type of medication to use.

"Antihistamines work best if your child has symptoms such as sneezing, itching and watery eyes," says David Tinkelman, M.D., clinical professor of pediatrics in the Department of Allergy and Immunology at the Medical College of Georgia in Augusta and an allergist in Atlanta. But antihistamines can make your child sleepy, decrease her ability to concentrate and cause dry mouth.

"Decongestants, on the other hand, will help open a stuffy nose, but won't help with a runny nose or sneezing. They may suppress appetite or cause insomnia, jitters or irritability," Dr. Tinkelman says.

Many over-the-counter preparations are antihistamine/decongestant combinations, which can provide more relief, but also more side effects. Your physician will tell you what to try or prescribe other treatment if the over-the-counter products don't work.

But never allow your child to use over-the-counter nose drops, warns Gail G. Shapiro, M.D., clinical professor of pediatrics at the University of Washington School of Medicine and in practice at Northwest Asthma and Allergy Center, both in Seattle. These drops cause the lining of the nose to shrink. This brings temporary relief, but the inflammation will soon recur, often worse than it was to begin with. There are prescription drops that work well, she notes, so consult your doctor if your child needs extra hay fever relief.

the problems. After your child's allergies are diagnosed, here's what you can do to help solve the problem.

For Dust Mite Allergies

Prepare to make changes. "Lots of kids are allergic to the droppings of the house dust mite, a microscopic insect that lives wherever dust collects, such as on upholstery, pillows, stuffed animals and carpeting," says David Tinkelman, M.D., clinical professor of pediatrics in the Department of Allergy and Immunology at the Medical College of Georgia in Augusta and an allergist in Atlanta. To decrease contact with dust mite droppings, you'll have to make some modifications in your furnishings—and probably change the way you clean the house.

Vinyl-wrap the bedding. Encase your child's mattress, box spring and pillow with vinyl-backed covers available at many discount and department stores. "Allergy supply companies make fancy ones that you can order, but for kids, the inexpensive vinyl covers are fine," says Gail G. Shapiro, M.D., clinical professor of pediatrics at the University of Washington School of Medicine and in practice at Northwest Asthma and Allergy Center, both in Seattle.

Tape the zippers. Dr. Tinkelman recommends finishing the vinyl treatment by putting tape over the zippers of all the vinyl covers. That way, the dust mites within the bed and pillow can't get out. Either duct tape or wide, heavy-duty plastic sealing tape will do the job.

Get rid of feathers and down. "Feather and down pillows and quilts are a haven for dust mites," says Rebecca Gruchalla, M.D., assistant professor of internal medicine in the Division of Allergy at the University of Texas Southwestern Medical Center in Dallas. "Instead, switch to cotton blankets and foam or polyester pillows that are washable."

Use hot water. Wash all of your child's bedding frequently in very hot water, says Dr. Shapiro. The hot water kills the mites and gets rid of the droppings. Use the hot water wash *and* rinse, and make sure you do all the bedding—mattress cover and blankets as well as sheets. It's best to launder bedding every one to two weeks.

Beware of floor coverings. Carpets and rugs are a favorite mite hideout. "Take the carpet out of your child's bedroom," says Dr. Gruchalla. "Instead, use a cotton scatter rug, which can be washed regularly in hot water."

Treat remaining carpets. It may not be practical to strip the carpets from your entire house, but you can keep them allergen-free. Treat your rugs and carpets with Allergy Control Solution, a 3 percent tannic acid solution, recommends Dr. Shapiro. It's often used along with Acarosan, a product that actually reduces the mite population in carpets, according to Dr. Shapiro. Both these products must be applied every three months to be effective, following instructions on the package. Both products are available by mail from Allergy Control Products, 96 Danbury Road, Ridgefield, Connecticut 06877.

Change vacuum cleaner bags. While it's important to vacuum frequently, you first need to make an important change. "Replace your usual disposable vacuum bag with one that's made of special paper that actually traps allergenic mite particles," says Paul V. Williams, M.D., clinical associate professor of pediatrics and allergy at the University of Washington School of Medicine in Seattle. "When you use a conventional vacuum bag, you're actually picking up the allergenic particles and blowing them into the air, making the situation worse." The allergen-trapping bags— one brand is Hysurf—can be found in a few stores where vacuum cleaners are sold or from National Allergy Supply, 4400 Georgia Highway, 120, P.O. Box 1658, Duluth, Georgia 30136.

Ditch the drapes. "Drapes and venetian blinds are big dust collectors," says Dr. LoGalbo. It's okay to replace them with washable curtains, but it's even better if you just install a pull-down shade that can be wiped off, says Dr. Gruchalla.

Rid stuffed animals of mites. Because dust mites can

abound in the fur of stuffed animals, it's best to move them out of your child's bedroom. But if your child is attached to one special toy, you can de-mite it with either the hot or cold treatment, according to Dr. Tinkelman. "Dust mites can't live in extremes of temperature," he says. "Treat the stuffed animal to a soaking in the hot water cycle of your washing machine, or put it inside a plastic bag and leave it in the freezer overnight."

You may want to let your child choose another stuffed animal occasionally, switching off between favorites. If you buy more, to make things easier, select ones that will withstand machine washing and drying.

Change sleeping arrangements. Sleeping on the bottom bunk of a bunk bed or under a canopy is a no-no, says Dr. Tinkelman. "Kids love canopies and bunk beds, but so do dust mites," he observes. Mites live both in the upper mattress of the bunk bed and in the dust that collects on top of a canopy.

Pay attention to closets. "Closets are rarely cleaned and aired, and they tend to be dust mines," notes Dr. LoGalbo. Any closet the child uses should be vacuumed every time the rest of the room is. If you have little-used closets with old toys or papers, keep the closet door closed all the time.

Dry up. "Mites love humidity," says Dr. Williams. "If you can keep the humidity below 50 percent, you can go a long way to reduce mite problems. Invest in a room dehumidifier for your child's bedroom."

For Mold Allergies

Buy a humidity gauge. Mold also flourishes anywhere there's high humidity, according to Dr. Williams. To stop mold allergens, measure the humidity in your home and use a dehumidifier, says Dr. LoGalbo.

Ventilate. "Get some fresh air circulating in the house, especially in the bathrooms and kitchen where mold tends to grow," says Dr. LoGalbo. Window fans or ceiling fans help to circulate air.

Take books out of the bedroom. "Mold spores are known to inhabit books," says Gilbert Friday, M.D., professor of pediatrics and chief of clinical services of the Asthma and Allergic Disease Center at the Children's Hospital of Pittsburgh. "For kids who are allergic to molds, it's best to keep books either in a glass-doored bookcase or out of the bedroom altogether. At the very least, dust the books frequently."

Use mold-killing cleaners. "Choose cleaners such as Lysol that inhibit mold growth," suggests Dr. LoGalbo. Also, you can make a mold-fighting mixture by adding a few spoonfuls of commercial bleach to a bucket of water. Just scrub damp areas and other surfaces with the bleach mixture to discourage mold. (Use rubber gloves to protect your hands.)

Lay off the leaves. There's mold aplenty in piles of fallen leaves. Discourage your allergic child from rolling in or playing near leaf piles, advises Dr. Shapiro.

For Pet Allergies

Move pets out. Kids can be allergic to dander, the dead skin from your pets. Cats, in particular, cause some of the worst problems because they lick themselves so often, says Dr. Friday, and when the saliva dries, the allergens from the saliva become airborne.

"Ideally, family pets such as cats and dogs should live outside," says Dr. Williams. If your pet can't live outside, you should consider finding it a new home.

Ban pets from bedrooms. If moving a pet outside isn't practical and your family can't bear to give up the animal, put some limits on its territory. It's most important to keep the pet out of the child's bedroom, says Jonathan Becker, M.D., a pediatrician and senior research fellow at the University of Washington in Seattle.

"Pets such as hamsters, guinea pigs and gerbils should be removed from the bedroom, too, because their droppings can get mold or fungi growing in them, which some kids are also allergic to," says Dr. Friday. "Even birds can pose a problem for allergic kids, because the flapping of their wings releases a fine powder of bird allergen into the air."

Keep Fluffy out of the basement. Don't relocate your cat to the basement if you have forced air heat, says Dr. Friday. "In a home that has forced air heat, the cat allergen, which is very light, would go right up through the heating system and be blown around the whole house," he says.

Wash your cat. "Preliminary research suggests that if you wash your cat every week for at least eight weeks with plain water or shampoo and water, you remove the surface allergens that come from its saliva. Unfortunately, you really must wash the animal every week—forever—to get continued benefit from this treatment," says Dr. Shapiro.

The problem is that it's difficult to get most adult cats to endure one bath, let alone a bath once a week. You'll have the most success with cat washing if you start when your pet is just a kitten.

For Pollen Allergies

Air-condition. Your child will not be able to avoid all contact with pollen, which is prevalent during the spring and late summer. But his nights *can* be more restful if you have an air conditioner in his room, according to Dr. LoGalbo. "It's hard to resist the temptation to keep the windows open when the nights are cool and fresh," he admits, "but that lets the pollen pour into your child's room, and he'll wake up miserable."

Schedule outdoor playtime. The middle of the day is the best time for hay fever-prone kids to play outside. "There is a higher concentration of pollen in the early morning," says Dr. Friday. "As the air heats up it rises and takes the pollen with it. In the evening, when the air gets cool again, the pollen settles back down, too. So the best time to let your kids play outside is somewhere in between."

Roll up car windows. "You get a higher concentration of pollen if you drive with the windows open," says Dr. Friday. "If your allergic child is in the car, it's best to use the air conditioner during the pollen season."

HEADACHES

How Doctors Spell Relief

If you're like many parents, you probably think of headaches as something kids give you, not something kids *get*. But research indicates that 50 to 70 percent of all school-age children have experienced a headache, according to Francis J. DiMario, Jr., M.D., assistant professor of pediatrics and neurology at the University of Connecticut in Farmington.

"The causes of children's headaches are very similar to the causes of adult headaches," says Dr. DiMario. "They get tension headaches; headaches associated with injury, illness or fever; and migraines." About 10 percent of children with headaches get chronic migraines.

All kinds of kids' headaches usually respond to the same treatments used for adult headaches, from over-the-counter pain relievers and warm compresses for occasional head-

---

MEDICAL ALERT

When to See the Doctor

Though rare, headaches can sometimes be symptoms of a serious problem such as meningitis, a brain tumor or bleeding in the brain, according to Loraine Stern, M.D., associate clinical professor of pediatrics at the University of California, Los Angeles, and author of *When Do I Call the Doctor?* She says you should call your doctor if your child's headache:

- Is accompanied by a fever, vomiting, stiff neck, lethargy or confusion.
- Follows a head injury.
- Occurs in the morning, accompanied by nausea.
- Increases in severity over the course of a day or from one day to the next.
- Is suddenly brought on by a sneeze or cough.
- Interferes with school or other activities.
- Is restricted to one side of the head.

aches to prescription drugs and biofeedback for chronic headaches. Even if your child's headache requires professional intervention, the experts say there are still measures you can take at home to help make the medical treatment more effective.

Before attempting any of these home remedies, however, read the "Medical Alert" to determine if your child's headache might be the symptom of something more serious.

Turn to a proven painkiller. "Simple analgesics such as acetaminophen [Children's Tylenol] are perfectly acceptable and effective for children's headaches, just as they are for adults'," says Dr. DiMario. Check the package directions for the correct dosage for your child's age and weight.

Apply a soothing compress. "Some kids like warm cloths on their heads, others like cold cloths. You just need to experiment," says William Womack, M.D., associate professor in the Department of Child Psychiatry at the University of Washington School of Medicine and codirector of the Stress Management Clinic of Children's Hospital and Medical Center, both in Seattle. "Keep the compress on for about 30 minutes, rewetting it as necessary," he says.

Head for bed. "Rest seems to be one of the most effective ways to reduce a migraine headache," says Dr. DiMario. "Many school nurses allow kids with headaches to lie down for half an hour. Often that is all that's necessary. They don't necessarily have to go to sleep. Just a half-hour of lying quietly can help." If your child is very sensitive to bright light during a migraine episode, you should draw the shades so he can rest in a darkened room, adds Dr. Womack.

Rub away the ache. Like adults, kids with tension headaches can often find relief by reducing stress. "If your child is stressed out, relaxing massage might help," says Alexander Mauskop, M.D., director of the New York Headache Center in New York City and assistant professor of neurology at the State University of New York Health Science Center.

"If the muscles around the scalp or temples are tender,

gently rubbing them can be helpful," says Dr. DiMario. "But some kids don't like it because the scalp is too tender to touch." If your child says stop, don't insist—but many children do like that soothing touch of a parent's fingertips.

Make meal-skipping a misdemeanor. Make sure your child doesn't skip meals, especially breakfast, which is the most important one, warns Dr. Mauskop. "Going all day without eating is a good way to get a headache or aggravate one you already have," he says.

Watch that egg roll, hold that pizza. By paying attention to what your child eats and when he gets his headaches, you may be able to spot a link. "In some susceptible children, headaches are triggered by certain things they eat, such as chocolate, peanuts, processed meat and aged cheese," says Dr. DiMario. "Pizza and Chinese food, if they contain monosodium glutamate, can bring on headaches in some children." If you think you've uncovered a connection, have your child avoid the suspect food and see what happens.

Curb the caffeine. Like grown-ups deprived of their customary morning coffee, kids can suffer from withdrawal headaches when they don't get their daily "fix" of caffeine. "Caffeine withdrawal headaches are common in children who drink cola and eat a lot of chocolate—both of which contain caffeine," says Dr. Mauskop. If your child is susceptible, you may need to strictly limit these items, offering them only as an occasional treat.

Chart those mood swings. Some kids' headaches have emotional rather than food triggers, says Kenneth Covelman, Ph.D., director of psychosocial services for the Pediatric Pain Management Program at Children's Hospital of Philadelphia and clinical assistant professor of psychology in psychiatry at the University of Pennsylvania School of Medicine, also in Philadelphia. "By charting not just your child's headaches but also his moods and activities for several days or weeks, you can sometimes see a pattern. For example, headaches may occur just before tests in school, or after arguments," says Dr. Covelman.

Have a plan to defuse tensions. "If you've identified an emotional trigger of your child's headaches," says Dr. Covelman, "help him formulate a plan for dealing with it." Your child may feel a lot better if he has more control over situations, he suggests.

"For example, if headaches occur after upsetting fights with his sister, talk about what he can do differently the next time they're playing together. Through role-playing, rehearse what he might say to her, such as, 'I don't like when you do this to me, so I'm not going to play with you until you apologize.' " Having a plan of action can help defuse the tension that leads to the headaches, says Dr. Covelman.

Don't rule out random events. If no dietary or emotional triggers emerge after a few weeks of charting your child's headaches, broaden the scope of your search, suggests Loraine Stern, M.D., associate clinical professor of pediatrics at the University of California, Los Angeles, and author of *When Do I Call the Doctor?* "Write down what the weather was like, how much your child slept the night before his headache . . . every possible factor you can think of.

"I had one child whose headaches seemed to come from the sunlight that shimmered on the surface of the family pool," Dr. Stern says. "Her parents noticed that if she went into the pool at a certain time of day, the light reflecting off the water gave her a headache. Often it's cockamamy things like that you might miss if you don't keep a record."

Reserve some time for fun. Many children who suffer from recurring headaches have fallen into the "all work and no play" trap, according to Dr. Womack. They need to schedule some fun.

"I see a lot of well-motivated, high-achieving, but overly intense kids in my clinic," he says. "They're in a lot of extracurricular activities, and they're preoccupied with getting good grades. They're perfectionists, type-A personalities who are really driven to achieve. For them, headaches have become a barometer of the stress in their lives."

If your child is like this, Dr. Womack suggests that you help your child decide which pursuits are most important and cut back on the rest. "That will free up some time for relaxation and fun," says Dr. Womack. "Children need to remember that things don't have to always be heavy and serious, and their efforts don't have to be perfect all the time."

Neutralize the Nintendo headache. Muscular tension headaches are often the result of mental stress. But sometimes they can have a purely physical cause, says Dr. Stern. For example, if your child plays a lot of video games or does work on a computer, he may be inviting a headache by holding his head in one position too long. Encourage him to roll his head occasionally or take frequent breaks.

Harness imagination's healing power. Visualization, biofeedback and other special relaxation techniques are often employed by professionals to help their patients head off headaches. But it's possible for parents to teach kids some basic relaxation skills at home, Dr. Womack says.

He suggests trying this technique: "Ask the child to imagine he's taking a warm shower and that everywhere the water strikes his body instantly feels more relaxed. Or have him picture himself stepping into a warm pool where the water gradually rises over his toes, his feet, his ankles and on up. This is a form of progressive muscle relaxation that kids find less boring than formal progressive muscle relaxation exercises."

Put yourself in the picture, too. If your child is learning relaxation techniques, you should also learn them, says Dr. Covelman. "Younger children may need some help practicing the techniques at home, and it's very helpful for parents to be able to do them, too," he says.

Support without nagging. Kids with chronic headaches need to practice their relaxation skills regularly, says Dr. Womack. "Unfortunately, many kids find repetitive practicing of any kind boring, like having to practice the piano." But if you nag them about it, he says, it's counterproductive—it just creates more stress. Be supportive instead.

"In addition to making space and time available for the child to practice," says Dr. Womack, "you need to remind him that this is something important that he should want to be doing for himself. If you give the child primary responsibility but make it clear that you want to help him to succeed, most kids will go along with it."

HEAT EXHAUSTION

How to Cope with Summer's Sizzlers

"Mad dogs and Englishmen go out in the midday sun." As that old line implies, running around in the heat is not exactly a wise thing to do.

But children love to play, and midday sun doesn't seem to faze them. That's why, if your child is on a team or loves playing outdoors in the summer, you need to be aware of a potentially hazardous condition: heat exhaustion.

Under normal conditions, the body keeps its cool by perspiring and by radiating heat through the skin. When it is really hot outside though, and your child is working or playing hard, this cooling system starts to break down. Your child may sweat so much that she gets dehydrated. She may complain of feeling weak, dizzy and nauseated. But when you take her temperature, you find that it's normal or only slightly above normal. These symptoms are all signals of heat exhaustion, which means your child definitely needs a good long break from the sizzling outdoors. And if the symptoms persist or become more serious, she may need a doctor's attention.

But with a bit of caution, you should never have to deal with this emergency. Here's how to avoid heat exhaustion or, if necessary, treat it until you can contact a doctor.

Dress infants for cooler comfort. "Use common sense and dress your baby lightly when the weather is warm," says Steve Sterner, M.D., a senior associate physician in the Department of Emergency Medicine at the Hennepin County Medical Center in Minneapolis. Babies may not be prone to overexertion, but if you bundle them up in warm clothing or wrap them in a heavy blanket on a hot day, heat exhaustion may result, Dr. Sterner cautions.

Keep them out of hot cars. If you leave an infant or child in a hot car—even for a brief period of time—it can lead to heat exhaustion. Worse yet, it can lead to heatstroke, which can be fatal. "Kids get very warm, very fast in that situation," says Dr. Sterner. "It is never a safe practice."

Offer more liquids. Make sure that kids are getting plenty to drink, even if they say they aren't thirsty, says David Keller, M.D., assistant professor of pediatrics in the Division of General and Community Pediatrics, University of Massachusetts Medical Center in Worcester. On a hot day when he's exercising, a seven- or eight-year-old child should have a six-ounce glass of water or juice every hour. Older

---

MEDICAL ALERT

When to See the Doctor

Heat exhaustion that is not treated may escalate and become heatstroke, a potentially fatal condition. It could be heatstroke if you see one or more of the following symptoms.

- Headache
- Weakness
- Disorientation, agitation or confusion
- Lethargy
- Coma or convulsions
- Fever of 105° or more

If your child shows *any* of these symptoms after being out in the sun, you should call for emergency medical treatment at once, according to Steve Sterner, M.D., a senior associate physician in the Department of Emergency Medicine at the Hennepin County Medical Center in Minneapolis.

"While you wait for help to arrive, get the child into the shade, undress him for maximum cooling and spray him with cool water," says Dr. Sterner.

"

children require even more. Always try to keep a water bottle full so the child can sip when he's thirsty.

Sneak them out of the heat. When the outside temperature is high, encourage kids to play in the shade, a cool room or a pool, says Ann DiMaio, M.D., director of the pediatric emergency room at the New York Hospital–Cornell Medical Center and assistant professor of pediatrics at Cornell University Medical College, both in New York City. And if they have to play on a sunny field, make sure they take frequent breaks from strenuous activity, she advises.

Douse them. "Turn a garden hose on your kids or give them a sprinkler to play in," says Dr. DiMaio. "Spraying kids with water will help keep their temperature down."

Chill out. If your child says she feels dizzy or sick to her stomach, she's showing signs of heat exhaustion. Take her into a cool room and give her plenty of fluids, says Dr. Sterner. It also helps to give a cool-water bath. If you don't have an air-conditioned room, turn on a fan. And meanwhile, call the doctor for further advice.

Skip the alcohol bath. You may remember getting a cooling alcohol bath as a child, but physicians do not recommend this practice today, notes Dr. Sterner. "Alcohol may aid slightly in cooling the body, but it is also absorbed by the skin. If you cover a lot of skin with alcohol by immersing your child in it, the alcohol absorption may have toxic effects," he says.

HICCUPS

Help Halt Those Hics

Hiccups may not be a major health calamity, but they sure can be annoying. At certain times, and for a variety of reasons, the diaphragm muscle separating the chest cavity from the abdomen goes into a bit of a spasm, and the vocal cords snap shut, making that "hic!"

sound. Hiccups may be triggered by indigestion, eating or drinking too fast, laughing on an empty stomach and fatigue—to name just a few culprits.

"There is a lot of opinion but very little scientific certainty about why hiccups occur," says Richard Garcia, M.D., a pediatrician and vice chairman of the Department of Pediatrics and Adolescent Medicine at the Cleveland Clinic Foundation in Ohio. Given that uncertainty, it's not surprising that the scientific community has yielded no surefire hiccup cure. But everybody has a suggestion, and many of them work, at least some of the time. The medical experts modestly admit, though, that your grandmother's cure may be as good or better than theirs. But the following recommendations can be added to your own list of family favorites.

For Infants

Pat baby on the back. If your baby has the hiccups, hold her upright against your shoulder and pat her back gently, suggests Dr. Garcia. "Some babies are prone to swallow a lot of air when they nurse or drink formula," he says. "And too much swallowed air distends the stomach, which can lead to hiccups. Some gentle pats may help bring up the air and stop the hiccups."

Check the nipple. "A baby may swallow too much air and hiccup if the hole in the nipple of the formula bottle is the wrong size," says Dr. Garcia. How can you tell? "When you turn the bottle upside down you should get a drip, drip, drip of formula that gradually stops, rather than a free flow or no dripping at all," says Dr. Garcia. He recommends experimenting with different bottle and nipple types to see what works best for your baby.

Go ahead and feed. Don't delay feeding your baby just because he has hiccups. "Hiccups won't interfere with your baby's eating. And eating just might make the hiccups go away," says Michael J. Pettei, M.D., Ph.D., associate professor of pediatrics at Albert Einstein School of Medicine of Yeshiva University in New York City, and co-chief of the Division of Gastroenterology and Nutrition at Schneider

MEDICAL ALERT

When to See the Doctor

Hiccups usually end within five or ten minutes, but some unfortunate people have suffered with hiccups for hours, weeks and, in very rare cases, years. "If your child's hiccups persist beyond a day or so, consult your doctor," says Michael J. Pettei, M.D., Ph.D., associate professor of pediatrics at Albert Einstein School of Medicine of Yeshiva University in New York City, and co-chief of the Division of Gastroenterology and Nutrition at Schneider Children's Hospital of the Long Island Jewish Medical Center in New Hyde Park, New York. In rare instances, hiccups—usually accompanied by other symptoms—may be a sign of an underlying disease.

Children's Hospital of the Long Island Jewish Medical Center in New Hyde Park, New York.

But don't overdo feeding either. During the first few months of life, if your baby always gets the hiccups *after* eating, overfeeding may be the culprit. "Try feeding your baby smaller portions, more frequently," advises Robert Wyllie, M.D., head of the Section of Pediatric Gastroenterology at the Cleveland Clinic Foundation in Ohio. "If you suspect that you've been overfeeding your baby, try feeding him on demand rather than on a schedule you've created, and never push him to eat more than he wants," Dr. Wyllie adds.

For Older Children

Break the cycle with a big drink. "If your child can swallow long enough to miss two or three hiccups, that should break the cycle and stop the hiccuping," says Dr. Pettei. Dr. Garcia suggests a variation on this cure: "Have your child take ten sips of water without stopping for air."

Try some sugar on a spoon. "If your child is older than two, a small amount of sugar or honey on a teaspoon

---

SOME BABIES GET A HICCUPING HEAD START

Here's a riddle. Someone is hiccuping for a half-hour on a crowded train and only one woman notices, but she is not the hiccuper. Who is hiccuping? Answer: the woman's fetus. Sound unlikely? It isn't.

In the second half of pregnancy, many babies get the hiccups several times a day, and the mother-to-be may feel her baby hic, hic, hiccuping for 20 minutes or more, notes Michael J. Pettei, M.D., Ph.D., associate professor of pediatrics at Albert Einstein School of Medicine of Yeshiva University in New York City, and co-chief of the Division of Gastroenterology and Nutrition at Schneider Children's Hospital of the Long Island Jewish Medical Center in New Hyde Park, New York. And the pattern may continue after the baby is born. "For the most part, such hiccups are perfectly normal and harmless," says Dr. Pettei.

---

may help," suggests Patience Williamson, R.N., a certified school nurse at the Rand Family School in Montclair, New Jersey. "This remedy may not work every time, but the kids sure enjoy it!" she adds.

Try the breath-holding challenge. Time how many seconds your child can hold his breath, and you can turn a breath-holding exercise into a game. "If your child can hold his breath long enough, the increased carbon dioxide in his lungs may get rid of the hiccups," says Dr. Wyllie.

HIVES

Giving Bumps the Bump-Off

If your child feels itchy, *really* itchy, have a good look at the area he's scratching. The good news about hives—those itchy, red raised bumps with pale centers—is that they usually go away on their own within 24 hours. The bad news is that it is very difficult to figure out why your child got them in the first place.

Hives may be a reaction to foods. The most common offenders are berries, chocolate, nuts, eggs, peanuts, fish and shellfish. But some children get hives when they're exposed to other allergens, such as penicillin, aspirin, pollen, some kinds of plants, a viral or bacterial infection, cold water or insect bites and stings. (Occasionally, these reactions can be severe and require emergency treatment. See "Medical Alert" on page 257.) In some cases, hives might be caused by an internal disease such as arthritis.

Hives may appear all over the body or just in one area. They may bloom and fade within a matter of hours, only to pop out somewhere new. Or they may persist for six weeks or longer—sometimes almost disappearing, only to recur. Although hives usually itch like crazy, occasionally they are not itchy at all.

Itching to do something about them? Read on.

Leave them alone. If your child has hives that don't itch, leave them alone, says Peter LoGalbo, M.D., assistant professor of pediatrics at the Albert Einstein College of Medicine of Yeshiva University in New York City and director of the Asthma and Allergy Center of Schneider Children's Hospital of the Long Island Jewish Medical Center in New Hyde Park, New York. "They may not be attractive, but if they don't itch, why worry?" Dr. LoGalbo says.

Give a soak. If the hives are the itching kind, have your child soak in a tub filled halfway with warm water and add ½ cup of cornstarch, baking soda or an oatmeal product known as Aveeno (available in drugstores), suggests Stanley I. Wolf, M.D., clinical professor of pediatrics at George Washington University School of Medicine in Washington, D.C., and an allergist in Silver Spring and Rockville, Maryland. Once a day may be enough, but do the soak more often if the hives persist or your child feels very uncomfortable.

Chill out. Applying an ice-pack or a cold compress on the itchy area frequently brings relief, says Dr. LoGalbo. You

MEDICAL ALERT

When to See the Doctor

There are two situations in which an allergic reaction involving hives can be serious, even life-threatening. If you notice any of the following symptoms, call for emergency medical help immediately, recommends Stanley I. Wolf, M.D., clinical professor of pediatrics at George Washington University School of Medicine in Washington, D.C., and an allergist in Silver Spring and Rockville, Maryland.

Angioedema is a hivelike reaction that causes swelling of the feet, hands, face and lips. Usually, it is no more serious than regular hives, but it can become acute in rare instances. "When your child has a severe reaction, her eyes and face become extremely swollen and grotesque looking. If the angioedema involves the tongue or the larynx, it can close off the airway unless your child gets a shot of adrenaline," says Dr. Wolf.

Anaphylaxis is a severe allergic reaction that causes difficulty in breathing or swallowing, according to Beth W. Hapke, M.D., a pediatrician in private practice in Fairfield, Connecticut. Dr. Hapke notes that anaphylaxis is not common in children. If your child gets hives and suddenly has difficulty swallowing, however, you should seek medical help at once, according to Dr. Hapke. (In infants, the warning signs include vomiting, excessive drooling or refusal to drink). The reason for urgency, according to Dr. Hapke, is that your child may stop breathing unless she gets a shot of adrenaline.

"If a severe reaction occurs, it will be within 30 minutes to an hour after your child has been in contact with an allergen," says Dr. Hapke. It will not occur hours or days after the onset of hives, she notes.

can apply this cool relief as often as necessary, for about ten minutes each time. But be sure to wrap the ice-pack in a towel so it isn't directly against the skin.

Use an antihistamine. "An oral antihistamine such as Benadryl or Chlor-Trimeton given every four to six hours as needed will usually ease the itching, but it may also cause

TRACKING DOWN THE CAUSE

"Finding the cause for chronic hives is really detective work. In some research studies, doctors were able to find an answer about 50 percent of the time. But in practice, any doctor who can pinpoint the problem in even 25 percent of the cases is doing a good job," says Stanley I. Wolf, M.D., clinical professor of pediatrics at George Washington University School of Medicine in Washington, D.C., and an allergist in Silver Spring and Rockville, Maryland.

Although there is no guarantee of success when you take your child to an allergist, it's worth trying to track down what is causing hives. Expect to give your doctor a detailed history about your child's diet, medication and lifestyle. If you are lucky, your doctor *will* be able to identify the source of the hives and be able to advise you about ways to prevent their recurrence.

your child to be tired and cranky," notes Beth W. Hapke, M.D., a pediatrician in private practice in Fairfield, Connecticut. These medicines are available without prescription at most pharmacies. Be sure to read package directions to make certain the product is recommended for your child's age. For the correct dosage, follow package directions or consult your physician. Some doctors don't advise Benadryl cream or spray because it could cause a reaction. Also, consult your doctor about alternative antihistamines if your child strongly dislikes taking a particular kind.

Consult an allergist. "Hives are usually nothing to worry about, but if your child has chronic hives that recur or persist for a period of six weeks or more, see an allergist," advises Dr. Hapke. The allergist can usually help you identify the specific allergens that are causing the hives and may prescribe medication that is more effective than over-the-counter medicines.

IMPETIGO

How to Stop the Spread

If your child has a cut, a skinned knee or a scratched-open mosquito bite, she may be putting out the welcome mat for a decidedly unpleasant visitor: impetigo. This contagious bacterial skin infection occurs when strep or staph bacteria gain entry into your child's skin. A frequent site for impetigo is around the nose and mouth, but it may appear anywhere on the body.

If impetigo is caused by staph bacteria, you'll see small, fluid-filled blisters that break easily and scab over into a honey-colored crust. If strep is the culprit (and yes, that's the same strep responsible for strep throat infections), there may not be blisters, but you will see crusting.

Impetigo remains contagious, spreading to other parts of the body and even to other family members, until it is treated with an antibiotic. Small areas can be cleared up

---

MEDICAL ALERT

When to See the Doctor

"Take your child to the doctor if he develops a fever along with the impetigo or if he has a blister that is larger than an inch in diameter," says Daniel Bronfin, M.D., staff pediatrician at the Ochsner Clinic and assistant clinical professor of pediatrics at Tulane University School of Medicine in New Orleans. A fever may indicate the presence of a deep skin infection such as cellulitis, which is more serious and must be treated with intravenous antibiotics. A large blister may indicate an abscess that needs to be drained, Dr. Bronfin says.

Also, impetigo due to strep bacteria may lead to a rare and potentially serious kidney disease. Alert your physician immediately if your child's urine becomes red or cola-colored, he warns.

by applying an antibiotic ointment available by prescription, but a large outbreak of impetigo needs to be treated with oral antibiotics. The antibiotics do a great job of stopping the infection, but your child may still be contagious for the first two to three days of treatment. During that time, she should avoid close contact with other kids, and you should be sure to keep her towel and washcloth separate from everyone else's.

Impetigo may cause scars that hang around for months, but these eventually fade away, says Daniel Bronfin, M.D., staff pediatrician at the Ochsner Clinic and assistant clinical professor of pediatrics at Tulane University School of Medicine in New Orleans. "In most cases, the worst part of impetigo is that it is itchy and unsightly, but if it is properly treated, it will go away in a week or two," says Dr. Bronfin.

To help speed your child's recovery and to prevent a repeat infection, try these simple suggestions.

Treatment

Keep it clean. "Wash the affected area with antibacterial soap three times a day," says Luisa Castiglia, M.D., a pediatrician in private practice in Mineola, New York.

Open it up. "If you keep the area covered up with a bandage or dressing, you may be encouraging more bacteria to grow. It's a better idea to leave the affected area exposed to the air. If your child is going out to play, you can cover it up temporarily," says Dr. Castiglia.

Encourage good hygiene. "Impetigo is often spread by scratching, so teach kids to wash their hands with soap and to keep their nails clean and short," says Fran E. Adler, M.D., a pediatrician in private practice in Upper Montclair, New Jersey.

Keep it cool. "Studies show that heat tends to increase itching, so keep your child comfortable with tepid baths," says Dr. Bronfin. The bath should be just about body temperature, not warmer. "In the summertime, it also helps to run the air conditioner," he adds.

Use a bit of antihistamine. If your child is very itchy, Benadryl Elixir, a liquid antihistamine product for children, can be a big help, says Dr. Bronfin. Be sure to read package directions to make certain the product is recommended for your child's age. For the correct dosage, follow package directions or consult your physician. Some doctors don't advise Benadryl cream or spray because it could cause a reaction.

Preventive Care

Catch it early. "An infection usually won't lead to impetigo if you catch it early. At the very first sign of any infection, wash the area well and apply an over-the-counter antibacterial ointment containing bacitracin. If the infection doesn't improve or if it starts to spread, see your doctor," says Dr. Adler.

Treat diaper rash seriously. "Impetigo can develop in a diaper area if your child's rash is not cleaned and protected," says Dr. Castiglia. One of the best ways to prevent impetigo in infants is to guard against diaper rash. (See page 150 for diaper rash remedies.)

Lubricate a sore nose. Impetigo is very common when a child has a runny nose, especially in the wintertime, says Dr. Adler. "A child's nose gets sore and chapped from all the rubbing and moisture, so keep the area lubricated with Vaseline so that the skin won't break down. Also, make sure that your child keeps her hands and face clean," says Dr. Adler.

INSECT AND SPIDER BITES

Antidotes for Pest Attacks

B uzzing mosquitoes and pesky flies are the bane of summer campers and picnickers. And while most spiders are as harmless as Charlotte, the heroine of E.

B. White's children's classic *Charlotte's Web,* a bite can produce annoying itching and minor pain for a few days.

Prevention is the best tactic. But if your child *does* get bitten or stung by a nonpoisonous creature, you can easily soothe the pain and itching if you follow the advice of experts. Here are the tactics that doctors recommend.

Treatment

Keep the area clean. For any insect or spider bite, wash the area with soap and water, says Gary Wasserman, D.O., a pediatric emergency medicine specialist, chief of the section of clinical toxicology and director of the Poison Control Center at The Children's Mercy Hospital in Kansas City, Missouri. "Continue to wash with soap and water two or three times a day until the skin is healed," he says. And make sure little fingers and hands get washed as well, to help keep germs at bay.

"For extra protection from infection, apply an antibiotic ointment or cream such as Polysporin or Neosporin after washing—not just on the surface, but by rubbing it in," says Dr. Wasserman.

Soothe with ice. To help quell the itch, apply an ice-pack wrapped in a towel, being careful to keep the ice-pack from direct contact with the skin, because of the danger of freezing. Or soak a washcloth in cool water, wring it out and press it on the itchy area, suggests says Dr. Wasserman.

Make a paste. Applying a paste of baking soda and water is the classic old-time remedy for itchy, painful bites, says Claude Frazier, M.D., an allergist in Asheville, North Carolina, and author of *Insects and Allergy: And What to Do about Them.* Mix just enough water with baking soda to make a paste that will cling to the skin, then spread it around the itchy area. Leave the paste on for 15 to 20 minutes, if possible.

Treat the pain. Acetaminophen (Children's Tylenol) can be given to help relieve pain, says Lloyd E. King, Jr., M.D., Ph.D., professor and chief of the Division of Dermatology at Vanderbilt University in Nashville. Check the package

MEDICAL ALERT

When to See the Doctor

There are two potentially deadly species of spiders, the black widow and the brown recluse, found primarily in warmer regions. If you can't identify the spider that bit your child, it's a good idea to take your child to a doctor for evaluation. And you *must* head for the doctor's office or emergency room if you see:

- A deep blue to purple mottled area around the bite, surrounded by a whitish halo with a very large outer ring of redness—known as the "red, white and blue" symptom. This is a good indication that your child has probably been bitten by a brown recluse spider, says Lloyd E. King, Jr., M.D., Ph.D., professor and chief of the Division of Dermatology at Vanderbilt University in Nashville. The brown recluse can also cause a body rash.

- Muscle spasms, tightness and stiffness, which are signs of a black widow spider bite. The black widow can also cause intense abdominal pain that mimics appendicitis, says Gary Wasserman, D.O., a pediatric emergency medicine specialist, chief of the section of toxicology and director of the Poison Control Center at The Children's Mercy Hospital in Kansas City, Missouri.

Other possible symptoms of poisonous spider bites include headache, fever, malaise, lack of appetite and joint pain. Also, take your child to the doctor if you see signs of infection around the bite (exaggerated swelling and redness) or if your child has pink- or red-colored urine, says Dr. Wasserman.

In the area of Arizona or New Mexico, an unidentified sting might be that of a scorpion. In some cases, that sting can be fatal to a child, especially under the age of ten, cautions Dr. Wasserman. Seek immediate medical care.

directions for the correct dosage for your child's age and weight. If your child is under age two, consult a physician. Aspirin isn't generally recommended for children because of the link with Reye's syndrome, a serious brain and liver ailment.

HOW SAFE IS THAT REPELLENT?

Insect repellents containing the chemical diethyltoluamide, otherwise known as DEET, work wonders when you need to repel flying nuisances such as bees and wasps, mosquitoes, biting flies and fleas.

But many parents are concerned—and rightly so—about using DEET-containing repellents on children. The products are not approved for use in children under two because very young children run the risk of absorbing a toxic dose through the skin. And doctors recommend that any insect repellent made with DEET be applied sparingly to the skin of children under ten.

"Technically you should avoid using DEET on children even up to age four," says Wayne Kradjan, Pharm.D., professor of pharmacy and associate dean for professional programs at the University of Washington School of Pharmacy in Seattle. "The alternatives are to keep the child covered as much as possible. But if you're in environment with a lot of mosquitoes or other insects, it's not always practical to keep the child covered up on hot days."

If you choose to use a product with DEET, select one with the lowest percentage of DEET, advises Dr. Kradjan. (They range from around 7 percent to 100 percent.) Use it very lightly on the child, applying the repellent to exposed skin and to clothing. Don't apply more often than every four hours, unless the child is in a situation that would cause the repellent to wash off or evaporate. Repellents don't actually repel insects, but will stop them from biting. So if an insect lands on your child but doesn't bite, the repellent is still working. Once your child's been bitten, it's time to reapply.

Do not, however, put DEET-containing repellents on areas of the body covered by clothing, warns Dr. Kradjan, because this will increase the amount absorbed.

Preventive Care

Repel flying insects. Avon's Skin-So-Soft bath oil can be an effective and safe mosquito repellent, says Dr. Wasserman. And commercial insect repellents containing DEET are very effective against biting flies and mosquitoes, he notes. However, DEET-containing products must be used sparingly on children under the age of ten and should never be used on children under two.

Stay away from Charlotte's web. Tell your children to avoid approaching spiders, particularly unusual-looking ones. And they should avoid playing with spider webs, says Dr. Wasserman. "Spiders become more dangerous when their webs are disturbed, especially when they have young ones to protect," he says. The web itself may also be irritating and itchy to some children.

Give shoes and clothing a shake. "Vigorously shake shoes and clothing that have been lying in the closet to dislodge any resting spider," says Dr. King. This is especially a good idea if the clothes are in a summer house where spiders have easy access.

LACTOSE INTOLERANCE

Handling the Dairy Dilemma

Your child's frequent diarrhea, bloating and gassiness have been a trial to both of you. But finally you've found out the cause: It's lactose intolerance, explains your doctor.

This may sound like a disease, but it isn't. It just means that your child has problems digesting lactose, the sugar in milk and dairy products. Normally this milk sugar is broken down by an enzyme called lactase that's produced in the small intestine, but some people don't produce *enough* lactase to do the job. So when your lactase-deficient child drinks milk or eats milk products, there isn't enough lactase to digest the lactose—and the intestines seem like a battle zone.

"Just about everyone is born with the ability to digest milk," explains Jay A. Perman, M.D., professor of pediatrics and director of pediatric gastroenterology and nutrition at Johns Hopkins University School of Medicine in Baltimore. "But for some, the ability to produce lactase declines once they're out of babyhood." Sometimes the decline is so gradual that symptoms don't pop up until adulthood, but others have problems as youngsters.

The good news is that, once diagnosed, lactose intolerance can be managed quite easily and successfully at home, says Dr. Perman. Managed so well, in fact, that children don't always have to say no to milk and cookies or birthday cake and ice cream. Here's how to handle your child's lactose intolerance to ensure smooth intestinal sailing.

Read labels. If your child has severe lactose intolerance, make scrutinizing food labels a habit. Foods other than milk, cheese, ice cream and the like can also contain lactose. "There are some kids who are so sensitive that even a bit of lactose found in processed meat can set them off," says Dr. Perman.

Study labels and look for lactose-containing ingredients such as casein, whey, lactose, milk solids or milk. In restaurants, check with the chef about the ingredients of the dish your child wants.

Keep a food journal. Use a daily diary of food and symptoms to keep track of what bothers your child and what doesn't, says Ana Abad Sinden, R.D., a pediatric nutrition support specialist in the Department of Nutrition Services at the University of Virginia Health Sciences Center in Charlottesville. "This lets parents get a better handle on what specific foods cause particular symptoms," she says.

In the diary, write down the quantity of lactose-containing food, the time when it was eaten and any symptoms that followed. That way you can tell at a glance if a bowl of ice cream caused gassiness, for instance, or a cup of milk produced diarrhea.

Experiment cautiously. "Everyone's tolerance level is different, and before you can manage a lactose malabsorption problem you need to identify its severity," says Dr. Perman. Start with small amounts of lactose-containing foods and gradually build up, suggests Sinden. Once you've established through the daily diary that your child can eat a half-slice of cheese without symptoms, for example, try a whole slice. And when you've found how much of one lactose-containing food your child can handle without problems, try another.

Check medications. Lactose can lurk where you least expect it. About one-fourth of both prescription and over-the-counter medications are made with lactose. "You should read the labels of medications your child needs to take, or ask your pharmacist whether there's any lactose in a particular drug," says Dr. Perman.

Don't go it alone. Encourage your child to eat lactose-

THAT INTOLERANCE COULD BE TEMPORARY

Most people who discover they are lactose intolerant will *always* be lactose intolerant. Their bodies will never make enough of the lactase enzyme to break down the sugars in milk products. But occasionally, lactose intolerance in babies and small children is a short-term condition, says Jay A. Perman, M.D., professor of pediatrics and director of pediatric gastroenterology and nutrition at Johns Hopkins University School of Medicine in Baltimore.

Temporary intolerance is called secondary lactose intolerance. "This is caused by an injury to the child's intestinal system either from a virus or a food allergy," explains Dr. Perman. Some children have problems digesting lactose for a period that may last as long as several months—but the problem may cease once the virus or allergy runs its course. Lactase deficiency can also be the result of an intestinal disease, however, and premature babies are sometimes temporarily intolerant until their lactase enzymes mature.

Any small child diagnosed as lactose intolerant should be monitored by a doctor, says Dr. Perman. The doctor will try to determine whether the lactose intolerance ceases—there's no point in avoiding lactose if you don't have to—*and* make sure there's not an intestinal problem that needs to be treated.

containing foods along with other foods, says Dennis Savaiano, Ph.D., professor of food science and nutrition at the University of Minnesota in Saint Paul. "Milk with cereal or cookies, for example, is tolerated better than milk alone," he says. "In fact *anything* with milk is better than milk alone." The other foods keep the lactase from arriving at the intestines all at once and overwhelming the few lactase enzymes your child does have.

Choose low-lactose foods. A glass of milk, with 12 grams of lactose, will be too much for many lactase-deficient kids, says Dr. Perman. "But hard cheeses have only a trace of lactose, while ice cream and cottage cheese have a moderate amount," he says. Yogurt with live cultures (check the container) is usually tolerated by lactose intolerant youngsters, because the bacteria in the yogurt has predigested much of the lactose.

Try lactase enzymes. Most drugstores carry a lactase supplement that makes up for the enzyme deficiency in your child's intestines. This product is sold as liquid, pills or capsules. Mix the liquid with regular milk 24 hours before use to break down 70 percent of the lactose, says Sinden. "That's usually all that's needed for milk to be tolerated," she says.

You can give your child a lactase pill before he or she eats the offending ice cream or cheese, says Dr. Savaiano. He also suggests opening up a capsule of the enzyme and sprinkling the contents on cereal and milk. "The amount your child will need depends upon the severity of her intolerance, and that's determined by experimentation," he says.

Consider calcium intake. If your child is severely lactose intolerant, there's a chance he or she may not be getting enough calcium—which is crucial for young, growing bones. Your child can get plenty of this essential nutrient by eating lots of yogurt, cheese and green vegetables, says Dr. Perman.

"But if your child is a finicky eater and eats no dairy products, then you may want to consider other sources of calcium," adds Dr. Perman. He suggests calcium-enhanced wafers you can find at health food stores or Tums, which also contain calcium. Check with your doctor about the dosage. Another option is calcium-fortified juice.

LARYNGITIS AND HOARSENESS

Clearing Up the Husky Whisper

Mommy! Mommy!" It's a call you're used to hearing—but this morning you hear only a faint whisper instead of a robust wail. Your child has lost his voice.

Laryngitis simply means that the larynx is swollen—that's the upper part of the windpipe that houses the vocal folds, commonly called cords. And as long as the larynx remains that way, your child will be very hoarse or unable to speak.

What causes the swelling? It could be a viral infection from a cold or flu, or an allergic reaction to dust or pollen. Or laryngitis could be the result of something as innocuous as overuse of the voice. If your child cheered hard at yesterday's hockey game, that could explain this morning's laryngitis.

But whether your child's voice is hoarse or whether he has lost it entirely, here's what you can do to help restore it.

Mum's the word. "The less your child uses his voice, the faster it will come back to normal," advises Mary Meland, M.D., a pediatrician with HealthPartners in Bloomington, Minnesota.

To encourage your child to stop talking for a while, try making nonverbal communication into a game. One way is to devise a system of hand signals for frequent expressions like "may I" or "give me." Also, provide a pad and pencil

MEDICAL ALERT

When to See the Doctor

Changes of voice in a small child can indicate a serious problem, says Michael Benninger, M.D., chairman of the committee on speech, voice and swallowing disorders of the American Academy of Otolaryngology/Head and Neck Surgery.

In older children, a swollen larynx may cause hoarseness or loss of voice, but it rarely interferes with breathing. In a child younger than four, however, the air passages are so narrow that if the tissues below the larynx becomes swollen, the air passage can become blocked with mucus, says Dr. Benninger. This difficulty in breathing is called croup, and it can be quite serious. (See page 130 for more information on croup.)

If your child displays any of the following symptoms, it may be a medical emergency and you should contact your physician immediately.

- A harsh, barking cough
- Labored breathing, with the chest visibly moving as the child tries to get air
- Noisy, gaspy breathing
- A sudden change in the sound of the voice, without evidence of a cold
- A deep, low voice
- Difficulty swallowing with lots of drooling

for your child. If she's too young to write words, have her draw pictures instead. And if your child can't stop using her voice entirely, at least call regular time-outs during the day to give the vocal cords a rest.

Avoid whispering. When your child does have to speak, have him use a soft, natural tone, says Michael Benninger, M.D., chairman of the committee on speech, voice and swallowing disorders of the American Academy of Otolaryngology/Head and Neck Surgery. A whisper strains vocal folds more than normal speech, he says.

Soothe with lozenges. Lozenges can help relieve a dry or irritated throat by stimulating saliva flow, says Dr. Benninger. "They're good for moistening and soothing the throat any time." He recommends avoiding those with anesthetic properties unless your child is uncomfortable. Sugarless lemon drops available at the pharmacy work well, too.

Give a warm drink. Hot herbal or decaffeinated tea, chicken soup or any warm liquid will help ease the discomfort of an irritated throat, says Dr. Benninger. Or you can dilute fruit juices with hot water to create a tasty, fruity hot drink.

Encourage frequent drinking. Keep a glass of water near your child, and encourage her to drink often. "Sipping water throughout the day can help your child break the throat-clearing habit, which can make hoarseness worse," says Dr. Benninger. Keeping the vocal cords moist is also soothing. Room temperature water is best because it's easiest on the throat.

But don't supply cold or iced water, he cautions, because cold water strains the blood vessels in the larynx by forcing them to warm the water.

Try steam from a sink. "Breathing steam for five minutes, several times a day is very soothing for a child with laryngitis or hoarseness," says Dr. Benninger. Fill a sink with hot water and have your child lean over it. Then drape a towel over your child's head and over the sink to form a "tent" where steam gathers.

Turn on the vaporizer. Your child's larynx may also be partly clogged with mucus. Use a humidifier or vaporizer in your child's bedroom to moisturize the air while he sleeps. "This loosens some of the mucus that's been deposited in the larynx," says Lewis First, M.D., a pediatrician and assistant professor of pediatrics at Harvard Medical School in Boston. "Diluting that mucus allows the child to cough it up or swallow it." Clean the humidifier or vaporizer often, following the manufacturer's instructions.

Avoid smoking near your child. Exposure to smoke can worsen inflammation of the larynx, so don't smoke around your child, says Dr. Meland. If someone in your household smokes, ask him to step outside the house to light up.

Keep nasal passages clear. You want your child to breathe through his nose instead of his mouth, because air that passes through the nose is warmer and moister, therefore less irritating to the vocal folds. "If a cold is keeping your child from breathing through his nose, use an over-the-counter decongestant," advises Dr. Benninger. A decongestant containing an antihistamine may dry the throat, however, so you need to counteract that by supplying plenty of warm liquids.

Try a gargle. If your child's throat is painful, a saltwater gargle can help, says Dr. First. "Gargling with saltwater can help reduce the pain and also thin out the mucus," he says.

But first make sure your child *can* gargle. "Children are usually capable of learning how to gargle by the time they are five or six," says Dr. First. Have your child practice

---

A REASON TO PIPE DOWN

It's no surprise that Junior's constant hoarseness or rough voice is the result of his shrieking at ball games and yelling at his little sister—but in some cases all that racket from your youngster can cause more than a swollen larynx.

Constant voice overuse may also cause tiny nodules to grow on the vocal cords, says Michael Benninger, M.D., chairman of the committee on speech, voice and swallowing disorders of the American Academy of Otolaryngology/Head and Neck Surgery.

Don't panic: This sounds more serious than it is. The only treatment required is that your child stop the overuse, whether it's screaming, yelling or talking loudly. "Nodules are like little calluses and will go away by themselves once the behavior that caused them is changed," explains Dr. Benninger.

gargling with plain water to see if she can manage. And before having her try the saltwater gargle, explain that the salt in it will make it taste unpleasant. To make the gargle, mix one teaspoon of salt in a glass of warm water.

Keep the volume down. Even after your child's voice has returned, he should be careful not to strain the vocal cords, so the problem won't return. "Encourage your child to talk quietly and not to scream while playing games," says Dr. Benninger. "And explain that trying to talk over loud background noise will only hurt his vocal cords."

If your child's voice problems are from constant overuse, try to find the reason your child is being so loud, suggests Dr. Meland. If he's shouting to get attention, explain gently that you'll only respond to him when he speaks in a reasonable tone. If he's talking loudly to be heard over a blaring television, turn the TV down or off, or consider moving it to a less central area of the house. If he's yelling because that's what he hears around the house, count to ten the next time you find yourself about to raise your voice.

LAZY EYE

Getting Vision Back on Track

Lately you've noticed that your child's one eye has been straying, looking off to the side while the other eye remains straight. In a newborn, it's common to see the eyes wander. But as a child gets older, his eyes should start focusing and work together—certainly before four months of age. So what's going on here?

A child with an eye that wanders may have amblyopia, or "lazy eye," a vision problem that may affect as many as 3 out of every 100 people, says Robert D. Gross, M.D., clinical assistant professor of pediatric ophthalmology at the University of Texas Southwestern Medical School in Dallas and a pediatric ophthalmologist at the Cook–Fort Worth Children's Medical Center in Fort Worth. While you may be concerned about what your child looks like when his eye drifts, there's much more to it than that. An amblyopic eye is actually a weak eye that has not developed normal vision, says Dr. Gross.

Amblyopia must be diagnosed by an eye doctor. Experts say early treatment by an eye specialist is critical.

To treat amblyopia, eye doctors often use a method called occlusion. By wearing a patch over the strong eye for a certain amount of time each day, the child learns to rely more on the weak eye. "The earlier you patch, the better," says Dr. Gross. "Parents may be unhappy patching a child at age two, but it may be more challenging to get the child to comply at age six. And besides, the older the child becomes, the harder it is to make a positive change in visual acuity."

Patching must be done under a doctor's supervision, and the instructions need to be followed to the letter. If your doctor recommends patching, here's how to make it easier for you and your child.

Help your child see the light. "Wearing a patch isn't much fun, but you can encourage your child by actively showing him why it's necessary," says Robert B. Sanet, O.D., a developmental optometrist and director of the San Diego Center for Vision Care in Lemon Grove, California, and associate professor at Southern California College of Optometry in Fullerton. "If your child is old enough to understand, cover his straight eye with your hand and ask him how it feels to see with the other eye. Explain that the eye is weak and that patching will make it as strong as the other eye."

Pick a patch time. Mark off a designated time for your child to wear the patch. "Call it patch time and make it the same time every day," says Dr. Gross. "That way, patching will become routine, and the child will know what to expect. If he needs to wear the patch for three hours a day, then he should get to pick which three hours."

Try to keep it on the home front. It may help to have patch time be during part of the day when the child is

MEDICAL ALERT

When to See the Doctor

If your child has a lazy eye, see an eye care specialist as soon as possible. "The earlier you get care, the less chance the problem has to become established," says Sherwin Isenberg, M.D., professor and vice chairman of the Department of Ophthalmology at the University of California, Los Angeles, UCLA School of Medicine and the Jules Stein Eye Institute.

"Even when there are no apparent problems, every child should have a complete eye exam between the ages of three and four," advises Kathleen Mahon, M.D., a pediatric ophthalmologist, clinical professor of pediatrics and surgery at the University of Nevada School of Medicine and director of the Mahon Eye Center in Las Vegas. "And if there is a family history of either amblyopia or the contributing factor of strabismus (crossed eyes), you should consider seeing a doctor much sooner."

The eye care specialist may be either an ophthalmologist or an optometrist. Both deal with vision problems like amblyopia, but the two types of specialists sometimes use different approaches. Ophthalmologists are medical doctors who are trained and licensed to provide total eye care—everything from examinations to surgery. Optometrists, on the other hand, are not medical doctors, and their orientation is non-surgical. But they are trained to examine eyes, diagnose problems and prescribe corrective lenses. Developmental optometrists also advocate a treatment method called vision training, which involves specially prescribed eye exercises.

Most medical doctors and optometrists treat amblyopia with patches or special eyeglasses. "The mainstay is patching, and glasses are used when necessary," says Dr. Isenberg. In some cases, when amblyopia is caused by other related eye problems, some medical doctors may advocate surgery after the vision has been improved by patching. "For children who simply won't wear a patch, special eyedrops are available that will blur the vision in the good eye, forcing the child to use the lazy eye to see," says Dr. Mahon.

home. "Encourage him to pick a time period like 3:00 to 6:00 p.m., when he's not at school or day care," says Dr. Gross. He'll be less self-conscious, and therefore more willing to wear the patch if he doesn't have to wear it in front of all his classmates, he points out.

Another important reason to patch at home is that you as a parent, can supervise the patching process. "Do not expect your babysitter or day care to enforce patching in your absence," notes Dr. Gross.

Take care to prevent peeking. Only an occlusion patch prescribed by your eye doctor should be used to treat amblyopia, according to Dr. Gross. These patches come in two sizes and have adhesive all around, so the patch can be firmly stuck to the face to prevent peeking. The Junior size is for children up to age five or so. Older children generally use the regular-size patch. It's important to securely fix the patch to the child's face and not to glasses, says Dr. Gross. "If the patch is attached to glasses, the child will be able to peek around the edges with the good eye, and the weak eye will not be challenged enough," he says.

Stick to your guns. Enforce patching to the best of your ability. "Both parents have to be absolutely committed to the process of patching. No matter what happens, the child has to comply," says Dr. Gross. "Be very consistent and very strict. Never make any exceptions. If you make one exception, that destroys your credibility with the child," he says.

Manage misbehavior. Dr. Gross offers three suggestions for dealing with kids who misbehave and refuse to wear their patch as prescribed. First, be consistent with your discipline. "Treat misbehavior with patching the same way you would treat any other type of misbehavior," he says. If you use a "time-out" or "go-to-your-room" tactic at other times, use it with patching mischief, too.

Second, deduct any time spent in patchless misbehaving from your child's daily patch-time quota. "That time doesn't count toward patch time, and the child will have

STRAIGHT TALK ABOUT CROSSED EYES

Crossed eyes might look funny on a teddy bear, but for a real-life child with this problem, it's nothing to laugh at. "An inward-turning eye is one of the most common forms of misalignment," says Sherwin Isenberg, M.D., professor and vice chairman of the Department of Ophthalmology at the University of California, Los Angeles, UCLA School of Medicine and the Jules Stein Eye Institute. "If left untreated for too long, the eye never develops full vision potential."

It's important to seek help early. "If your child is born with an eye that crosses all the time, see your doctor right away," says Dr. Isenberg. If an ophthalmologist determines that surgery is necessary, he will probably recommend that the operation be performed relatively soon, according to Dr. Isenberg.

Sometimes, a family photograph can help you detect strabismus (crossed eyes) in a young child, according to Kathleen Mahon, M.D., a pediatric ophthalmologist, clinical professor of pediatrics and surgery at the University of Nevada School of Medicine and director of the Mahon Eye Center in Las Vegas. If you see a photograph of your child in which her eyes appear to be different colors, it may indicate that one eye is slightly crossed. Get it checked, suggests Dr. Mahon.

---

to make it up. As soon as he realizes that, the behavior should stop," says Dr. Gross.

Third, if a child takes the patch off for an activity, then that activity should not be allowed. "If a child takes the patch off when he's watching TV, for example, then don't let him watch TV," says Dr. Gross.

Go down for the count. Don't skimp on patch time. "If a child removes the patch even a little bit before the designated time, have him put it back on. If you're not sure how long it's been off, have him start over," says Dr. Gross. "And if patching is not completed one day, then make up for the lost time by adding time the next day."

Talk to the teacher about teasing. A patch can make a

kid the butt of many a joke. So if patch time must be during the school day, enlist the aid of your child's teacher, says Dr. Sanet. "The teacher can give a lesson on how we are all different, that there are short people and tall people, fat people and thin. He can make the point that differences, such as wearing glasses or patches, are just differences, and do not make people better or worse than others."

Alert the school nurse. Send the school nurse a "patching report card," suggests pediatric ophthalmologist Kathleen Mahon, M.D., pediatric ophthalmologist, clinical professor of pediatrics and surgery at the University of Nevada School of Medicine and director of the Mahon Eye Center in Las Vegas. It should explain what the child's vision problem is and note the hours that the child should be patching. "Ask for the nurse's and the teacher's assistance. It helps to have someone at school who checks on the child," she says.

LICE

An All-Out Attack to Clear the Hair

Yes, any child—even yours—*can* get a case of lice. And, no, it does not necessarily mean that your child is unclean. Lice, in fact, are almost as easy for kids to get as the common cold. There's a potential for lice whenever children are in a group.

"About 10 million cases of head lice occur each year, and three-quarters of them are in children under the age of 12," says Edward DeSimone, Ph.D., a pharmacist and associate professor of pharmacy and administrative and social sciences in the School of Pharmacy and Allied Health Professions at Creighton University in Omaha.

The first clue that your child may have lice is an itchy scalp. But to see the real evidence, you have to take a close look at your child's head. While you seldom see the lice themselves, their eggs, or nits, are easily visible. These gray-ish-white oval eggs attach firmly to the hair shaft. They're

---

MEDICAL ALERT

When to See the Doctor

Just about everyone can be treated at home for head lice, says Deborah Altschuler, president and cofounder of the National Pediculosis Association in Newton, Massachusetts, and adjunct assistant professor of preventive medicine and biometrics at the Uniformed Services University, F. Edward Hébert School of Medicine in Bethesda, Maryland.

The exceptions? Always check with your doctor before using a home lice treatment on:

- A child under two.
- Someone with allergies or asthma.
- A person with lice or nits in the eyebrows or eyelashes.
- A pregnant or nursing woman.

The doctor may prescribe a different medication or want to supervise the treatment for these people.

Also, if you are pregnant or nursing and need to use a lice treatment on someone else, contact your doctor first.

---

tiny, about the size of a sesame seed, and won't wash or blow off, as a flake of skin would.

Effective remedies are as near as the corner drugstore. Here's what the experts suggest you do.

Offer reassurance. Battling lice *does* require some time and effort, but approach the problem calmly so your child doesn't panic or feel ashamed. Explain to your child what lice are and how you're going to get rid of them, suggests Dr. DeSimone. Be sure to assure your child that you don't blame her for getting lice, he says.

Buy an OTC head-lice product. You can banish the invaders with many over-the-counter products such as RID, A-200, R & C and NIX, says Dr. DeSimone. "All these products are similar," he explains. "They're either a combination of two chemicals—pyrethrins and piperonyl butoxide—working together or they contain a synthetic pyrethrin." The products come in shampoo, liquid or gel form.

The instructions on the package should be followed explicitly because all of these products are pesticides, says Dr. DeSimone. (And experts advise against buying lice sprays because they expose your child to too much pesticide.

Consider a trim. Although it's not necessary to cut a child's hair just because she has lice, shorter hair can be easier to deal with, says Deborah Altschuler, president and cofounder of the National Pediculosis Association in Newton, Massachusetts, and adjunct assistant professor of preventive medicine and biometrics at the Uniformed Services University, F. Edward Hébert School of Medicine in Bethesda, Maryland. Remember, however, you cannot take a child with lice to a barber or hairdresser.

Wash hair over the sink. This way you can confine treatment to the scalp, says Altschuler. You don't want to use lice products in the shower, where the rinsed-off solution can cascade over the body. "These products are pesticides and should be used with caution," she says.

Before you begin, remove your child's shirt and provide a small towel to cover her face. If the product gets in your child's eyes, flush them thoroughly with water right away. Don't be alarmed if some mild skin irritation and itching results from the lice killer, however, and don't mistake this itching for re-infestation.

Be a nit-picker. The lice product will kill the lice, but not all the nits, says Mary Meland, M.D., a pediatrician with HealthPartners in Bloomington, Minnesota. "The more nits you can remove, the less likelihood there is of a recurrence a couple of weeks later," says Dr. Meland. Also you won't run the risk of mistaking an old nit for a new nit, adds Altschuler.

For nit removal, use a nit removal comb. While there will be a comb packaged with the lice-control product, some work better than others. If the comb is not effective, you can remove the nits with a pair of baby safety scissors (with rounded ends) to cut off the hair that has nits attached.

After the delousing treatment, when your child's hair is dry or only slightly damp, comb it out, then use an old tooth-brush and water to remove the nits from the nit comb. If your child used a towel or bathrobe, pop these items into a hot-water wash right away, along with any clothes he was wearing before the treatment, then dry them in a hot dryer.

Treat everyone who's infested at the same time. It only takes one little louse to infest a child (they lay up to ten eggs a day), and lice can easily spread from one person to another. So to get rid of these critters you need to exam-ine everyone in the household for signs of lice, says Altschuler, and treat those who are infested.

Make a clean sweep. Once you've detected the lice and treated your children, you need to tend to the household. First, gather up everything washable that has come in con-tact with your child's head. "This means hats, scarves, hooded coats, hair bands and any clothing your child may have worn in the past few days," says Altschuler. Enlist your child's cooperation in doing this. Don't forget sheets, pillowcases and towels. Wash all items in hot water and dry in a hot dryer.

What you can't wash, you can vacuum or send to the dry cleaners. Vacuum sofas, sofa pillows, mattresses and rugs (especially around the beds), and then put the vacuum cleaner bag in a plastic bag and throw it away. To clean combs and brushes, soak them in hot (not boiling) water for ten minutes.

Take care of Teddy. Yes, the stuffed animals your child hugs and plays with also have to be treated. You can care-fully vacuum your child's favorite animals so she'll have them to keep her company, and pop the rest into a large plastic trash bag. Seal the bag tightly with a twist-tie and put the bagged toys away where your child can't get at them.

Generally, lice can't survive off the scalp for more than 24 hours, but it takes the eggs 7 to 10 days to hatch. There-fore, keep the bag sealed for 14 days, says Dr. DeSimone. "After that time, any lice or nits that may have been on the toys will be dead," he says. Any items such as headphones that can't be thoroughly washed or vacuumed should be given the same two-weeks-in-a-bag treatment, according to Dr. DeSimone. Just be sure to keep all bagged items away from small children because of the hazard of choking.

Check daily. Inspect every child in your house for nits every day for at least seven to ten days after treatment, in case you missed a few. "Check for nits throughout the hair, but pay particular attention to behind the ears and the nape of the neck," says Dr. Meland. If you see new evidence of lice, you'll need to give your child another lice treatment. However, "If you need a second treatment, it should be given seven to ten days after the first treatment," says Dr. DeSimone.

It's a good idea to make nit-checking part of a regular daily routine even after the lice are long gone, to watch for recurrences. It's easier to vanquish lice if you catch them early.

Teach your child not to share *everything*. All it takes is one hitchhiking louse to make its way from a hat or brush onto another child. "We all want our children to share their belongings," says Dr. DeSimone. "But children should be taught *never* to share combs, brushes, hats, hair ornaments and headphones." Explain to your children why they shouldn't share these items, and make sure each child has his own comb and brush. In fact, your child should have an extra comb and extra brush to take along to school so he won't be tempted to borrow them.

MARINE STINGS AND CUTS

Remedies for Seaside Perils

Nothing's more fun than a day at the beach—unless you or your child has a close encounter with a stinging jellyfish, Portuguese man-of-war, sea urchin or coral.

Though most plentiful in warm climates, jellyfish and their cousin, the Portuguese man-of-war, are common to just about every North American beach area. They drift along on top of the water with their tentacles trailing, ready for the unwary swimmer. But these creatures and any broken-off tentacles can still sting when they're just lying around on the beach or floating in the water, even after a couple of days.

Sea urchins don't actually bite or sting, but they have spines that can puncture the skin and release venom. And while coral may look like exquisite rock, it's really a fragile colony of tiny creatures that can cause a painful wound if a child happens to step on it or scrape a leg against it.

It's best that all these injuries be seen by a physician. But here's what you can do before you reach the doctor.

Jellyfish and Portuguese Man-of-War

Get to dry land. "If the child is stung in water, take him out of the water," says Kenneth W. Kizer, M.D., M.P.H., professor of emergency medicine and medical toxicology at the University of California, Davis, School of Medicine and a specialist in wilderness medicine. Depending on how much venom is released, a sting can be quite serious. Because the child may panic or even lose consciousness, it's crucial to get him out of the water.

Reach for your credit card. Jellyfish and Portuguese man-of-war tentacles have tiny parts that resemble miniature harpoons. When these venom-filled "harpoons," called nematocysts, puncture the skin, the result is painful. You want to get the tentacles and nematocysts off as quickly as possible, says Glenn G. Soppe, M.D., a physician in San Diego, California, who lectures on aquatic bites and stings.

Although you can't see the nematocysts, you can scrape them off with a credit card, says Dr. Kizer. Just brush the edge of the card across the sting area. "If possible, wear surgical gloves while you're doing this," says Dr. Kizer. "You want to be sure you don't get stung, too."

Rinse with salt water. "Use only salt water to rinse the

MEDICAL ALERT

When to See the Doctor

Jellyfish and man-of-war stings may cause pain, cramps, nausea and tingling as well as a hivelike rash, says Kenneth W. Kizer, M.D., M.P.H., professor of emergency medicine and medical toxicology at the University of California, Davis, School of Medicine and wilderness medicine specialist.

For these stings, it's imperative to seek medical attention if the child complains of tightness in the throat or if he experiences shortness of breath or difficulty breathing. Children with any underlying health problems, such as diabetes, arthritis, and/or immune problems should be taken to the nearest medical center immediately, says Dr. Kizer.

Coral injuries can lead to infection: "The problem with coral is that it's sharp, jagged and fragile," says Dr. Kizer. "Little pieces of coral tend to break off in the wound, making it very prone to infection. And some of the coral secretions can be toxic." These wounds demand special attention by a doctor who is familiar with coral injuries, according to Dr. Kizer.

Puncture wounds from sea urchins, stingrays and any spiny fish should also be treated by a doctor as soon as possible, although you should immerse the wound in hot water (110° to 115°F) immediately to relieve pain.

---

wound," says Dr. Kizer. Fresh water can actually cause the little "harpoon cells" to fire off and inject more venom, he cautions. Don't rub the skin and *never* rub it with sand because this will cause the nematocysts to fire off more venom.

Neutralize them. You also want to neutralize the nematocysts so they don't inject any more venom. The best neutralizer is vinegar, but you can also use a slurry of baking soda and water or a mixture of rubbing alcohol and meat tenderizer blended into a liquid paste, says Dr. Kizer.

"In Hawaii, where I used to practice, we used alcohol mixed with meat tenderizer all the time," he says. "The alcohol keeps the nematocysts from firing, and the meat tenderizer breaks down the venom." He recommends that you mix just enough alcohol to the meat tenderizer to make a thin paste, like ketchup. Apply this paste to the wound and leave it there until the pain goes away, usually anywhere from 5 to 30 minutes. (Because some children's skin may be sensitive to ingredients in meat tenderizer, it's best to monitor your child to see if irritation or an allergic reaction occurs.)

Use painkillers. "Because many of these injuries cause inflammation, over-the-counter products such as acetaminophen [Children's Tylenol] can be helpful," says Dr. Kizer. Check the package directions for the correct dosage for your child's age and weight. If your child is under age two, consult a physician.

Give a jellyfish lesson. "The best treatment for jellyfish stings is prevention," says Dr. Kizer. Point out jellyfish lying on the beach and warn your child not to touch them. "Jellyfish can remain venomous for at least a day or two after they've washed up on the beach," he points out.

Coral and Sea Urchins

Remove spines with tape. If your child steps on coral, you can remove the fine, hard-to-get pieces by applying a piece of adhesive tape to the abrasion site and then removing it, says Constance L. Rosson, M.D., of the Good Samaritan Hospital in Portland, Oregon. When you pull the tape off, you pull up the tiny spines. Then bathe the area with vinegar, suggests Dr. Rosson.

Clean it out. If the wound is bleeding, apply pressure for a few minutes to stop the bleeding. Then use salt water or fresh water to clean out the wound. "Remove any obvious foreign material," says Dr. Kizer. "And remember that these kinds of injuries are at very high risk for infection," he says.

Get into hot water. The toxins released by sea urchins can be broken down by heat. For these wounds, soak the body part in hot water, around 110° to 115°F, 30 to 90 minutes, says Dr. Kizer. That's warmer than body temperature, but not hot enough to scald. (This treatment also works for other stinging fish such as scorpion fish, lionfish and catfish.)

Raise the limb. Swelling may occur with both coral and sea urchin wounds. Elevate the area, if possible, to discourage swelling, says Dr. Kizer.

Check tetanus records. "The bacteria that cause tetanus live in the ocean, and this may be a problem for coral and spine puncture wounds," says Dr. Kizer. After the child's first shots, she should get them every ten years, plus a booster if she has a nasty injury and the last shot was more than five years ago, he says.

Prepare with protection. To help your child avoid sea urchin stings, point out tide pools or rocky areas where these creatures are often found, suggests Dr. Kizer. He recommends reef shoes or aquatic shoes with hard, spine-proof soles and mesh tops for any child who's walking or swimming in a beach area that has sea urchins or coral.

MEASLES

Going the Distance with the Virus

Measles is a viral infection that was once one of the most common childhood illnesses. But thanks to the measles vaccine, it is relatively rare in the United States today. Kids still do get the measles, though, if they aren't immunized. So if your child did not get the vaccine, he may very well come down with this unpleasant virus.

Measles starts out like the common cold, with a cough, runny nose, red and watery eyes and a mild to moderate fever. But you should suspect your child has measles rather than a cold if you detect tiny white spots on the inside of the cheeks. Give the doctor a call.

Usually, the progression of measles is fairly predictable. After two to three days of fever, a whole-body rash breaks out, the cough worsens and the fever pushes higher, into the 103° to 104° range. The fine red spots on the body may join together to form larger splotches. But the rash, which lasts from five to eight days, is not itchy.

Sometimes children with measles develop an ear infection, pneumonia or neurological complications. Most of the time, though, kids with measles just feel really sick for seven to ten days. There's not really much you can do about it, except to try to relieve some of the symptoms.

Ease the fever with medication. Give your child a non-aspirin pain reliever such as Children's Tylenol or Tempra to help reduce fever and irritability, says Blair M. Eig, M.D.,

---

MEDICAL ALERT

When to See the Doctor

Measles can be complicated by a bacterial infection such as pneumonia or by an ear infection. If your child develops either of these infections, he needs to be treated with doctor-prescribed antibiotics. You should call the doctor immediately if your child complains of an earache, if he has yellow discharge in the eyes or if he develops a nasal discharge which becomes yellow and stays yellow for more than 24 hours, say Betti Hertzberg, M.D., a pediatrician and head of the Continuing Care Clinic at Miami Children's Hopital.

"If your child has fever after the fifth day of the rash, or any symptoms of pneumonia such as labored breathing, wheezing, chest pain or severe coughing, you need to contact your child's pediatrician as soon as possible," she says.

Your child will need immediate medical attention if he has any neurological symptoms such as a seizure, delirium or weakness or spasm of an arm or a leg, adds Blair M. Eig, M.D., a pediatrician in private practice in Silver Spring, Maryland. And if you can't wake him from a nap or from sound sleep, you should call for emergency assistance.

a pediatrician in private practice in Silver Spring, Maryland. Check the directions on the package for the correct dosage for your child's age and weight. If your child is under age two, consult your physician. "If your child has a high fever that is really debilitating, your pediatrician may prescribe some ibuprofen," adds Dr. Eig. (But ibuprofen should not be given to children unless you have a doctor's recommendation.)

Try a sponge bath. A sponge bath may also help your child feel more comfortable when the fever is high, says Richard Garcia, M.D., a pediatrician and vice chairman of the Department of Pediatrics and Adolescent Medicine at the Cleveland Clinic Foundation in Ohio. Have your child sit in a tub that's partially filled with lukewarm water, and gently sponge the water over his neck and shoulders.

Be generous with beverages. "Give your child plenty of liquids, as much as she can tolerate, preferably juice, Gatorade or Jell-O, which turns to liquid in the stomach," says Betti Hertzberg, M.D., a pediatrician and head of the Continuing Care Clinic at Miami Children's Hospital. "Beverages are important—with high fever and sweating, kids tend to get dehydrated more quickly," Dr. Hertzberg says.

Control the cough when necessary. You can try a mild cough suppressant that contains dextromethorphan to relieve the cough, especially if it's interfering with your child's sleep, suggests Dr. Eig. Over-the-counter products such as Triaminic-DM contain dextromethorphan. Be sure to read

---

IMMUNIZATION IN BRIEF

Measles immunization, recommended when a child is 15 months old, gives lifelong protection for most people. But with some kids, one dose of the vaccine is not enough. Doctors recommend a second dose for children 11 to 12 years of age or older who have not had measles. Check with your school district to see when re-immunization is advised in your area.

package directions—or check with your physician—for the correct dosage for your child.

Make the most of mist. "A cool-mist vaporizer will put some humidity in the room air and make it easier for your child to breathe freely," Dr. Garcia says. If you do use a vaporizer, though, you must clean it often, following the manufacturer's instructions. "Otherwise, bacteria and mold could grow in the still water," he cautions.

Keep the lights low. With measles, the eyes can become very irritated and sensitive to light. "Keep the lights dim in your child's room, or give him sunglasses to wear," advises Dr. Hertzberg.

Flush and wipe the eyes. "Rinsing the eyes with plain saline solution—available at drugstores—may be soothing," says Dr. Eig. Use an eyedropper to put several drops in the corner of each eye.

If your child's eyes get crusty, wipe them with cotton balls that have been wrung out with boiled water, says Dr. Hertzberg. "Be sure to wipe from the inside corner of the eye to the outside, and use a different cotton ball for each eye," she says.

Restrict activity. Be sure that your child stays indoors, preferably in bed, says Dr. Hertzberg. "With the measles, he'll probably feel too sick to do much else," she says.

MOTION SICKNESS

Taming the Upsets

I t's one of life's mysteries. Some kids can rocket through the air upside down on amusement park rides, screaming with glee and without a twinge of discomfort, while other kids get pale, clammy, dizzy, nauseated and thoroughly sick just riding in a car.

Some kids, unfortunately, are more susceptible to motion sickness than others. And for parents of kids who are prone to motion sickness, that long vacation trip can turn into a series of roadside stops. Some families don't dare go anywhere without a sickness bag handy.

But what causes the sickness-prone kid to feel this bad?

Motion sickness occurs when the brain receives conflicting messages from the inner ears (which control balance and equilibrium) and the eyes, says Mark D. Widome, M.D., professor of pediatrics at Pennsylvania State University Children's Hospital in Hershey. A child reading a book in the backseat of a car, for example, will feel the motion of the car but will not see the motion, since her view is focused on the printed page on her lap.

Even babies may experience motion sickness, although they won't be able to tell you about it, adds Robert Mendelson, M.D., a pediatrician and clinical professor of pediatrics at Oregon Health Sciences University in Portland. "If your baby is unusually fussy on long car rides—most babies tend to be lulled to sleep—it could be caused by motion sickness," he says.

As unpleasant as motion sickness is, it has no lasting effects. Treatment varies from child to child, and therapies fall into a category that Dr. Mendelson calls WW—whatever works. The WW options may also work if you're traveling in a plane or boat—but car travel is the most common troublemaker. So here are some tactics for the open road.

Crack the window. Fresh air seems to make a queasy child feel a bit better. So open the window a bit on car trips, even if it's cold outside, advises Dr. Mendelson.

Make frequent stops. Since many kids don't get sick during the first 30 minutes or so of a car trip, the more stops you make, the less likely your child will become ill. So stop *before* you hear the first cry of, "Mommy, I don't feel so good," Dr. Widome advises. "When you stop, have the child get out of the car to get some fresh air and walk around a bit."

Pass up heavy, greasy meals. A bellyful of greasy French fries or a double cheese pizza is just asking for motion sickness. And once your child is nauseated, points out Dr. Mendelson, the sight or smell of any food may be more than he can tolerate. Carry along some sandwiches, crackers and crunchy vegetables rather than relying on fast food. And avoid any grease-laden meal before the trip begins.

Learn what your child can stomach. Try feeding your child *something* before one trip and *nothing* before another, then see which works better. Some children travel better with an empty stomach, while some do better if they've had dry toast or crackers or something to drink, says Dr. Mendelson.

Be glad for that car seat. For young kids, the car seat is not only a necessary safety measure, it's also a great nausea-prevention device. The seat lifts children up higher, and they're always less nausea-prone if they can see out the window, according to Dr. Widome.

Furnish a front-row seat. Move the child into the front seat and encourage him to look at cars and buildings far ahead or to look at the horizon. "This way your child will 'see' the same motion that his body and inner ears 'feel,' " says Dr. Mendelson. The other advantage of moving up front is that backseats tend to bounce and sway more, which just may be the final straw for an upset stomach. If kids must sit in the backseat and they're beyond the car seat stage, play some roadside games (like "I see something green") that get them to look out the window.

Nix the printed word. Reading, playing cards or doing homework in the car can prompt motion sickness. Although books with large pictures and only a few words may be okay, your best bet is entertaining your child with music or stories on a tape recorder, says Dr. Mendelson. If you don't have a supply of tapes at home, you can stock up on music and stories at your public library before a long trip.

Beware of fumes. Cigarette, pipe or cigar smoke can make an already queasy child lose his lunch. But Dr. Widome notes that any perfumes or automobile or bus exhausts can also be offensive to your child. If you're following diesel trucks down a busy highway, adjust the ventilation or air conditioning to keep road fumes *out*.

Go for the OTCs. Many over-the-counter antinausea medicines such as Dramamine and Marezine may be effective with your child. These products are primarily antihistamines, and many come in children's formulations as chewable tablets or liquids. These are given *before* the trip.

"Talk to your pediatrician to find out if one of these is appropriate for your child and what dosage to give," says Dr. Mendelson. These work for many children but may make your child drowsy. Never give your child an antinausea medication without a doctor's approval, especially if the child is taking any other medication, because the drugs could interact and cause problems.

Try a syrupy solution. Emetrol is another over-the-counter medication that's sometimes helpful, says Dr. Mendelson. It contains the essence of coke syrup, that time-honored remedy from years ago, and it won't make your child drowsy as the antihistamine-type drugs do. "I recommend giving it to susceptible children just before getting in the car and then giving them a small dose every 15 to 20 minutes while en route," says Dr. Mendelson.

Scopolamine is a no-no. Even if you have a scopolamine patch on hand, under no circumstances should a child be allowed to use it. (A scopolamine patch is an antinausea skin patch available by prescription only.) "These are meant strictly for adults," warns Dr. Widome. Scopolamine has side effects that may be tolerable for adults, but not for children.

Be prepared. No matter what treatment you try, it's best to be prepared, says Dr. Widome—and sometimes just knowing that you're ready for the worst can help calm a nauseated child. Have a supply of sturdy plastic bags for emergencies, plus a damp washcloth in a plastic bag for cleanups and a fresh change of clothing for your distressed child.

MUMPS

Help for the Pain and Swelling

Remember having the mumps when you were a kid? Along with feeling weak, headachy and feverish, your parotid glands, located in front of each ear, swelled up on both sides of your face. The swelling was tender and painful, too, and may have lasted from three to seven miserable days.

Most cases of the mumps are unpleasant but not serious. It is possible, however, for mumps to have serious complications, such as infection of the spinal cord and brain, deafness or a painful inflammation of the testicles in teenage and adult males.

The best way to deal with mumps is with prevention.

MEDICAL ALERT

When to See the Doctor

Mumps should always be diagnosed by your doctor, because other illnesses can cause swelling of the glands near the face. "Most of the time, when parents think their child has mumps, the swelling is due to swollen lymph nodes which may be caused by a different viral or even bacterial infection," notes Blair M. Eig, M.D., pediatrician in private practice in Silver Spring, Maryland. "The parotid glands cause swelling above the jaw line, in front of the ears, while lymph node swelling occurs below the jaw," Dr. Eig adds.

Once mumps has been diagnosed, consult your doctor again if your child is vomiting; has a stiff neck, a severe headache, swelling or pain in the testicles (in teenage boys), abdominal pain, a fever higher than 101°; or acts and looks very sick, advises Dr. Eig. If any of these symptoms are present, your child may have one of the complications of mumps that need immediate medical attention.

The MMR vaccine protects children from three of the once-common childhood diseases—measles, mumps and rubella. It is now recommended that children receive two doses of MMR, the first at 15 months of age and the second later in childhood. Unfortunately, not every child gets the necessary immunizations, and if yours is among them, it is quite possible that she'll contract the disease.

If your child does come down with mumps, the only thing you can do, besides checking with the doctor, is keep her comfortable. Here's how.

Treat the pain. "Give your child acetaminophen [Children's Tylenol] for fever and discomfort," suggests Lorry Rubin, M.D., chief of the Division of Pediatric Infectious Diseases at Schneider Children's Hospital of the Long Island Jewish Medical Center in New Hyde Park, New York, and associate professor of pediatrics at the Albert Einstein School of Medicine in New York City. Check the package directions for the correct dosage for your child's age and weight. If your child is under age two, consult a physician.

Make meals moist. "The parotid glands produce saliva, but during the mumps, they can't work as efficiently to moisten the food your child is eating," says Jack H. Hutto, Jr., M.D., chief of pediatric infectious disease at All Children's Hospital in St. Petersburg, Florida. "If chewing is a chore, offer your child foods with a high liquid content: soup, ice cream, pudding, a slush drink or Cream of Wheat," suggests Dr. Hutto.

Don't be tart. "Avoid giving your child citrus fruits or juices, or any other food that is high in acid," says Dr. Rubin. "Acidic foods stimulate the parotid gland to secrete saliva, a painful process during the mumps."

Shower some extra affection. Spend as much time with your child as you can. "Reading a story, talking, singing or rocking can help make her feel better," says Dr. Hutto.

MUSCLE ACHES AND CRAMPS

Soothing Action That Brings Relief

For a child, occasional muscle aches or cramps seem to come with the territory. Whether it's general soreness in your daughter's back and shoulders from overdoing her butterfly stroke or a painful cramp in the calf muscle that awakens your son from a sound sleep, the pains that plague kids can range from mild to severe.

Frequently, muscle aches strike active kids who like to exert themselves. But sedentary children can be troubled by muscle aches, too. "When kids who are unused to exercise try to push themselves to keep up in gym class or at play with their friends, they often overuse their muscles," says George H. Durham II, M.D., a pediatrician at the Bryner Clinic and a clinical associate professor of pediatrics at the University of Utah School of Medicine, both in Salt Lake City.

Muscle aches can afflict kids any time of the day or night. Children who exercise in extreme heat sometimes get painful (but not serious) "heat cramps" in the calf, thigh or abdomen. Other painful cramps in the calf, foot or thigh

---

MEDICAL ALERT

When to See the Doctor

A muscle pain or cramp is rarely cause for worry, according to Flavia Marino, M.D., a clinical instructor in pediatrics at New York University Medical Center, Tisch Hospital, and a pediatrician in New York City. But she says you should alert your child's physician if the pain is very severe, is recurrent or is accompanied by fever, sore throat, a rash, abdominal pain, joint swelling, weight loss or a loss of strength in the muscle.

occur at night and awaken kids from sleep, adds Dr. Durham.

"Night cramps happen to well-nourished, healthy, active children," he says. "They may be the result, according to some studies, of very active leg movements during certain portions of the sleep cycle." You can't prevent all muscle aches and cramps, but by following these steps you can help your child feel more comfortable.

Fight heat with a stretch-and-chill. "If a heat cramp has already hit, give your child something to drink, stretch out the muscle and apply an ice-pack to it for up to 20 minutes," advises Brian Halpern, M.D., clinical instructor of sports medicine at the Hospital for Special Surgery in New York City and fellowship director of Sports Medicine at the University of Medicine and Dentistry of New Jersey, Robert Wood Johnson Medical School, in New Brunswick. Be sure to wrap the ice-pack in a towel so it won't freeze the skin.

Beat the heat with liquids. Heat cramps are preventable, doctors say. But you need to take along a water bottle to your child's summer soccer game. "Your child can avoid cramping by drinking plenty of liquids during exercise, especially in the hot weather," says Dr. Halpern. For very active sports like soccer, tennis or football, he should drink a few ounces every 10 to 20 minutes or so in hot weather—and have a cupful of water or sports drink whenever there's a break in the game.

Plan to build fitness gradually. A child who pushes his muscles harder than they want to go will surely feel the pain. "In Utah, many of our school programs encourage kids to run half a mile to a mile every day under the direction of the teacher," says Dr. Durham. "That can put a lot of pressure on the child who is overweight or not as athletic as the others. When these kids force themselves to keep up, they often suffer leg aches from doing too much, too soon.

"A better approach is to encourage your child to build up strength and endurance gradually. Exercising that way is less intimidating to him, and less stressful to the muscles," Dr. Durham says.

After a tough workout, coddle the muscles. Even active kids may have muscle pain as a result of strenuous physical exercise. "When the muscles are stressed, there is some tissue swelling and an accumulation of metabolic waste products," explains Flavia Marino, M.D., a clinical instructor in pediatrics at New York University Medical Center, Tisch Hospital, and a pediatrician in New York City. This causes a little soreness, which is nothing to worry about, Dr. Marino says.

"Some rest, perhaps a warm compress over the sore muscle, and some acetaminophen [Children's Tylenol] should do the trick," says Dr. Marino. Check the package directions for the correct dosage for your child's age and weight, or check with your physician.

Be reassuring about night cramps. "Night cramps can be very frightening to kids, particularly when they are in that pre-adolescent stage when they tend to be very concerned about their bodies. They may be worried that there's something horrendous going on," says Dr. Durham. He recommends that you reassure your child that cramping is normal. If this is something that you, too, have experienced, tell your child about it—and let him know it's probably a passing phase.

Rub away the knot. "Massaging the cramped muscle in the direction that it runs should unknot it and make the pain go away," says Dr. Marino. "But your child may get some additional comfort from a hot-water bottle or a warm compress," she adds.

NAIL-BITING

Backing Off a Nervous Habit

M any children bite their nails, says Paul Kechijian, M.D., clinical associate professor of dermatology and chief of the nail section at New York University Medical Center. Usually they grow out of the habit, and nagging them about it only makes the situation worse.

What can you do if your child can't or won't keep her nails out of her mouth? First, understand why she does it.

"Nail-biting is a nervous habit that's often a symptom of anxiety or insecurity," says William Womack, M.D., associate professor in the Department of Child Psychiatry at the University of Washington School of Medicine and codirector of the Stress Management Clinic of Children's Hospital and Medical Center, both in Seattle. "It's your child's way of comforting herself."

Figure out what's eating your child, and you're halfway to getting her to stop eating her nails. Eventually, most children stop biting their nails when they start to care how their nails look—or when their friends start to notice. Meanwhile, try some of these creative solutions.

Help your child understand. Enlist your child's cooperation by helping her understand why she's biting her nails. "Explain that sometimes people bite their nails because they worry a lot or are upset and nervous," says Dr. Womack. For example, ask her if she does it when relatives visit, when she's meeting new friends or when she's trying hard to learn something new. Your child may be better able to control the habit if she can talk about the stresses she's experiencing, according to Dr. Womack.

Nail down a deal. Ask your child if her nail-biting bothers her. If, and only if, your child wants to stop biting her nails, you and she can talk about a "contract," suggests Dr. Womack.

For instance, would she consider not biting her nails for a dime a day? Or for a week—in exchange for a visit to an amusement park? Would she appreciate a new watch of her own for not biting her nails for a month?

Keep a chart of successful non-biting days, then reward her for compliance with the "deal," says Dr. Womack.

Trim off some stress. If you teach your child relaxation techniques, she can counter the stress that usually leads to nail-biting, suggests Dr. Womack. "Say to her, 'When you

MEDICAL ALERT

When to See the Doctor

If all your child does is bite off the tips of her nails, it's not a medical problem, says Paul Kechijian, M.D., clinical associate professor of dermatology and chief of the nail section at New York University Medical Center.

It only becomes a problem when children bite their nails more aggressively—particularly if they tear off their nails and cause their fingers to bleed. The cuticle area is especially important because the nail forms under the whitish half moon (usually seen only on the thumb), then grows out from underneath the cuticle.

"Theoretically," says Dr. Kechijian, "you could bite your nail tips for 25 years and never have permanent deformity because you're not injuring the nail root. But the cuticle has an important function, which is to act as a barrier to keep bacteria, yeast and liquids from getting underneath the skin of the finger. When children bite the sides and cuticles of their nails, or peel, tear and rip the cuticle off, they can get a low-grade infection of the finger and the nail root." And that can lead to permanently deformed nails.

If you see any sign of infection—fingers that are chronically swollen and red, or nails that are bumpy—see a dermatologist, says Dr. Kechijian.

feel like biting your nails, think of something pleasant, like playing on a beach or having fun with friends, suggests Dr. Womack.

Offer a manicure. "Have your child get a manicure," says Frances Willson, Ph.D., a clinical psychologist in Sherman Oaks, California, and chairman of the Health Psychology Committee of the Los Angeles County Psychological Association. "It's better if she gets it professionally than if you give it; then she'll have an investment in someone outside of you. But she has to want it."

Suggest a substitute. Have your child try substituting a sugarless lollipop (available at health food stores) for biting her nails, suggests Bobbi Vogel, Ph.D., a family counselor in Woodland Hills, California, and director of the Adolescent Outpatient Program at Tarzana Treatment Center in Tarzana. "Your child may find it easier to stop nail-biting if she has a substitute means of oral gratification, at least temporarily," says Dr. Vogel. Besides a lollipop, you can also offer sugarless gum or a crunchy carrot stick.

Try positive distraction. If a child is ready to give up nail-biting, you can help her learn to keep her hands otherwise occupied, says Dr. Vogel. For example, if your child habitually bites her nails while staring at the TV set, keep a supply of drawing materials near the TV and encourage her to color or draw while her favorite shows are on. Or buy her a special "worry bead" bracelet she can wear and play with when she's tempted to bite her nails.

Annoy the taste buds. With your child's cooperation, and if she's over four years old, put something bitter on her nails, suggests Dr. Vogel. One over-the-counter product, Thum, contains cayenne pepper extract and citric acid. "This will do more harm than good, however, if your child feels she's being punished for being bad," points out Dr. Vogel. Only use it if she agrees.

NEGATIVITY

Upbeat Ways to Brighten an Outlook

S occer's stupid. I don't want to play."
        "I don't want to go to the party. It's not going to be any fun."
    "I don't see why I have to take math. I'm not going to Harvard."
    "I can't do that."
    Sound familiar? If so, you probably have a child who travels with his or her own personal black cloud. Some

children are born looking on the negative side. They're temperamentally slow to warm, uncomfortable with new situations and hesitant to tackle anything for the first time. Many use a negative attitude—"I can't, I won't, I don't"—to avoid all those things that make them anxious or afraid.

Whether it's something they're born with or something they acquire, negative children can benefit from a dose of confidence-building. Here are a few things that can jump-start the building process, according to experts.

Catch your child being positive. Look for what excites him and what makes him feel good about himself, especially if he doesn't seem to notice. Comment on the fact the he's having a good time, suggests Thomas Olkowski, Ph.D., a clinical psychologist in private practice in Denver. "Chances are these will be times when the child is involved and feeling sure of himself. Once he experiences confidence, he'll be more willing to try other things."

Don't push. "Allow your child to go at his own pace," says Dr. Olkowski. "Just keep an eye and ear open to the things he's really interested in and attracted to." For example, if your child is glued to the karate championships on "Wide World of Sports," you might want to take him to the nearest karate studio "just for a look." You may have to go back a few times to look some more before suggesting he sign up, but by then he may even ask.

Offer an "out." Often, a child will be more willing to try something if he knows he can bail out when he wants to. "Just say, 'try it for a little while—for 10 or 15 minutes,' " suggests James Bozigar, a licensed social worker and coordinator of community relations for the Family Intervention Center at Children's Hospital of Pittsburgh. "Often, once kids get *into* something, they find they really enjoy it. But negative kids need to know from the start that the new activity is time-limited."

Be supportive. Rather than berate your child for being so negative, encourage him to talk about why he feels the way he does, says Lynne Henderson, Ph.D., director of the Palo Alto Shyness Clinic in Menlo Park, California. "Listen to his feelings and be reassuring and soothing, all the while encouraging him to keep going. Tell him things like, 'Let's just get through this class and see how you feel then.' Even if children don't like an activity, they can feel good about the fact that they finished."

Have a family story hour. This is the time to talk about how you never wanted to run relays because you were the shortest kid in the freshman class, or about how you got sick to your stomach the morning of the math test because you were the original number bumbler.

"Kids have this false notion that their parents are perfect. They need to hear about what we were like as kids, so they can see that we struggled with the same fears, problems and screw-ups," says Dr. Olkowski. "They need to know that the 'terrible things' happening to them also happened to other people."

Laugh it up. It helps to laugh at our own mistakes, so our kids learn to laugh, too. One child who felt she couldn't do anything right loved hearing the story of her mother's first job interview: "At the end of that interview, I got up from my chair, picked up my briefcase and walked into a closet," her mother told her. Laughter is often the best medicine for a negative attitude born of fear. "If we don't take ourselves so seriously, our kids are going to learn they can make mistakes and laugh about them and still regroup and go on with their lives," says Dr. Olkowski.

Chart negative behavior. "Every time negativity occurs, make a note of it and what was going on at the time," advises Bozigar. This will help you identify triggering situations. One mother who charted her son's negative behavior discovered that he was resisting attempts to get involved in after-school activities because he preferred spending that time with her. When she made clear plans to spend time with him on weekends, he felt better about staying late at school. Another mother found that her daughter was only negative about the activities in which her older sibling was involved. By planning activities without "big sister" around, her daughter was much more willing to participate.

Use a secret signal. Use a thumbs-up or an A-Okay sign to signal your child when you notice he's approaching something positively. This serves two purposes, says Dr. Olkowski. It's a simple, secret way to show your child you're proud of his positive behavior, and it may help you learn something about your child you didn't know. "I had one mom who came back two weeks later and said about her son, 'I can't get over how many things he was doing right!' "

Don't label. There's no quicker way to ensure your child will remain negative than to label him that way. "Most of us follow the adage, if you say my name I'll play the game," says Dr. Olkowski. "If you tell me I have a crummy attitude about things, and that attitude is working for me, then I'm going to continue to have that crummy negative attitude. Focusing on the positive is always more effective with kids."

NIGHT TERRORS AND NIGHTMARES

Taking the Fear Out of Bedtime Hours

You're awakened by a blood-curdling scream. You race to your child's room to find her sitting bolt upright in bed, howling, her eyes wide open and filled with terror. You call her name but she stares right through you, as if you aren't there. She may begin thrashing and striking out. She may even try to get out of bed. Then as suddenly as it began, the "spell" is over and she's sound asleep.

"Most parents who witness this say the child looks like she's possessed," says Barbara Howard, M.D., assistant clinical professor of pediatrics at Duke University Medical Center in Durham, North Carolina. "But there's a perfectly rational explanation. The child is experiencing a night terror."

Though night terrors may sound like something that requires professional help, they are actually normal and fairly common in children. Experts say they occur during the deepest part of the sleep cycle, about an hour or two after the child falls asleep.

"Normally, this is the point where the child cycles into a lighter sleep where dreams occur," says Ronald Dahl, M.D., director of the Children's Sleep Evaluation Center at Western Psychiatric Institute and Clinic in Pittsburgh and associate professor of psychiatry and pediatrics at the University of Pittsburgh Medical Center. "But particularly if the child is very tired, a split may occur. Part of the system says it's time to go into light sleep, but another part says, 'No, I'm still tired.' So part of the brain stays deeply asleep while another part goes into a high-arousal state."

The child who is having a night terror is not awake, yet not quite asleep, notes Dr. Dahl. And the "terror" aspect of this phenomenon really only registers on the parents. The child herself is not conscious, nor does she remember playing out this scene from *The Exorcist* the next day, says Dr. Dahl.

Nightmares, on the other hand, are very frightening for children. "A nightmare is essentially a dream that is sufficiently scary to wake a child up," says Dr. Dahl. "In fact, the child may wake up quickly, become fully awake and have trouble getting back to sleep. He may be a little confused, but he'll probably be coherent. A nightmare is likely to occur late in the night or early in the morning, in the second half of the sleep period."

Both night terrors and nightmares tend to run their course and disappear overtime. But there are a few techniques you can use to make things easier for your child.

Night Terrors

Stay calm. "Remind yourself that although a night terror looks scary, it's not a seizure. It's not a terrible thing," says Dr. Dahl. "Night terrors are very common and normal, especially in kids between the ages of three and five."

Stand by until it's over. Though it may be difficult to watch your child screaming, there's really nothing you can do to stop a night terror, says Dr. Howard. "But you can make sure the child is safe when it's happening by re-straining her if necessary. Children do sometimes hurt themselves thrashing or running around. And it's almost impossible to wake them."

Don't mention it. "Don't talk to your child about the episode the next morning," says Dr. Howard. "And don't let siblings talk to her about it either. Kids don't remember night terrors. But if they find out later what they did, they may get upset about being out of control."

Try a preventive wake-up call. "If your child is experiencing terrors, you could try waking her up about 30 minutes after she goes to bed, and then letting her go back to sleep," says Dr. Howard. "That breaks up the sleep cycle and tends to interrupt the pattern of the night terrors."

Make sure your child is getting enough sleep. "Increase the total amount of sleep your child is getting," suggests Dr. Dahl. "If she's fairly young, it might mean letting her go back to taking daily naps. For an older kid, try letting her sleep longer in the morning or put her to bed a little earlier."

The reason for this, Dr. Dahl explains, is that the more tired a child is, the more difficult it will be for her to switch from deep sleep to light sleep. "The classic time for night terrors to occur is when young children first give up their daily naps," he says. "The first time a kid stays up for 12 hours or more, there's more pressure on her sleep system than she's ever had, and it drives her deeply into sleep, deeper than she's ever been. At the end of that first deep sleep cycle is when she's most likely to have a night terror."

Think happy thoughts. "If kids are worried, anxious or a little bit more fearful than usual as they fall asleep, they're more likely to have these events," says Dr. Dahl. "Ask your child if anything's worrying her just before she falls asleep. Often a child who is well-behaved, but shy and inhibited by temperament, will get into the habit of lying in bed and worrying.

"Helping the child establish a positive routine at bedtime

HOW TO STOP A SLEEPWALKER

Sleepwalking, like night terrors, usually occurs during a child's transition from very deep to light, dreaming sleep, says Ronald Dahl, M.D., director of the Children's Sleep Evaluation Center at Western Psychiatric Institute and Clinic in Pittsburgh and associate professor of psychiatry and pediatrics at the University of Pittsburgh Medical Center.

"This is a very difficult transition for young children to make, and they often do strange things, like sleepwalking or talking in their sleep," says Dr. Dahl. If you have a sleepwalker, safety is the primary concern. Here's what the experts recommend you do.

Wake the child up. "You can often wake a child up from sleepwalking and guide him back to bed," says Barbara Howard, M.D., assistant clinical professor of pediatrics at Duke University Medical Center in Durham, North Carolina.

Increase sleep time. "Being overtired is a major factor in sleepwalking," notes Dr. Dahl. "Ninety-nine percent of children experiencing these partial arousals do better after increasing the total amount of sleep."

Install a gate. "Install a portable, folding gate or a screen door to block the doorway so he can't get out," suggests Dr. Howard. "These are better than locking the door and you can hear him if he gets up." You should also place a gate across any stairways.

Change bed arrangements. "If your child is sleeping in a bunk bed, make sure you take him off the top bunk," says Dr. Dahl.

can reverse that," he says. Have her focus on positive thoughts about the good things that have happened to her that day. Help her feel safe and secure. That seems to cut down on night terrors."

Talk over fears during the day. "Help your child express her worries and fears during the day rather than letting them surface at night," says Dr. Dahl. "Often a child who gets night terrors has a small, specific but irrational fear that's worrying her. As soon as she expresses her fear and understands that it's not worth worrying over, the night terrors go away."

Don't make it a habit. "Be careful to avoid what's called secondary gain, which means the child gets some benefit from having had a night terror," says Dr. Howard. "Even though the night terror was unintentional, if the child wakes up and finds the parent there, concerned about her and giving her a lot of attention, it can seem like a reward. That can reinforce and perpetuate the problem. So it's important not to coddle the child too much—by waking her and giving her something to eat or drink, for instance."

Nightmares

Turn on the light. If a child wakes up with a nightmare and comes running to your room, be prepared to listen and find out why the child is afraid.

"Most kids want their parents around," says Dr. Dahl. "Some don't need much more than your reassurance that everything is all right." But sometimes, you may have to go back to the child's room, turn on the light and show him there's nothing there. "The child really needs to spend more time with you until he winds down," says Dr. Dahl.

Break the rules now and then. Your child may want to spend the rest of the night in your bed, even if it's not usually allowed. "It's okay to occasionally break the rules if the child is badly frightened," says Dr. Dahl, "though you may have to nip that behavior in the bud before it becomes a bad habit. Most kids will go back to their bed without protest the next night if you remind them of the rule."

Give the child a nightmare protector. A flashlight or a "protective" stuffed animal can be very soothing to a child plagued by nightmares, says Sheila Ribordy, Ph.D., a clinical psychologist specializing in treating children and families and professor of psychology and director of clinical training in the Department of Psychology at De Paul University in Chicago.

"For a child, it's important to feel he has some control

over his nightmares," she says. "Children need to have a sense that they are powerful people so things aren't so scary for them."

Have a bedside chat. "If a child is having a lot of nightmares, you may need to help him relieve some of the stress that comes up during the day," says Dr. Howard. "Children these days are under enormous stress. Often they're watching violent movies or TV programs. Sometimes they're subjected to a bully at school or at day care. Or they're being asked to toilet train or deal with a new sibling or give up their room." Since these stresses can lead to nightmares, it helps if you can talk to your child about what's happened during the day, according to Dr. Howard.

Follow a calming bedtime routine. "Your child's experience at bedtime should be a calming one," says Dr. Howard. She suggests including a story, a song or cuddly animals in the routine.

Children who are having nightmares may develop a fear of falling asleep, and a bedtime routine that includes books or music can help. "Playing music or story tapes gives them something to focus on other than the fear of nightmares that might be coming," says Dr. Ribordy. "Often these activities are distracting enough to help them fall asleep easily."

NOSEBLEEDS

Staunch Techniques to Stop the Flow

I t can be a horrifying experience for a small child—*and* for a parent. Small noses can produce alarming amounts of blood, and all that unexplained blood can scare the bravest of kids.

"Once my five-year-old son woke up in the middle of the night to find his pillow, pajamas and face covered with blood," recalls Cynthia Sloan, a suburban Philadelphia mother of three. "His screams brought me running. It only took a second to know why he was so terrified—it looked like a massacre had occurred in his bed."

But nosebleeds are seldom anything to worry about. "They almost always look worse than they are," says Oval Brown, M.D., associate professor of otolaryngology and chairman of the Division of Pediatric Otorhinolaryngology at the University of Texas Southwestern Medical Center in Dallas.

Most nosebleeds in children are the result of too-vigorous blowing, an accidental smack in the nose during rough-and-tumble play or some reckless picking with a sharp-nailed finger. "The scratch that causes all that blood is usually minor," says Jonas Johnson, M.D., professor of otolaryngology and vice chairman of the Department of Otolaryngology at the University of Pittsburgh School of Medicine, and most nosebleeds can be stemmed easily at home.

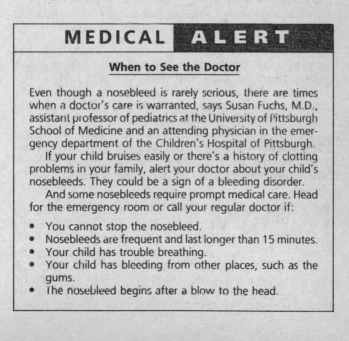

MEDICAL ALERT

When to See the Doctor

Even though a nosebleed is rarely serious, there are times when a doctor's care is warranted, says Susan Fuchs, M.D., assistant professor of pediatrics at the University of Pittsburgh School of Medicine and an attending physician in the emergency department of the Children's Hospital of Pittsburgh.

If your child bruises easily or there's a history of clotting problems in your family, alert your doctor about your child's nosebleeds. They could be a sign of a bleeding disorder.

And some nosebleeds require prompt medical care. Head for the emergency room or call your regular doctor if:

- You cannot stop the nosebleed.
- Nosebleeds are frequent and last longer than 15 minutes.
- Your child has trouble breathing.
- Your child has bleeding from other places, such as the gums.
- The nosebleed begins after a blow to the head.

But once the bleeding has stopped, your job still isn't over. "Complete healing requires seven to ten days," says Dr. Johnson. During that time you'll want to take preventive steps to help keep the scab in your child's nose intact and avoid another nosebleed.

Here's what the experts recommend to stop the flow and help prevent recurrences.

Treatment

Reassure your child. First, make sure *you* remain calm. "If your child sees that you're upset and scared, he will be, too," says Dr. Johnson. Explain to your child in calm tones that the nosebleed isn't serious and that you can stop it quickly with your child's help.

Try a nasal spray decongestant. If you have one on hand, you could try an over-the-counter product such as Neo-Synephrine or Afrin. These are vaso-constrictors that shrink blood vessels and help a scab form, says Dr. Johnson. "This may help speed up the process," he says.

Pinch the nose shut. With your child upright in a chair or in your lap, gently squeeze the soft part of the nose shut with a tissue or clean washcloth, says Dr. Johnson—or have your child do it. "Holding the nose shut firmly for ten minutes will almost stop the bleeding," he says. "The aim is to get a clot to form at the site of the injury."

Be sure that your child doesn't lean back, which can cause blood to flow down the back of the throat. This not only tastes bad and can initiate a coughing fit, but the blood can also irritate the stomach and cause vomiting, says Dr. Brown.

Be a clock watcher. When you're holding a child and pinching his nose shut, ten minutes can seem like a long time, admits Dr. Johnson. But don't give up too soon. "To be sure you've pinched your child's nose long enough, set a timer or sit near a clock," he suggests. If you don't hold the nose long enough, the bleeding will start again shortly after you let go.

Chill out. In addition to holding the nose shut, a cold cloth against the back of the neck or bridge of the nose can constrict blood vessels and help stem the flow, says Susan Fuchs, M.D., assistant professor of pediatrics at the University of Pittsburgh School of Medicine and an attending physician in the emergency department at the Children's Hospital of Pittsburgh.

Distract your child. "To help keep your child sitting that long with a pinched-shut nose, talk to him about what you're doing and why you're doing it," suggests Dr. Johnson. Other ways to distract him: Read a favorite story aloud, or watch a television show or video together.

Preventive Care

Don't blow it. After your child has a nosebleed, "don't let her blow her nose, no matter how stopped-up it feels," says Dr. Fuchs. "The simple act of blowing the nose can dislodge the delicate clot and start the bleeding all over again."

Curb physical activity. For several hours after the nosebleed has stopped, keep your child quiet and inactive. And ask your child *not* to run hard or to do things like hang upside down from the monkey bars until the damaged nose is completely healed—at least a week later. "Strenuous activity increases the pressure on blood vessels and can cause the nosebleed to start up again," says Dr. Johnson.

Discourage picking or rubbing. "Picking is probably what started the whole mess," says Dr. Fuchs, admitting that keeping a child from nose-picking is no easy task. "Even rubbing the nose, which will feel itchy as it's healing, can start the bleeding again," she adds. You *can* trim your child's nails to lessen the damage. If your child tends to pick in his sleep, slip socks or gloves on the hands at bedtime to help prevent another bleeding episode.

Humidify your home. Homes with dry heat can also dry out the nasal passages, making nosebleeds more likely. "A vaporizer can help in those cases," says Dr. Fuchs. Make sure you clean the vaporizer often, following the manufacturer's instructions.

Keep it moist. To humidify your child's nose directly, use a saline solution, suggests Dr. Brown. "Add ¼ teaspoon of salt to a cup of warm water, and put it in a nasal spray bottle that has been washed out," he says. Warm the bottle under running hot water until it's body temperature, and then spray three or four spritzes inside your child's nose. You can also purchase saline nasal spray at the drugstore, says Dr. Brown. The only drawback of the homemade solution is that it won't keep more than three days.

OVERWEIGHT

How to Handle Chubbiness

Baby fat was adorable on your infant—but now that he's older you're starting to worry about his pudginess. Perhaps you can remember how cruelly children taunted overweight classmates when you were a child, and you don't want your child to suffer.

So you take your child to the doctor, who confirms that Junior is a bit heavier than average for his size and reassures you that he doesn't have a hormonal problem.

Now what? Is your child's chubbiness a natural phase he'll grow out of or the result of genetics? You just can't tell. But trying to force your child to lose weight will frustrate both you and your child. What you can do is ensure that your entire family eats right and stays fit and help your chubby child feel good about himself. Here's what the experts recommend.

Forget about diets. Forcing a child to diet or limiting portions could encourage the eating problem you want to avoid, says Alvin N. Eden, M.D., associate clinical professor of pediatrics at the New York Hospital–Cornell Medical Center, chairman of the Department of Pediatrics at

Wyckoff Heights Medical Center, both in New York City, and author of *Positive Parenting* and *Dr. Eden's Healthy Kids*. Your child may resent your interference and begin to hoard food or eat all he can when you're not around, for example. Older children, particularly girls, can become obsessed with weight loss and develop eating disorders.

If a child is tremendously overweight and concerned about it, doctors recommend that the child not try to lose weight too rapidly. Slowing down weight gain as he continues to grow makes the most sense.

Be positive. Don't tell your child he is fat or nag him about his weight. All that does is undermine his self-esteem, says Barton D. Schmitt, M.D., professor of pediatrics at the University of Colorado School of Medicine, director of consultative services at the Ambulatory Care Center at Children's Hospital of Denver and author of *Your Child's Health*. "In fact, don't discuss his weight at all, unless he brings it up." If your child expresses concern about being chubby, explain that what's important is that he eat plenty of nutritious foods and get lots of exercise to help him grow up strong and healthy.

Help your child like his body. Reassure your child that you love him just the way he is, says Dr. Schmitt, and explain that people come in all shapes and sizes. And never talk disparagingly about your own hefty thighs or make rude comments about a fat person on television.

Have family and friends clam up. Well-meaning family and friends can make both you and your child miserable by saying things like, "My Susie is getting chubby!" or "I can't believe you're letting her eat dessert!" Politely but firmly tell the do-gooder that Susie looks fine to you, suggests Dr. Schmitt—and give Susie a big hug if she happens to overhear.

Make all changes a family affair. "Any dietary changes should be made for the whole family, not an isolated individual," says Jodie Shield, R.D., a spokesperson for the American Dietetic Association and an instructor of clinical nutrition at Rush University in Chicago. That way, you're not singling out one child by putting her on a diet—rather, you're instituting a healthier way of eating for everyone.

And if you want to discourage your plump child from eating certain foods such as potato chips and soda, then it's best not to bring those foods into the house, she says.

Switch habits slowly. When you're changing your child's diet, "small steps work best," says Gail Frank, R.D., a registered dietitian, professor of nutrition at California State University in Long Beach and a spokesperson for the American Dietetic Association. "You want to develop a new habit pattern, which, if done slowly, becomes ingrained. If you try to make changes too quickly, it will always seem like a sacrifice," she says.

Eat at the table. "Eating becomes almost unconscious if it's done while watching TV or reading," says Frank. That's how excess calories wind up in your child before he knows what's happened, she says.

Make it clear to your child that he should only eat when he stops all other activities. "Create an atmosphere for eating that focuses only on eating," says Frank.

Slow down the pace. In these fast-paced times, many families develop the habit of gobbling meals. And children who eat fast tend to pack in more food than those who take longer, says William J. Klish, M.D., professor of pediatrics and head of the section of nutrition and gastroenterology at Baylor College of Medicine in Houston.

Encourage the whole family to eat slowly and enjoy their food. Slower eating gives the brain a chance to tell the stomach that it's full.

Feed a hungry child. In general, you want your child to learn to set his own limits on how much he eats. "Withholding food from a child who is hungry will just lead to overeating whenever he gets a chance," says Dr. Schmitt. You also don't want your child to fear becoming hungry or not having enough to eat.

Furnish healthy snacks. Most children need refueling between meals, says Dr. Eden, and a midmorning or midafternoon snack can keep your child from being ravenous and overeating at mealtime. But be sure to serve nutritious snacks such as plain popcorn, fruit or vegetables or a slice of low-fat cheese, and always serve them at the table.

Limit television viewing. "Too much television viewing is one of the leading factors contributing to rapid weight gain and obesity," says Dr. Schmitt. "This usually becomes a problem at the age where children are allowed to watch

---

CHOOSE LOW-FAT, LOW-CALORIE PRODUCTS

You can easily trim fat from your family's diet by switching from high-fat foods to their low-fat or fat-free counterparts, suggests Gail Frank, R.D., a registered dietitian, professor of nutrition at California State University in Long Beach and a spokesperson for the American Dietetic Association.

Ice cream, milk, yogurt, cottage cheese, sour cream and cream cheese now come in low-fat and even no-fat varieties. And baked snacks such as pretzels and crackers have less fat than fried ones such as chips, she says.

Exception: Don't reduce the milk or fat in the meals of children under the age of two, as they have special dietary needs.

To lower the caloric punch of your family's meals, "Look for whole-grain foods, because fiber can help fill you up without piling on the calories," says Jodie Shield, R.D., a spokesperson for the American Dietetic Association and an instructor of clinical nutrition at Rush University in Chicago. "Breads, bagels, pastas and rice are all good choices. But be careful about what you put on them. Don't use creamy sauces, which are high in fat." Instead use simple tomato sauce, for example, or a sauce made with low-fat meat.

Other calorie-cutting suggestions: Serve jelly instead of butter, preferably the fruit-only variety with no added sugar. Use steamed or stir-fried vegetables instead of deep-fried ones. Choose the leanest cuts of meats, such as sirloin, tenderloin, round and flank cuts. Remove skin from chicken before cooking. And rather than frying foods, roast, broil or barbecue them instead.

TV without checking first with a parent—probably around school age." The more time children spend watching TV, the less time they're jumping rope, playing hopscotch or riding bikes.

And to make matters worse, kids routinely snack on junk food while they watch the tube. "It becomes a knee-jerk reaction," says Dr. Klish. "In other words, as soon as your child sits down in front of the TV she gets hungry and wants a snack."

Remove temptation. Some people are "cue sensitive" and want to eat whenever they see a reminder of food, says Dr. Eden, who recommends "fat-proofing" your house. Clearing your house of bags of chips and putting away items such as candy dishes or cookie jars will make your child less likely to eat just because the food isn't right in front of him.

Beware of breakfast traps. Take a look at the label of your children's favorite breakfast cereal—it may be packed with sugar. Slowly wean your kids off high-sugar cereals and onto low-sugar, high-fiber cereals, adding fruit instead of sugar if they miss the sweetness. Or serve homemade oatmeal, whole-grain muffins or yogurt. For a treat, says Frank, give your kids whole-wheat pancakes or pancakes with fruit. These are low in fat, unlike eggs and bacon or sausage.

Take your child food shopping. "The supermarket is a learning laboratory," says Frank. By taking your child along on shopping trips, you can teach her all about foods and how to make healthy choices. And if your child is allowed to select foods (within limitations, of course), he will be more likely to eat them. Point out some healthy snack or breakfast items, for example, and let him choose which ones he wants.

Encourage exercise. "I try to get every child involved in some team sport or some form of physical fitness," says Dr. Schmitt. "Encourage your child to walk or bike to a friend's house instead of driving her there. Ask her to walk the dog every day. See if there's an aerobics class she might join at school or the Y, or a swimming program," he says. But don't push your child into a sport she isn't interested in.

Plan active family outings. Family outings *don't* have to center around a meal in a restaurant or a trip to the ice cream store. "Go to the zoo," suggests Shield. "Or organize a game of softball for neighborhood families."

And remember that children copy the behavior they see. The more your child sees you being active, the more likely he will be active, too.

PINKEYE

Chasing the "-itis" Out

As you tuck your daughter into bed you notice her eyelids are a bit pink and swollen. The next morning they're even redder, and she complains that they're itchy.

Chances are good you're looking at pinkeye—a fairly common infection that tends to spread among small children, who generally can't resist rubbing their eyes and touching everything in sight. Pinkeye is the infectious form of conjunctivitis, a swelling of the membrane inside the eyelids. In more severe cases, the membrane oozes pus and the whites of the eyes are reddened.

The cause? It could be wayward bacteria or the same viruses that cause colds, sore throats or measles. Most often your child will get pinkeye at the same time as a cold, says Barton D. Schmitt, M.D., professor of pediatrics at the University of Colorado School of Medicine and director of consultative services at the Ambulatory Care Center at Children's Hospital, both in Denver, and author of *Your Child's Health*.

But there's also a form of conjunctivitis that isn't infectious. It can be caused by allergy, injury or even a bug that's flown into your child's eye. (Technically, this isn't pinkeye at all, but many people call all types of conjunctivitis pinkeye.)

You'll want to describe symptoms to your doctor, who may want to see your child, says Dr. Schmitt. The viral form of pinkeye goes away on its own, just as the cold that likely caused it does. Noninfectious conjunctivitis also seldom requires treatment, although if it's caused by an injury or allergy your doctor may treat the eye. For a bacterial infection the doctor is likely to prescribe antibiotic drops or ointment to hasten the recovery time.

But whatever kind of pinkeye your child has, those swollen eyes are probably itchy and uncomfortable. Here are some tips to help make the recovery time shorter and more comfortable.

Soothe with compresses. One of the best ways to make your child feel better is by putting warm compresses on the eyes. "Use a washcloth that's been warmed up to a little above body temperature," advises Robert Mendelson, M.D., a pediatrician and clinical professor of pediatrics at Oregon Health Sciences University in Portland. "Lay the cloth on the affected eye or eyes and as it cools, replace it with another one that's been warmed up." Do this for five to ten minutes three or four times a day.

Take care with stuck eyelids. When a child has the bacterial form of pinkeye, her eyes may ooze quite of bit of pus during the night. Sometimes the eyes get stuck shut and need to be soaked open. It's important to remind your child at bedtime that this could happen, just so she won't be frightened the next morning when she can't open her eyes easily.

"Warm, wet compresses are the best way to get the crusted material to soften," says Francis Gigliotti, M.D., associate professor of pediatrics, microbiology and immunology at the University of Rochester School of Medicine and Dentistry in New York. Soak a washcloth in warm water and apply it to the infected eye or eyes. Just be sure no one else uses the washcloth afterward, or they may get pinkeye, too.

Read to—or feed—a resistant child. If a toddler doesn't want that warm compress over her eyes, it helps to read a favorite book while you're giving the treatment, advises Dr. Mendelson. For a baby, try applying the compress while feeding your infant.

"Reading to children or feeding them often distracts them enough to get the job done," says Dr. Mendelson. "Older kids, on the other hand, figure out right away that the compresses feel good, so they are usually quite cooperative."

Reduce the risk. The germs that cause pinkeye are easily spread among other members of a household, says Dr. Gigliotti. Towels, sheets, pillowcases and washcloths used by the infected child should be laundered immediately in hot water. After you've dropped the items in the washer, wash your hands thoroughly so *you* won't get infected.

Out with those contacts. Children who wear contact lenses should remove them at the first sign of pinkeye, says Dr. Mendelson. Then they should wear their glasses until the condition clears up. The combination of pinkeye and contacts could cause a serious cornea irritation.

Consider sterile saline drops. A drop or two of saline solution, available at most pharmacies, can be very soothing for infected eyes, says Dr. Gigliotti. "But if you have a toddler who won't cooperate, it's better not to force the issue," he adds.

Older kids are usually willing to put up with the strange feeling of eyedrops just to get the soothing relief they offer. To help keep your child from blinking at the moment you squeeze the dropper and sending the drops rolling down the cheeks, tell your child to concentrate on looking up rather than focusing on the moving dropper, says Dr. Mendelson. Then gently pull down the lower lid and place the drops into the pocket this creates.

Don't touch the eye with the tip of the dropper. "If you touch the dropper to the eye and then insert it into the bottle, you'll get bacteria growing in the saline," warns Dr. Gigliotti. "This can cause a second infection down the road."

MEDICAL ALERT

When to See the Doctor

Although it's a good idea to discuss any case of pinkeye with your doctor, there are a few instances when consulting a doctor is a must, says Francis Gigliotti, M.D., associate professor of pediatrics, microbiology and immunology at the University of Rochester School of Medicine and Dentistry in New York.

Consult your pediatrician for:

- Any sign of pinkeye in an infant.
- Excessive pain or blurred vision, which could be caused by a scratched cornea or an inflammation of the iris, and would need different treatment.
- Pinkeye that still produces pus after 48 hours on medication.
- Pinkeye that hasn't cleared up after seven days.

If you think you've contaminated the tip of the dropper, wipe it immediately with sterile gauze. You can use the dropper again after wiping it clean, but make sure you don't share the saline solution with anyone else in the family. And after the infection has cleared up, discard the dropper, dispenser bottle and remaining solution.

PINWORMS

When an Itchy Bottom Signals Problems

There's a voice coming from the darkness next to your bed and it doesn't belong to the morning radio newscaster. "I can't sleep," it says in that whining pitch you know oh-so-well. So you turn on the light and find your child standing there, scratching his pajama bottoms.

This is the third morning in a row that he's been a walking alarm clock, rousing you before 6:30 A.M. with complaints of itching.

If this scenario sounds familiar, your child may have pinworms.

Pinworms are a type of intestinal nematode (a round worm) that live only in people. In the United States, they are the most common worm infection. "Pinworms are quite prevalent," says Robert Pond, M.D., physician with the Epidemic Intelligence Service at the Centers for Disease Control and Prevention in Atlanta. "Studies show that between 10 and 30 percent of children get them."

Because pinworms lay microscopic, infectious eggs that can spread from person to person, the problem is easy to pass along, says J. Owen Hendley, M.D., professor of pediatrics and head of pediatric infectious disease at the University of Virginia School of Medicine in Charlottesville. Pinworms take up residence in the large intestine of an infected child. At night or in the early morning, the female worms travel down to the anal opening and deposit their eggs on the surrounding skin. When the child scratches the itchy area, pinworm eggs get on his hands and under his fingernails.

Then, if he doesn't wash his hands, the pinworm eggs get on whatever he touches, including toys and other household objects. Other children come along, touch what the infected child touched, and get the eggs on their hands, too. If they stick their hands in their mouth without washing them first, says Dr. Hendley, they can swallow the eggs, get infected, and the next thing you know, those kids have itchy bottoms, too.

Once your doctor has confirmed that your child has pinworms, he'll probably prescribe medication. And, meanwhile, here's what to do yourself.

Reassure your child. The thought of having worms could upset anybody, especially a youngster. So it's important to explain to your child that this does not mean that he is bad or dirty, and that he does not have to be embarrassed. Lots of children get worms.

"These worms do not have much of a mouth. They have

MEDICAL ALERT

When to See the Doctor

One of the recommended ways to get rid of pinworms is with a medication that must be prescribed by your physician, says J. Martin Kaplan, M.D., professor of clinical pediatrics at Hahnemann University in Philadelphia. So you should take your child to the doctor when the telltale signs appear.

The prescribed medication, mebendazole (Vermox), is a pill that your child will take once or twice, depending on your physician's advice. The medication causes the worms to be expelled with bowel movements. "Treatment with mebendazole usually does the trick," says Janice Woolley, M.D., a pediatrician in private practice in Mercer Island, Washington.

In very rare instances, pinworms can enter the vagina and cause vaginitis, says Dr. Kaplan. If your little girl has pain or discharge, be sure to tell your physician.

---

no teeth and they can't bite," says J. Martin Kaplan, M.D., professor of clinical pediatrics at Hahnemann University in Philadelphia. He recommends saying to your child, "There is nothing to be afraid of. You can't be hurt. The only thing you will be bothered by is some itching, and the medicine the doctor has given you should take that away."

Put water to work against itching. If your child has a lot of itching, taking a bath or wiping the anal area with a moist cloth can bring some temporary relief, says Janice Woolley, M.D., a pediatrician in private practice in Mercer Island, Washington. But be sure to keep that cloth away from other members of the family—and wash your own hands thoroughly if you touch it.

Buy cartoon-y soap. To stop pinworm from spreading and to prevent re-infection, you should take steps to emphasize cleanliness. Good hand-washing habits are particularly important, says Dr. Kaplan. If your child is potty training, encourage hand washing by overseeing her. Buy a soap that

THE DETECTIVE WORK IS UP TO YOU

Experts say that the best way to pin the rap on pinworms is for parents to collect the hard evidence themselves.

While your child is sleeping, spread the cheeks of his buttocks and look at the anal opening with a flashlight. Sometimes you can see the female worms, which are a whitish color and about ¼ to ⅓ inch long. "They look like a small piece of cotton," says J. Martin Kaplan, M.D., professor of clinical pediatrics at Hahnemann University in Philadelphia.

If you can catch one with a pair of tweezers, stick it in a bottle or small plastic bag and take it to your doctor, says Dr. Kaplan. But even if you're not quick enough to nab a worm, be sure to tell the doctor that you've seen one, he says.

You may be able to collect a sample of pinworm eggs from a sleeping child by pressing a piece of cellophane tape against the skin around the anal opening. You can't see the eggs, but if they're there, the tape will pick them up. Seal the potential evidence onto the tape by placing it on a glass slide (which you can get from your doctor or buy at the drugstore), sticky side down. Take this to your doctor who will look for the presence of eggs under a microscope.

Usually, the detective work doesn't even wake kids up, says Dr. Kaplan. You can also check when your child comes to you complaining of itching, or first thing in the morning before your child has had her bath.

she will relate to and want to play with, such as soap in the shape of a cartoon character, he says.

Keep nails cut short. Regularly trimming back your child's fingernails can also help, adds Dr. Woolley. Long fingernails provide convenient hiding places for eggs in transit. If you cut them short, it's easier for the child to wash up thoroughly—and wash away those eggs.

Practice moderation. Emphasize good hygiene, but don't go overboard. "You can wash your child's anal area, but don't scrub too hard in an effort to achieve ultra-cleanliness," says Donald Gromisch, M.D., professor and chairman of the Department of Pediatrics at Nassau County

---

IT'S A FAMILY AFFAIR

Because pinworms are so mobile, there's a chance that if one member of your family gets infected, others will, too. "I usually treat the entire family the first time around because it is so common for others to get infected," says Janice Woolley, M.D., a pediatrician in private practice in Mercer Island, Washington. The usual treatment is for each family member to take a mebendazole (Vermox) pill.

Other doctors treat only the infected child at first. But if the worms make a repeat performance, the entire family is then checked. "If reinfection occurs, everyone in the household should be examined, because you can get a Ping-Pong infection, where pinworms just move from one person to the next," says Donald Gromisch, M.D., professor and chairman of the Department of Pediatrics at Nassau County Medical Center in East Meadow, New York, and professor of pediatrics at the State University of New York at Stony Brook.

Since thorough hand washing helps prevent reinfection, be sure all the children in the family lather up. Also, remember that being infected once does not "vaccinate" you from being infected again, says Dr. Woolley. So keep up the good habits.

Medical Center in East Meadow, New York, and professor of pediatrics at the State University of New York at Stony Brook. Scrubbing can be counterproductive if it irritates the child's behind, he says.

POISON IVY, OAK AND SUMAC

Stopping the Scratching before It Starts

You tuck your tired kids into bed, all worn out from an afternoon's play in the park. The next morning you hear plaintive cries from their bedrooms, and when you investigate, you discover unhappy children with red itchy patches on their hands and legs.

Looks like poison ivy—or poison oak or poison sumac. Regardless of which of the three your children encountered, the cause of the trouble is the same: an oil called urushiol. "It oozes out when any part of the plant—the roots, leaves or flowers—is crushed," explains William Epstein, M.D., professor of dermatology at the University of California, San Francisco, School of Medicine.

If one child escaped the wrath of the plant, that doesn't imply lifelong immunity. Children under seven are rarely sensitive to this oil, say experts, and it takes at least one exposure to develop a sensitivity. (Some people don't become sensitive until after several exposures—and about 30 percent of the population never does.)

You'll know if your child is sensitive within 12 to 48 hours after he comes in contact with the plant's leaves, roots or stems. "The area first becomes red and itchy, and blisters appear a few days later, then oozing and crusting," explains Dr. Epstein. You can expect a week to ten days of uncomfortable itching, he says.

What can a parent do? Here are some things to help soothe the misery—and ways to avoid exposure to these plants in the future.

Treatment

Try some ice. Applying an ice cube wrapped in a plastic bag to the itchy area for one minute can help cool the itch, says Bill Halmi, M.D., clinical assistant professor of dermatology at the Thomas Jefferson University Hospital in Philadelphia. If an ice cube isn't available, use cold running water.

Coat with calamine. Yes, the same stuff you likely used as a kid. "This old over-the-counter lotion is still a good choice," says Dr. Epstein. "It helps the itch and it helps dry up the blisters." Be sure to check the expiration date on any calamine bottle that you may have in your cabinet, since after the expiration date it's no longer effective.

Take a soothing bath. A warm—but not hot—bath with

MEDICAL ALERT

When to See the Doctor

Poison ivy, oak or sumac is little more than an obnoxious nuisance for most kids. But some children—about 10 to 15 percent of those who are sensitive—have reactions so severe that a trip to the doctor is imperative, says William Epstein, M.D., professor of dermatology at the University of California, San Francisco, School of Medicine. "It's one of the few true emergencies in dermatology," he says, and may require immediate treatment with corticosteroids.

Here are signals that you should head for the emergency room or call your doctor immediately.

- Your child gets red and itchy and starts to swell within 4 to 12 hours after exposure (normally, a reaction doesn't occur for 12 to 48 hours)
- Your child's eyes are swollen shut
- Your child's discomfort is so intense that she is unable to go about daily routines
- Your child is itching and oozing so much that clothes stick to the skin

---

either baking soda or oatmeal can provide relief for an itchy child. Fill the bathtub with warm water and stir in about ½ cup of baking soda. Then let your child lie down and soak for a while, says Dr. Epstein. For an oatmeal bath, use ground colloidal oatmeal, such as Aveeno, advises Robert Rietschel, M.D., chairman of the Department of Dermatology at the Ochsner Clinic and clinical associate professor of dermatology at Louisiana State University and Tulane University School of Medicine, all in New Orleans. This product is available at most drugstores. Directions for use are on the package.

Cool the flame with a fan. Seat your child in front of a fan, lay a dampened washcloth across the itchy area and switch on the fan, suggests Dr. Rietschel. "This tends to dry up the ooze by causing evaporative cooling," he explains. "As the skin cools, the blood vessels compress, which in turn helps cut down on the ooze." Try this four times a day during the two to three days the blisters are at their worst.

Reach for OTC antihistamines. An over-the-counter antihistamine such as Benadryl can help cut down on the itch, says Dr. Rietschel. "What's more, since it tends to make kids drowsy, it can be particularly helpful if your main problem is getting the child to sleep through the night," he says. Be sure to read package directions to make certain the product is recommended for your child's age. For the correct dosage, follow package directions or consult your physician. Some doctors don't advise Benadryl cream or spray because it could cause a reaction.

DEBUNKING THE BLISTER MYTH

The blisters that you get from poison ivy, oak or sumac sometimes ooze—and the ooze is infectious-looking stuff. But it's actually harmless and *doesn't* spread the rash, according to Robert Rietschel, M.D., chairman of the Department of Dermatology at the Ochsner Clinic and clinical associate professor of dermatology at Louisiana State University and Tulane University School of Medicine, all in New Orleans.

"Inside those blisters is simply your own serum, a clear liquid from your blood," says Dr. Rietschel. "Once the blisters have formed, the poison oils that caused the rash are long gone."

Because the blisters can continue to appear over a week's time, however, many people assume that scratching the blisters has caused the ooze to spread the rash, says Dr. Rietschel. In fact, the skin only breaks out in the area where it initially came in contact with the poisonous oil from the plant.

It takes longer to react to a small amount of poison than a large amount, Dr. Rietschel explains. "Where the poison was most concentrated is where the skin erupts first," he says. "Places where only a little bit of oil touched the skin erupt days later."

Smear on the hydrocortisone. "This topical cream may tone down the itch a bit," says Dr. Reitschel. You'll find hydrocortisone cream at your drugstore, and Dr. Reitschel recommends the 1 percent dosage.

Avoid these two topicals. You *shouldn't* use a topical antihistamine such as Caladryl or a topical anesthetic containing benzocaine, such as Solarcaine Medicated First Aid Spray, according to Dedee Murrell, M.D., dermatologist and junior faculty member at New York University School of Medicine in New York City. Your child could become sensitized to these drugs, causing a completely different rash to develop.

Preventive Care

Learn the enemy. An ounce of prevention is worth a pound of cure when it comes to itch-producing plants like poison ivy, oak and sumac. Point out these poisonous plants to your children so everyone can identify them, suggests Dr. Murrell. Libraries, nature centers and schools have books and pamphlets to help children identify poisonous plants of the region.

Try a barrier cream. Before setting out on a hike or other excursion where you might come in contact with poisonous plants, coat the exposed areas of your child's skin with a barrier cream. Three good choices are Stoko Gard, Hydropel or Hollister Moisture Barrier Skin Ointment, which were found to be more effective than other barrier preparations in studies at Duke University Medical Center in Durham, North Carolina.

"The difficulty is that all exposed parts of the body need to be covered," says Dr. Murrell. "If one square inch is left unprotected, your child can break out there." She recommends applying the cream an hour before your child goes out. If you live in an area with a lot of poisonous plants, it's advisable to reapply the cream every hour or so.

Limit Rover's romping. You may be carefully steering your children clear of all poisonous plants, but in the meantime your pooch is running gleefully through the woods—

and if he romps through a patch of poisonous plants, he'll likely come back with oil-coated fur, says Dr. Epstein. The dog won't be affected by that oil, but it will transfer to you or your children when you pet the dog or he rubs up against one of you. If your dog *does* get away from you—and you suspect he's been near such plants—hose him down to help remove the oil.

Wash the skin. If your child has just leapt into a patch of poison ivy to retrieve a Frisbee, quick intervention may prevent a reaction. "You have about ten minutes to wash it off before it's too late," says Dr. Rietschel.

Plain water will do the job, but it's better to use soap, says Dr. Halmi. Any kind of soap will do, but *don't* use a washcloth. The cloth might spread the offending oil around.

Wash everything. The oil from poison plants can stick to *anything*, and it can remain active for months. If your child has been exposed, promptly wash his clothes and towel in hot water, says Dr. Epstein. Also wash hiking boots, toys and tools. Rubber and cotton gloves offer some protection, but only for a short time. After you've hosed down or washed the contaminated articles, drop the gloves in the washer and immediately wash *your* hands, says Dr. Halmi.

Break out the alcohol. While soap and water are best at eliminating the oil, in a pinch you can use rubbing alcohol. "If you use it immediately, rubbing alcohol will dissolve the poison plant oils," says Dr. Epstein. This can be harsh on sensitive skin, but it's still better than living with an itchy outbreak.

Never, ever burn it. If you burn your yard debris, make sure you never get any of these poisonous plants mixed in. Getting near the smoke or fire from burning plants can have disastrous effects, says Dr. Epstein. "Not only does the oil splatter like grease in a hot pan, it can even become airborne," he says. The result can be an outbreak that looks like you rolled in a patch of poison ivy. Worst of all, if you inhale the smoke, you can get an outbreak in your nose or throat.

POSTURE PROBLEMS

Straight Talk about Slouching

Considering the power of gravity and the flexibility of young bodies, it's no wonder kids slouch around and drape themselves over the furniture. But as sure as there will always be slouching kids, there will always be parents to holler *"Stop slouching!"* Trouble is, that parental war cry usually falls on deaf ears. Gravity has the upper hand.

But how important is good posture?

"We are born with normal curves in our spine, and the intention of good posture is to support those natural curves and maintain them," says Eli Glick, a physical therapist at Phycare Physical Therapy in Bala Cynwyd and Flourtown, Pennsylvania. "If your child slouches when he walks—and leans back in a chair when he sits—he's increasing his chances of injuring his spine."

The postural behavior your children are learning now will stay with them throughout their adult lives, according to Glick. Poor posture as a child can mean back pain as an adult.

But how can you help your kid straighten up when "Quit slouching!" doesn't seem to be doing the trick? Here are some posture-improvement tips from the professionals.

Get your kid moving. "Probably the best thing for every kid is to be active in some kind of nontraumatic athletic activity," says Scott Haldeman, M.D., Ph.D., D.C., a chiropractor and associate clinical professor of neurology at the University of California at Irvine. "My personal preference is swimming, since it's the least traumatic and exercises all muscles of the body, including those that could help improve posture." Other good sports for posture improvement include soccer, basketball and running, according to Dr. Haldeman. But he doesn't recommend football.

Practice some sitting stretches. To improve her posture, your child should try some exercises while she's in a sitting position, according to Sharon DeCelle, a physical therapist

MEDICAL ALERT

When to See the Doctor

Sometimes, a child's slouching is the result of a growth problem rather than an actual posture problem, according to Scott Haldeman, M.D., Ph.D., D.C., a chiropractor and associate clinical professor of neurology at the University of California at Irvine. This may be the case if a child has scoliosis, an abnormal side-to-side curvature of the spine.

If scoliosis runs in your family, you'll want to keep an eye on your children through adolescence for signs of abnormality.

"Look for one shoulder being higher than the other, or one hip that appears higher than the other. Notice if clothing never fits your child right or if hems are always uneven. Those are tipoffs to get professional screening. When in doubt, see an orthopedist who specializes in scoliosis," says Dr. Haldeman.

---

in private practice in Memphis and Director of Physical Therapy at Hillhaven-Raleigh, a skilled nursing facility, also in Memphis. Have your child sit erect in a chair, well away from the back of the chair. Ask her to pull her shoulders together toward the back. She should then try to push her shoulders downward to bring them out of the slouch position.

Then ask your child to raise her arms over her head with her palms turned to the outside. She should move her arms down, bending her elbows, as though she were trying to put them into her back pockets, then hold for five to ten seconds.

"Have your child do this exercise several times in a row, three times a day," suggests DeCelle. Even better, she says, do the exercise with your child, since most of us don't have optimal posture.

Talk about what's going on. "At puberty, girls sometimes slouch to hide their development," says DeCelle. "Since girls grow faster than boys, they are often self-conscious about their height and their breasts," points out DeCelle. Talk to your daughter about the changes she's experiencing, she suggests. Help her feel good about herself, and reassure her.

Go the sign-up route. One of the best things you can do to help your child overcome poor posture is to sign her up for some type of movement class: dance, gymnastics, ice skating or swimming lessons—anything the child enjoys and wants to learn, says DeCelle. "These classes will help promote the child's awareness of her body, teach motor skills and instill self-confidence."

Add motion to sitting. "It's really important to encourage children *not* to stay seated in a chair for hour after hour," points out Glick. Since long periods of sitting motionless puts a lot of stress on the spine, a child should stand up and move about as often as possible, preferably changing positions every half-hour.

When your child *has* to stay in his seat (in school, for instance), suggest that he take a "stretch break" every 15 to 30 minutes, adds Dr. Haldeman. "The child can stretch by leaning forward to touch the floor or leaning backward and stretching his legs out in front of him," he says.

Raise the book. A child isn't doing his spine any good if he's hunched over a desk looking down at a book. "When your child is doing homework, he should raise his book to an angle," says Glick. It's handy to have a book stand on the desk. But if he doesn't have one, he can just lean the book he's reading against another pile of books.

Buy a child-size chair. The best furniture for children is a size that fits their bodies, notes Dr. Haldeman. "If you sit in a chair that is either too big or too small, you're more likely to be squished into an uncomfortable position that could affect posture." He encourages parents to get child-size chairs and tables that kids can use comfortably.

Have his eyesight checked. Poor eyesight can also contribute to bad posture if your child is forced to bend over his books just to see the print, says Glick. If your child hunches over his desk to peer closely at the page, have his vision checked.

Adjust the computer angle. If everyone in the family uses one computer, the screen may be set at a convenient height for adults rather than children. Show your child how to adjust the monitor so he can view it comfortably, suggests Glick.

Position a pillow. "Proper seating is important for good posture," says Glick. The best kind of chair provides support up and down the entire spine, including the small of the back. A straight-backed chair can be improved if you place a pillow behind the child's lower back for better support. If a regular bed pillow is too big, try a smaller sofa pillow or purchase a special back pillow.

Say okay to bare feet. Recent research has shown that children are more likely to have good posture if they go without shoes as often as possible and is safe, according to Janet Perry, a physical therapist with Rehabilitation Network in Portland, Oregon. "That way they get more 'sensory information' from their feet and will have better walking and postural skills." Children should be allowed to go shoeless around the house—and in other places where it's safe to walk barefoot—as a way to improve their posture, according to Perry.

Remind him to stop slouching. As simple as it may sound, "You have to tell your child to stop slouching when he's slouching," says Dr. Haldeman. Your reminders may be viewed as a hassle, but your child will get in the habit of standing up straight—at least when you're around.

Change your TV pose. "Set a good example," suggests Glick. If the parents and older siblings slouch, younger children are likely to slouch, too. "Lying on the couch in front of the TV is a poor setup," says Glick. If that's what Daddy and Mommy do, it will be hard to convince Junior to sit up straight.

Put a foot up. "If your child has to stand somewhere for a long period of time, teach him to put one of his feet up on something for a while, and then switch back and forth, putting one foot up for a while, then the other," says De-Celle. Standing with one foot up takes some strain off the back.

PRICKLY HEAT

An Array of Rash Approaches

You are taking your two-week-old for her first ride in the stroller on a mild spring day. Although the thermometer is registering 61°F, the breeze feels chilly. So you carefully dress your baby in a long-sleeved T-shirt, overalls and a lovely pink angora hat and jacket knitted by Great Aunt Edith. You also tuck her under a blanket.

Your walk goes well, and you both enjoy the fresh air. But when you get home, it's a while before you divest your daughter of all those extra clothes. When you do, you notice a fine, pink rash on her neck and upper back. What you're looking at is called prickly heat, the end result of too much heat with no place to go.

"When a baby gets hot, sweat must evaporate off the skin in order to cool her body down," says Scott A. Norton, M.D., a staff dermatologist at Tripler Army Medical Center in Honolulu. "If you interfere with this process by covering the skin with lots of clothing, plastic pants or even heavy moisturizers, the sweat that needs to get out becomes trapped beneath the surface of the skin, resulting in an itchy rash."

Newborns are particularly vulnerable to prickly heat because their sweat ducts are not mature, which makes it easier for the beads of moisture to be trapped, says Dr. Norton.

Although prickly heat is common in babies, who are unable to complain about being overdressed, older kids can get the rash, too. Fortunately, it's easy to treat and even easier to prevent. Here's how.

Don't overdress your child. "While prickly heat can some-times occur as the result of fever, the most common cause is overdressing or swaddling a baby tightly in warm blankets," says Dr. Norton. Dress your baby sensibly—preferably in lay-ers that can be peeled away as conditions change—and you'll likely avoid the problem altogether, he says.

Avoid heavy moisturizers. Tender newborn skin tends to be dry and in need of moisturizing. But heavy, oil-based creams can be a problem, notes Dr. Norton. "Moisturize with a light, water-based lotion instead," he advises. Mois-turel, Lubriderm and Alpha-Keri body oil are some of the moisturizers you can use.

Keep cotton in contact with skin. Plastic is a great mate-rial for keeping wetness out, but it also traps moisture in the skin. "Let your child's skin breathe by using cotton rather than plastic diaper wraps, and by covering plastic mattress and playpen covers with cotton ones," says Sam Solis, M.D., chairman of the Department of Pediatrics at Children's Hospital, assistant professor of pediatrics at Tu-lane University School of Medicine, both in New Orleans, and a pediatrician in Metairie, Louisiana.

Bring the temperature down. The first step in treating

MEDICAL ALERT

When to See the Doctor

Properly treated, prickly heat should disappear within a few days, according to Betti Hertzberg, M.D., a pediatrician and head of the Continuing Care Clinic at Miami Children's Hos-pital. But there could be complications if bacteria get trapped under the skin, she says. This can occur when your child scratches the itchy rash. Dr. Hertzberg suggests you make sure that your child's nails are short and clean, and that you see a physician if there is pus, inflammation, red streaking or fever associated with the prickly heat. These are all signs of a secondary infection.

prickly heat once it develops is to get your child to stop sweating. "Remove some clothing, take her into an air-conditioned room or sit her in a tub of tepid water," suggests Dr. Solis. (The water should be just a little warmer than skin temperature.)

Soak away the itch. To counter the itching that accompanies prickly heat, add some baking soda or a colloidal oatmeal product such as Aveeno Bath Treatment to a tub of tepid water, suggests Betti Hertzberg, M.D., a pediatrician and head of the Continuing Care Clinic at Miami Children's Hospital. "Have your child splash around in the tub for a while," says Dr. Hertzberg. "A good soak will soothe the skin and take away the itching."

Try a cool compress. While a thin coating of mild, water-based moisturizing lotion may help stop the itching, cool compresses sometimes work better. Make a compress by dipping a washcloth in a mixture of one teaspoon of baking soda per cup of cool water, suggests Dr. Hertzberg. Apply to the rash for five to ten minutes or as long as your child can tolerate it. This should be done four or five times a day, Dr. Hertzberg says.

Bed down with an antihistamine. If your child is extremely itchy, give her an itch-relieving antihistamine such as Benadryl Elixir before she goes to sleep, suggests Dr. Hertzberg. (Be sure to read package directions to make certain the product is recommended for your child's age. For the correct dosage, follow package directions or consult your physician. Some doctors don't advise Benadryl cream or spray because it could cause a reaction.) "Kids are much more sensitive to itchiness at night, and more likely to scratch the rash, which can lead to infection," she says.

Apply a hydrocortisone cream. "For kids aged three or older, soothe the itch with a light coating of 1 percent hydrocortisone cream," says Dr. Norton. "You can apply this over-the-counter remedy twice a day for two days to soothe itching and relieve inflammation and redness," he says.

Screen the sun without grease. Older kids tend to get

prickly heat when they use a heavy, oily sunscreen that clogs sweat pores, notes Dr. Norton. The answer to the problem is *not* to stop using sunscreen, however. "Because of the problems associated with sun exposure, children should always use sunscreen, but it's best to avoid the oily, cocoa butter-laden preparations," says Dr. Norton. In his practice in Hawaii, he advises his patients to use less greasy lotions that are hypo-allergenic, block UVA and UVB sunlight and are marketed for young children.

RINGWORM

A Round-Up of Remedies

Bathtime can be filled with wonderful discoveries. Your child learns to blow bubbles, she says the word *boat* or she grabs the washcloth and exclaims, "Mine! I do it!"

But bathtime is not so wonderful for the parent who discovers a curious, round patch on a child's scalp or skin. Typically, the patch starts out looking just a little dry and flaky. But a day or two later, you may notice that the patch is larger, and it's clearly circular, with a flat center and a raised, reddish border. Your doctor's diagnosis: ringworm.

Named for the characteristic circular shape of the patches, ringworm isn't actually caused by worms. Instead, it's the result of a fungus infection. This particular type of fungus comes in a variety of forms, but the two that occur most often in children are on the scalp and the body.

If your child has scalp ringworm, first you'll see either flakes or little bumps on the child's head, says Bernard A. Cohen, M.D., director of pediatric dermatology at Johns Hopkins University School of Medicine in Baltimore.

Sometimes the symptoms can resemble severe dandruff.

AVOID MAJOR HAIR FALLOUT

If your child has scalp ringworm, he's likely to lose some hair. But if the ringworm is treated early and properly, this loss is only temporary and the hair grows back, says Bernard A. Cohen, M.D., director of pediatric dermatology at Johns Hopkins University School of Medicine in Baltimore. You should, however, be aware of warning signs and take prompt action to avoid more serious or extensive hair loss.

Permanent hair loss can happen if the child who gets scalp ringworm has an allergic reaction to the fungus. In these cases, a crusted area called a kerion can form. Often about the size of a fifty-cent piece, a kerion has pustules, or raised swollen plaques. Not only is it tender, the kerion can also break down, and you may see some oozing and weeping. Later, scar tissue may form.

"A kerion is not a common problem," says Dr. Cohen, "but when it does occur, if it is not treated early, there is a significant risk of scarring." When scarring occurs there can be a permanent bald spot in that area, he says. So the bottom line is to get your child's ringworm treated promptly.

As the infection progresses, the marks spread out, forming circles or ovals with flat centers and raised, red borders, says Dr. Cohen. Sometimes there's itching, and you may see areas with broken hair shafts or definite hair loss.

A child with body ringworm develops similar-looking patches, but they occur only on hairless areas of the body. These can be flaky and itchy, too.

"Between 3 and 5 percent of kids in the United States get ringworm," estimates William L. Weston, M.D., chairman of the dermatology department and professor of dermatology and pediatrics at the University of Colorado School of Medicine in Denver. "Nationwide, ringworm of the scalp predominates because the majority of kids live in cities, and scalp ringworm prevails in urban areas," Dr. Weston says. "Ringworm of the body is seen more often in rural areas."

Scalp Ringworm

If your doctor determines that scalp ringworm is the problem, he'll probably prescribe an oral medication (usually griseofulvin or ketoconazole). While you're waiting for the medicine to work, here are some additional steps you can take at home.

Pair the medicine with milk, not juice. "Griseofulvin is best absorbed when it is taken along with something that contains fat," says Dr. Cohen. "So your child should take it with a meal, ice cream or a glass of whole milk, not juice or water."

Segregate combs, brushes and hats. The fungus that causes ringworm can be transmitted via contaminated objects, says Dr. Cohen. So don't let your child share personal items with any other kids when she has ringworm. Keep her combs, brushes and hats on a high shelf so other children in the family don't use them. And because the fungus can also be spread through hand-to-hair contact, try to keep little girls from braiding or playing with each other's hair, says Dr. Cohen.

Settle for a little less scratching. There is nothing you can do to stop your child from scratching her head during the night, says Sandra Hurwitch, R.N., a dermatology nurse at the Dermatology Clinic of Children's Hospital in Boston. But during the day, try to distract your child from the itching by engaging her in activities. Give her something to occupy her hands, such as crayons or paints, she suggests.

Talk to the teacher. Experts agree, there's no reason to keep a child out of school just because she has ringworm. But you should tell your child's teacher about the problem, explain where the infection is located and discuss what to tell other kids in the class. Being careful not to single out the child, the teacher should take the opportunity to reinforce good personal hygiene habits, which include not sharing combs, brushes and hats. "Children may get frightened about catching the fungus from someone else," says Hur-

SHAMPOO WITH SPECIAL SUDS

If your child has scalp ringworm and is taking the oral medication griseofulvin, she should also wash her scalp with a lotion containing selenium sulfide, says A. Howland Hartley, M.D., associate professor of dermatology and pediatrics at the George Washington Medical Center and head of dermatology at Children's National Medical Center in Washington, D.C. "Selenium kills fungus spores and seems to expedite the therapy," he says.

Your physician may prescribe Selsun Rx, a lotion that contains 2½ percent selenium sulfide. If the scalp is crusty and oozing, he may advise shampooing every day. For less serious cases, two or three shampoos per week are sometimes recommended. And other members of the family can also use the selenium sulfide shampoo as a preventive.

Over-the-counter shampoos with selenium sulfide are available, but some of them contain less than 2½ percent selenium sulfide, cautions Dr. Hartley. You should check with your physician before using these nonprescription products because they may be less effective than prescription formulas, he says.

witch. "But ringworm won't spread from one person's scalp to another's unless there is close contact."

Top it off with a cap. If your child is embarrassed by the appearance of her patchy scalp, or if people overreact to seeing it, send her out with a hat, suggests J. Martin Kaplan, M.D., professor of clinical pediatrics at Hahnemann University in Philadelphia. Covering ringworm will not encourage the growth of the fungus. You can buy your child a cap that has a favorite cartoon character or sports team logo on it, or a stylish hat from a kids' clothing store.

Don't rely on OTC creams. The experts agree that trying an over-the-counter antifungal cream to treat scalp ringworm can do more harm than good. "Tinea capitis is not something to be treated with OTCs," says A. Howland Hartley, M.D., associate professor of dermatology and pediatrics at the George Washington Medical Center and head of dermatology at Children's National Medical Center in Washington, D.C.

If you apply a topical ointment, it can kill the fungus on top of the skin, but it won't reach the fungus below the scalp at the hair follicles, Dr. Hartley says. That could make it harder for your doctor to detect the fungus and diagnose the problem.

Consider a communal checkup. That childhood saying, "There's a fungus among us" is all too appropriate here. Ringworm is contagious. And if your child has scalp ringworm, it's possible that other family members could get scalp *or* body ringworm. "If one child in the family is infected, I recommend other family members get checked, too," says Dr. Cohen.

Body Ringworm

"Because ringworm on the body can be confused with other skin disorders such as eczema, you need a physician to diagnose it," says Dr. Kaplan. But once it's been positively identified, treatment can begin.

Rub on some relief. Your doctor may prescribe a topical antifungal medication. But it's also possible to treat body ringworm with over-the-counter ointments, according to Dr. Cohen. Among the nonprescription creams recommended by doctors are the miconazoles, such as Micatin, and the clotrimazoles, such as Lotrimin.

Generally, these ointments are applied to the affected area two or three times a day for six weeks—but check the package label for specific directions. "Don't expect to see results for at least a week," says Janice Woolley, M.D., a pediatrician in private practice in Mercer Island, Washington. "And even if you see good results within two weeks, continue using it until the last sign of ringworm disappears," she says.

One sign that the area is getting better is if the rash begins to flatten out and the blisters start to dry up, says Dr. Cohen. The skin may get flaky and peel off, he adds.

"If the area is so flat that you can close your eyes and run your finger over it without feeling a thing, then the ringworm is gone," he says.

(If over-the-counter products let you down, however, ask your doctor about topical ointments that are available by prescription only, suggests Dr. Cohen.)

Leave cortisone combos on the shelf. When selecting an over-the-counter ointment, read the labels carefully and steer clear of products that contain both an antifungal agent and cortisone. "There is no role for combination medications in treating ringworm," says Dr. Cohen. Cortisone suppresses the redness so it looks like the problem is getting better faster than it really is, he explains. "But as soon as you stop the medication, the fungus comes back," he warns.

Say yes to school. Kids with body ringworm, like those with scalp ringworm, can go to school, Dr. Kaplan says. But he warns that other children should not touch the affected area. Be especially sure to tell your child not to share clothing, such as sweatpants or sweatshirts, that may have touched the affected area.

RUNNY NOSE

Drying Up the Drip

A mong kids, runny noses are as common as sticky fingerprints on the woodwork. And when kids get together, wet noses often outnumber dry ones. That's because a runny nose is usually a sign of the common cold. And experts say the average child is likely to catch a cold virus about eight times a year. Figure in the fact that colds are spread fastest by busy hands, multiply this by all the times children handle the same books and playthings, and it adds up to a lot of drippy noses.

And viruses aren't the only cause. Runny-nose problems

MEDICAL ALERT

When to See the Doctor

If you have an infant, you should contact your doctor if your baby's runny nose is accompanied by a fever, or if it prevents him from eating or drinking, says Lee D. Eisenberg, M.D., assistant professor of otolaryngology at Columbia University College of Physicians and Surgeons in New York City.

For an older child, check with the doctor if his runny nose is accompanied by coughing or a fever of 103° or more. If the nasal discharge persists beyond two weeks, or the mucus is yellowish or has a strong odor, you'll also need to check with a physician. "Color, odor and a cough can all indicate an infection that should be treated with antibiotics," says Dr. Eisenberg.

can also be prompted by cold air or by allergens like dust, animal dander and pollen.

Of course, there's a good side to mucus. It's nature's cleansing mechanism, according to Ted Kniker, M.D., professor of pediatrics, microbiology and internal medicine in the Division of Pulmonology, Allergy and Critical Care Medicine in the Department of Pediatrics at the University of Texas Health Science Center in San Antonio. "A runny nose has some utility because it helps flush out bacteria, viruses, irritants and tissue debris associated with inflammation," he says.

But even a good thing can be overdone. A nose that runs too heavily or too often can make both you and your child uncomfortable. If that's the case, here's what the experts suggest to do.

Encourage blowing with tissues. "The only trick to nose blowing is getting your child to do it," says Bob Lanier, M.D., a pediatric allergist and immunologist in private practice in Fort Worth, Texas, and host of the nationally syndicated radio and TV program "60 Second House Call." One way you can encourage a child to blow more often is by giving her some personal tissue packs. Add some stickers with her favorite cartoon characters—like the Little Mermaid, for example.

Teach toss-'em-out habits. Used tissues should go straight into the trash, or your child could pass on her cold virus to other kids, says Dr. Lanier. Make sure your child has a wastebasket nearby, and stress the importance of using it.

Teach her to wash her hands afterward, too. Studies show that contaminated hands spread viruses faster than sneezes do, says Dr. Lanier. Remind your child to wash her hands after using tissues, and after a while she'll get into the habit.

Buy a tube of lip balm. "A child may resist nose blowing because her upper lip is raw from wiping away mucus," says Helen Baker, M.D., clinical professor of pediatrics at the University of Washington in Seattle. An older child can carry lip balm in his pocket and use it as needed to soothe the irritated area. Toddlers are too young to carry lip balm, but a thin coating of petroleum jelly may help. "Try to smear a coating of Vaseline on your child's upper lip whenever you get the chance," says Dr. Baker.

Give a salty squirt. Over-the-counter saline (saltwater) drops and sprays, such as Ocean, can help flush out irritants that may be causing the nose to run, says Dr. Kniker. To put the drops in your child's nose, have him lie on his back on the bed, with his head over the edge, advises Dr. Baker. Place two drops in each nostril and let them seep in for two to three minutes.

Prop up the head of the bed. Tuck a strong support under the head of the bed, to elevate it, suggests Dr. Baker. In addition, you can use extra pillows to prop up the child's body even more. The prop should be about 18 inches high. That way, you enlist gravity's help so mucus can drain better. You also help prevent seepage down the back of the throat, which can lead to coughing fits, he says.

THE "SNIFFLE SALUTE" MAY SIGNAL ALLERGY

"If your child's runny nose lasts more than two weeks, there's a good chance it's caused by an allergic condition," says Ted Kniker, M.D., professor of pediatrics, microbiology and internal medicine in the Division of Pulmonology, Allergy and Critical Care Medicine in the Department of Pediatrics at the University of Texas Health Science Center at San Antonio. An obvious clue is if he constantly rubs the tip of his nose with his palm in an upward fashion—what some doctors refer to as the allergic salute. Other signs include intense sneezing, burning, itchy and watery eyes, and bluish circles under the eyes (known as allergic shiners).

A doctor can perform skin tests to help identify the sniffle trigger. For hay fever-like symptoms, your doctor may also suggest an over-the-counter antihistamine to help your child through the sneezing season. For more persistent symptoms, a prescription steroid nasal spray or allergy shots may be needed.

Another possible cause of runny nose in children under two is an allergy to a food such as cow's milk. "Five percent of all babies have cow's milk sensitivity, which can cause nasal allergy, asthma, colic, vomiting, diarrhea and skin rashes," says Dr. Kniker. When milk is removed from their diets and a formula with low allergy potential is substituted, he says, often the runny nose and other symptoms vanish. But this change in diet should only be made with a doctor's recommendation.

Fend off cold air with a scarf. If your child's nose drips when she's in cold, windy air, she probably has nonallergic rhinitis, says Lee D. Eisenberg, M.D., assistant professor of otolaryngology at Columbia University College of Physicians and Surgeons in New York City. This is a harmless, common condition that can be remedied by wearing a scarf over the nose to warm the incoming air, he says.

Suction away those secretions. A baby may have so

much excess mucus that it interferes with his breathing and he can't drink or eat comfortably. "He'll kick up a fuss until you clear his nose," says Dr. Baker. The fastest way to do this is with a rubber ear bulb, purchased from the drugstore. (She prefers it to a nasal aspirator because it has a longer, easier-to-use tip.)

Place the baby on his back. Squeeze the bulb, then insert the long, tapered tip in one nostril, and gently release the bulb to suction up the mucus. Withdraw the tip and squeeze the secretions out in a tissue. Repeat with the other nostril. When you're done with the ear bulb, boil it before you use it again.

SCHOOL REFUSAL

Help for the Reluctant

His first month in middle school, Stephen started missing the school bus routinely.

When Jane entered the first grade, she began having painful stomachaches every school morning.

Three-year-old Tyler screamed with anguish whenever his mother left him at preschool.

All these children shared a problem that occurs in many children: They didn't want to go to school. The possible causes range from simple separation anxiety at leaving their parents to serious problems with school, classmates or teacher.

After you've ruled out actual physical ailments, here's how you can deal with the child who doesn't want to go to school.

For All Children

Explain the facts. Whatever age your child, you need to explain why the child must go to school, says David Waller, M.D., pediatrician, child psychiatrist and chief of child and adolescent psychiatry at the University of Texas Southwestern Medical Center and Children's Medical Center in Dallas.

For the preschool child, keep it in simple terms: "This is a place where people will take care of you and you can play while we are at work" or "Mommy and Daddy want you to meet new friends, and this is a good place to do it." But make it clear that you're not angry at your child or punishing her.

For older children, explain that it's a law that they attend school. Dr. Waller recommends that you tell them the consequences of missing school or constantly being tardy. If the child knows he may receive poor grades, get detention or possibly have to repeat a year, he's more likely to climb on that morning bus.

Visit the school. For the child just starting preschool or kindergarten or transferring to a new school, arrange a visit before the first day.

"Spend some time in the classroom with your child," says Karen Smith, Ph.D., a pediatric psychologist and associate professor of pediatrics in the School of Medicine at the University of Texas Medical Branch in Galveston. "Talk to the teacher, too, so that your child can see that Mom and Dad like this new person, that she's not someone to be afraid of. You might need to do this more than once for very anxious children," she says.

Supply a map. Children can worry a great deal about finding their way around a strange place. Draw a map of the school in bright colors for your child and point out places such as the art room, bathroom and lunchroom. Hang the map on the wall of your child's room.

"It's important for your child to become familiar with the physical layout of any new school," says Leah Klungness, Ph.D., a psychologist in Locust Valley, New York. "Not being able to find the bathroom can upset a child who is already shaky about new beginnings."

Tantalize with descriptions. Find out what types of activities your child's preschool or school will have, and describe them to your child. "Talk to your child about the kinds of things he'll be doing there and the friends he'll make," suggests Dr. Smith. "Try to find something of interest that will happen in that setting that might not happen at home." For example, if your child will learn to fingerpaint at preschool or have recess every day at kindergarten, explain that to him.

Just for Preschoolers

Depart cheerfully. This means no prolonged leave-takings with smothering hugs and kisses and syrupy reassurances. "Don't tell your child, for example, that he shouldn't be afraid or that nothing bad will happen to him," says Dr. Waller. "If a child reads anxiety in a parent, he's bound to think that there must be something to be anxious about."

Give a quick kiss and a hug, tell your child when you will return and leave with a smile on your face—whether or not your child is screaming and beseeching you to come back.

Leave openly. Although it may seem easiest to sneak off while your child is playing quietly, don't do it. "Whether your child is howling or playing quietly, never just disappear," says Cathleen A. Rea, Ph.D., a clinical child psychologist at Riverside Regional Medical Center and the Behavioral Medicine Institute in Newport News, Virginia, and an assistant professor in the Department of Psychiatry and Behavioral Science at Eastern Virginia Medical School in Norfolk. "That's traumatic to a child; Mommy or Daddy disappearing is his worst fear. You need to let him know when you're leaving."

Plant a lipstick kiss. Preschool children may find a lipstick imprint from Mom comforting. "Cover your lips with lipstick and then kiss your child on her hand or wrist where she can see the lipstick imprint," suggests Dr. Klungness. "Lipstick doesn't wash off so easily, so it's a constant reminder of your presence."

Supply pictures of Mom and Dad. A small photo of his parents tacked into his cubby or locker may be immensely comforting. "A picture showing you in your office or workplace is particularly helpful," says Dr. Klungness. "Looking at that picture, the child sees you in a particular physical environment, and he won't feel as if you've disappeared."

Arrange for a greeting. It's important that you don't just drop your child off in a crowd of children, says Dr. Rea. "When you walk into the day care center, you want to have a teacher or aide come over immediately to greet you and your child. She should get down to eye level and help with the transition from parent to day care setting," she says. At a busy day care center, you may have to make a request in advance, but most caregivers will be happy to cooperate with this greeting arrangement.

Provide a time framework. Very young children often don't have a good sense of time, so telling your child a specific activity you will do together that evening will help her realize that day care isn't forever. "You could tell her that you'll stop for a snack on the way home, or that you'll read her favorite book while dinner is cooking," suggests Dr. Rea.

Take Teddy along. It can make day care far less frightening to take along a favorite toy, says Dr. Rea. "Bringing any special transitional object from home is often comforting to an anxious child," she says.

Ask about your child's behavior. After a few weeks you may feel that things aren't getting any better. Your child still screams and cries when you leave. But once you're out of sight—unknown to you—he may be playing happily the rest of the day.

"Check with your child's teacher to find out if there's a decrease in the intensity and the duration of the emotional distress your child experiences," suggests Dr. Smith. If your child adjusts rapidly after you leave, stop worrying.

For Older Children

Talk it out. Talk gently with your child to find out what is bothering him about school, suggests Dr. Klungness. If you can't discover the problem, arrange a conference with the teacher. There could be a bully who has been picking on your child. Other children could be taunting your child because of the style of his clothing. Your child may be anxious because he feels he's not doing well in school.

Or something could have happened that embarrassed your child. Dr. Rea counseled one child who refused to go to school after he dropped his lunch tray in the cafeteria. "It can be as innocuous as that," she says.

Think about things at home. A sudden change in your child's school-going behavior can sometimes be traced to events at home. "Consider if there is something going on at home that might have precipitated your child's refusal to go to school," advises Dr. Waller. "Sometimes a child who has experienced a death or illness in the family—or notices her parents' marital problems—feels that she is 'needed' at home and will do what she has to to remain there."

If there is a problem, don't lie to your child about it, but don't go into great detail either, says Dr. Waller. Explain that it is Mommy and Daddy's job to deal with the problem. Your child should understand that it's *her* job to go to school and try to do well. Reassure her that you will be honest with her so she doesn't feel she needs to stay home to know what's going on.

Take charge of real problems. While your child needs to know that every school day won't be perfect and that she has to learn to deal with problems, she also needs to know you will help when needed, says Dr. Klungness.

For instance, if your small child is being tormented or hit by other kids on the bus, talk to the bus driver or principal. If your child is having trouble with schoolwork, set aside time when the two of you can work together on problem areas. And if you become convinced that the teacher has taken a dislike to your child or doesn't want to help solve your child's problems, you should arrange a meeting with the principal to consider transferring your child to another class.

Accentuate the positive. For the child with minor problems; acknowledge what your child dislikes about school, but try to identify some things at school that she does like. Remind her of the music lessons she loves or a friend she sees only at school, says Dr. Smith.

Seek guidance. Talk to the school's guidance counselor or nurse and ask if your child can visit the nurse during the day if she suddenly becomes anxious, suggests Dr. Waller. You don't want to encourage frequent visits, but if the anxious child knows she has someone to turn to, it gives her reassurance. "It's better than coming home early, which would only reinforce the school refusal behavior," says Dr. Waller.

Give praise to your child. Sometimes the best reward is a big hug and a word of praise from Mom and Dad. Be sure to acknowledge your child's efforts. "Your child should be complimented every time she stays through the school day or goes to school without protest," says Dr. Smith.

SEPARATION ANXIETY

Parting without Such Sorrow

For all of us, life is filled with good-byes—sometimes tearful—but none are so poignant as those experienced by our children. At various developmental stages, preschoolers may exhibit what's known as separation anxiety, usually expressed by crying—even screaming—as we leave them at day care, at school or with a babysitter. Separation anxiety is not only normal, it's also a positive sign that your child is attached to you. But there are ways to take some of the pain and tears out of parting.

Let your child know you're always coming back. "If a mom tells me her child screams every time she leaves, I tell her, 'You don't get away often enough,' " says Robert Mendelson, M.D., a pediatrician and clinical professor of pediatrics at the Oregon Health Sciences University in Portland. "A child who screams every time his mother leaves may not be sure she's coming back." After several short absences, though, even the most anxious child should get the message that Mommy can leave and come back, too.

Prepare the child. Let your child know you will be leaving, even if it causes a little anticipatory anxiety. It's better than a surprise, says Jay Belsky, Ph.D., professor of human development at Pennsylvania State University in University Park. However, he cautions, don't belabor it. "Say simply and casually, 'Mommy and Daddy are going out and the babysitter is coming to stay with you.' If you keep talking about it," says Dr. Belsky, "it will sound like you're anxious, too, and you'll communicate that to your child."

No long good-byes. "At the point of departure, make it clean and crisp," says Dr. Belsky. "Standing in the doorway cajoling and explaining is the worst thing you can do because it creates more anxiety. Remind yourself that the distress you see at the point of separation is most likely not going to continue after you are gone."

Since it's short, make it sweet. Leaving the child with an "I love you" and a kiss may be helpful. Dr. Belsky suggests that you tuck a "kiss" into the child's pocket as a good-bye ritual.

Acknowledge the child's feelings. Instead of saying, "Now don't cry" or "Don't feel that way"—which betrays your own anxiety over having caused your child's distress—acknowledge how the child is feeling and reassure him. "Say 'I know this is difficult for you, but you're a big boy and I know you can do it,'" suggests Dr. Belsky. "Make sure you tell the child that it's okay to feel the way he does."

Leave something of yourself. Whether you give the child something personal, like a piece of jewelry or article of clothing, or start a project that you promise to finish when you return, you're sending the message "I am coming back," says Dr. Belsky. "Anything that sends that message, that preserves continuity and preserves the relationship is a good thing."

Plan some activities. "For the older child—five or so—it's often helpful to structure the time you're going to be away with games and activities because distraction can help children not obsess on the experience," says Sheila Ribordy, Ph.D., a clinical psychologist specializing in children and families and professor of psychology and director of clinical training in the Department of Psychology at De Paul University in Chicago.

Leave them with someone they know. Children feel much more secure with a familiar face than with a strange one. If you're using a new babysitter, ask her to come over at least 45 minutes before you leave. And be sure to sit and talk with the babysitter and your child before you walk out the door, suggests Dr. Belsky. "Parents should have a nice friendly conversation, maybe do some laughing with this person. Children usually feel that any friend of Mommy's is a friend of theirs."

SHYNESS

Guiding the Way to Social Skills

J ust as some kids seem born to be wild, others are born to be shy. "Shyness is often a symptom of a cautious temperament, which is hereditary, like blue eyes and curly hair," says Jerome Kagan, Ph.D., a leading shyness researcher and professor of psychology at Harvard University in Cambridge, Massachusetts.

"Unless shyness is interfering with your child's life, don't think of it as a problem," says Dr. Kagan. "Many children outgrow their shyness as they have more social experiences. You don't want your child to believe you are disappointed in him."

But what if shyness has grown to the point where your

child is having trouble making friends, is turning down invitations to classmates' parties and never volunteering in class? Then his shyness is a problem that can result in both academic problems and an unhappy social life.

"Shy kids have a hard time asking for help," says Lynne Henderson, Ph.D., director of the Palo Alto Shyness Clinic in Menlo Park, California. "A study of college students found that the shy ones were less likely than their non-shy peers to seek information or use the career placement service. They had a disadvantage that was handicapping their careers."

The experts agree: If your child's shyness is a real problem, the best time to start intervening is as early as possible. Here are some helpful techniques they recommend.

Don't put a label on it. "If you label a child as shy, you only see his shy behavior and tune out what is not shy," says Dr. Henderson. That affects the child's behavior and also affects your perception of him, she notes. Instead, point out the child's strengths, says Dr. Henderson. "Focus on the times when a child is being more social, rather than when he's being shy." Also, use some descriptive words that accentuate the strong points of his behavior, she suggests. For example, a shy person might be better described as cautious, careful or a deep thinker.

Ask for his feelings. Rather than scolding a child for being shy, reflect back to him in a neutral way what he may be feeling, suggests Dr. Henderson. "If he's hiding behind your leg instead of playing with his friends, say, 'It seems like you're not sure you want to play right now.' Something like this might be an accurate reflection of the child's experience but not a negative label," says Dr. Henderson.

Create safe social encounters. Allow the child to invite a schoolmate over after school. Or let him pay a visit to the home of a child he seems to like. "The more comfortable social experiences shy children have, the less anxious they become," says Dr. Kagan.

Be sociable yourself. "When your child is little, work on having people in the home," says Dr. Henderson. Invite friends for a weekend barbecue or a games night. Have another parent and her child over for lunch. "This is often difficult in homes where both parents work, but a shy child needs to get used to an environment with other people in it, so it doesn't seem so frightening."

Stay on standby with your child. For a shy child, large gatherings can be terrifying. "Don't just walk into a room full of people and leave the child standing there," says Dr. Henderson. "Hold onto the child's hand until she gets established. Wait for her to let go." Dr. Henderson recommends that you walk over to another child or a group of children and start talking to them until the child starts talking, too. "A shy child needs to feel secure and to know you're there if she needs you," he notes.

Encourage your child to talk at home. Establish a daily "good news" time. At dinner or bedtime, allow your child to share some good news of the day, suggests Dr. Henderson. "Listen in a nonjudgmental way to what he describes as the high point of his day and then acknowledge his feelings. You might ask what he enjoyed about the experience, but don't load him up with praise. "This is not a chance to give him an 'A' but a chance to share himself," says Dr. Henderson. "Being listened to and acknowledged with respect helps build self-confidence."

Follow the child's lead. Don't force your child into situations, says Dr. Kagan. Instead, listen carefully to what he says so you can help steer him toward activities and people he's shown an interest in. "You're trying for gentle desensitization, and that only works if the child is doing something he really wants to do."

Add the spice of variety. You never know what activity can spark the interest of a shy child. So be sure to explore the variety of activities available in your community, from swimming lessons to children's theater, suggests Dr. Henderson. This will help you and your child learn where his interests lie. "It's like food. You provide all the basic food groups and the child then can pick and choose."

Enlist the help of a teacher. A receptive, empathetic teacher can help lure your shy child out of the corner into the thick of things or pair him with a friendly classmate who is more outgoing, notes Dr. Henderson. Be sure to let the teacher know you're trying to find activities that will help your child feel good about himself. And show your appreciation for the teacher's help. "If you're really appreciative to a teacher who looks out for your child, she'll do more of it," says Dr. Henderson.

Have a dress rehearsal. Novel situations are a nightmare for shy people, because they generally tend to overestimate danger, says Byron Egeland, Ph.D, professor of child development in the Institute of Child Development at the University of Minnesota in Minneapolis. If your child is going to a party, starting in a new classroom or moving to a new neighborhood, talk about what is going to happen and go over some of the things he may see, hear or do, recommends Dr. Egeland. If possible, visit the new neighborhood or school with your child, talk to his new teachers and also have him meet the other children. "The more you can familiarize your child with a new situation, the less there is to fear," he says.

Stay cool, calm and casual. Even if you feel anxiety about a new situation, don't reveal that to your shy child when preparing him for new situations, suggests Dr. Kagan. "Many parents who were shy themselves are really worried their child will relive their unhappiness. They can get so tense that their anxiety is communicated to the child," he notes.

Share your experiences. Since 93 percent of the population acknowledges feeling shy at least once in a while, you no doubt have a story or two to tell about your insecurities. And those stories help a shy child to feel more confident in similar situations.

"Everybody feels shy sometimes. It's the human state," says Dr. Henderson. Share the ways you overcame your insecurities, she says. "Children need to see that this is just part of the everyday human struggle and that you can cope."

Don't demand perfection. "One of the problems we frequently have to work on in the shyness clinic is the belief
that being good socially somehow means being perfect all
the time," says Dr. Henderson. Shy children need to find
out that they can make friends without being perfect. "People think they need to act like movie stars," he notes. "But
kids need to know that being friendly doesn't mean being
perfect."

SIBLING RIVALRY

Suggestions to Stop the Slugfest

So, your kids don't exactly get along like the Waltons.
Okay, so they get along more like the World Wrestling
Federation. This is normal, right?

Wrong. Although parents can't necessarily recreate the
warm, fuzzy feelings the siblings on Walton's Mountain
had for each other, there are certainly many ways to avoid
full-scale warfare among brothers and sisters. "You can
easily make their interaction a better experience by what
you do," says child and family psychologist Barry Ginsberg,
Ph.D., executive director of the Center of Relationship En-
hancement in Doylestown, Pennsylvania.

"There are no easy answers, but it's important to remember that some conflict can be constructive—provided it
doesn't get out of hand," says Dr. Ginsberg. "Stresses and
fights occur because that's how we negotiate a new, more
stable level of relationship. But kids tend to be clumsy at
this, and so they need their parents' help."

Here are a few ways to maintain the peace in your household.

Set clear limits. You may not be able to stop your children
from arguing, but you can keep disagreements from escalat-
ing into brawls, says James Bozigar, a licensed social worker
and coordinator of community relations for the Family

Intervention Center at Children's Hospital of Pittsburgh. "Make it clear that hitting and the behaviors that often provoke it—name calling, taunting, attacking personal weaknesses—are off limits," he says. "You can say, 'You don't have to love your baby sister, you don't even have to like her, but you must stop hitting her.' "

Call a family powwow. If you're trying to establish new guidelines for behavior, it's better if the siblings themselves play a role in figuring out what those guidelines would be, says Adele Faber, coauthor of *Siblings without Rivalry*. Faber, who conducts nationwide workshops on sibling relationships, recommends calling a family meeting to do just that.

"Open the floor to discussion," she says. "When it's a rule the child has helped fashion, he'll want to try to make it work. But if it's a rule imposed from on high, he'll be more likely to test or challenge it."

Reinforce the family's new guidelines. If the rule is "no hitting," the disciplinary action for infractions should be a time-out, says Mark Roberts, Ph.D., a professor of psychology at Idaho State University in Pocatello. Dr. Roberts and his colleagues have studied which techniques are most effective in stopping sibling aggression. "Calling time-out wins hands down," he says. "When the kids begin to fight, parents should say, 'No hitting in this house. *You* sit on this chair, and *you* sit on that chair.' The chairs should be up against walls and around the corner from each other so the kids can't see each other. Wait two to five minutes, then talk with the kids about their argument. They will probably have cooled off, so this is a good time to discuss alternatives to fighting."

Substitute words for fists. Brothers and sisters who fight often don't know how to share, take turns, consider others' feelings or negotiate—all skills they're going to need to form relationships outside the home, says Faber. "So one of the rules that is especially helpful is, 'Say it with words, not with fists,' " she says. By using language to express their anger, siblings take the first step on the road to mutually respectful relationships.

Says Faber: "The sweetest thing I heard was from a mother who had tried this method. She called me and said, 'I passed by the kids' room today and saw my older child with his fists raised about to clobber his younger sister. She looked up at him and said, "Michael, use your words." He stopped, with his fists in mid-air, and said, "Get out of my room!" She said, "I'm going." I was so pleased.' I told that mother, 'Now, *that's* civilized behavior.' "

Don't ask who started it. The usual response to the question, "Who started it?" is a two-parter: "He did." "No, she did." But you don't want to play judge or jury, says Faber. "You won't get to the bottom of it. The bottom is bound to be murky. Often you'll hear, 'I had to hit him because I could tell he was about to hit me.' " It's better to say, "Boy, you two sound angry at each other!" That statement diminishes rage and provides an opening for a discussion of the children's real grievances. "So, Adam, you're upset because you want to watch TV. And, Jim, you're upset because you need quiet to study. What can be done in a case like this?"

Reflect feelings back to the child. Very few kids are really happy about sharing their parents' love and attention with someone else, even if that someone else is related to them. Negative feelings toward siblings are normal, says Faber. "It's important to allow those negative emotions to surface. Feelings that are banished don't vanish. They either go underground and get expressed in dreams, nightmares, headaches and stomachaches, or they're acted out in punches or pinches," she says.

Faber suggests listening to your child's feelings and then reflecting them back in a way that acknowledges the child's mixed emotions about a sibling—who is, after all, both an interloper and a playmate. "A father in one of my workshops listened to his son's long list of objections to his new baby sister. Then he reflected back to the boy, 'Sounds to me as if part of you wants her out of here forever. And part of you is sometimes glad she's here.' Periodically over the next few weeks, the little boy said, 'Daddy, tell me again about my two feelings.' I think that child is well on his way to emotional health," says Faber.

Create a special time for one-to-one parenting. "When a new sibling arrives, reserve special times when you can fully commit yourself to being with the older child," says Dr. Ginsberg. "Don't allow any external events to change this. The older child needs to be confident that he will have his special time alone with the parent."

Ask the older child to give you a hand. An older sibling will feel more involved in things if you give her a simple job to do, like bringing you diapers. "This will increase the child's sense of importance and responsibility," says Dr. Ginsberg. "You can say, 'Now that we're busier with the new baby and you're older, you can have this job that will help out around the house." Just be sure the task is meaningful—not some busy work invented simply to make the child feel better. "That's phony, and kids can see right through it," Dr. Ginsberg says.

Look for patterns. Sometimes, sibling fights exhibit a pattern, says Dr. Ginsberg. "Once you see the pattern, you can head off clashes by structuring—that is, shaping the situation in advance for the best kind of interaction possible," he observes.

"For example, if your children always fight when they get home from school, it may very well be to get your attention," Dr. Ginsberg says. "They've been away from you all day. If you're busy in the kitchen when they get home, they may feel this is the only way to get to you." So what can you do? "You can structure things differently by preparing dinner before your kids come in, and giving *them* your time and attention," he says. "Or include them in the meal-preparation process so they're there with you."

Figure out a way to say "you're special." "Children need to be seen and enjoyed as separate individuals," says Faber. "If you were to say to your husband, 'Who do you love more, your mother or me?' and he replied, 'Honey, I love you both equally,' he would be in big trouble. But if he said, 'Honey, there's no comparison. My mother is my mother and you're my beloved wife,' he'd be on safe ground."

The same policy works for kids. For example, when little Amy asks, "Who do you love best?" you can answer, "Each of my children is special. You are my only Amy. No one has your thoughts, your feelings, your smile, your way of doing things. Boy, am I lucky you are my child."

Respect sibling differences. While it may seem "fair" to give each child the same number of pancakes in the morning, this "fair" treatment doesn't recognize that each child's appetite may be different, says Faber. "If you hear, 'Hey, you gave him three pancakes and you only gave me two,' respond with, 'Oh, are you still hungry? Do you want a whole pancake or just a half? A whole? Well, one whole pancake coming up.' What you've done is shift the message from 'You are getting as much as your big brother' to 'I am meeting your individual needs.' "

SIDE STITCHES

So Long to the Pain

S ide stitches don't give much warning. One minute your kid is fine and the next minute he's doubled over with a sharp pain in the side. These unpleasant little pains can grab hold when your child is running after a soccer ball, sprinting for third base or just walking fast.

What causes a side stitch? No one knows for sure, but it apparently occurs when the diaphragm, the muscle that helps us breathe, doesn't get all the oxygen it needs. When the diaphragm or the abdominal muscle in front of the diaphragm begins to spasm—that is, tighten and release in short, spasmodic bursts—the child feels a painful side stitch.

You can help prevent or stop your child's side stitch quickly with these tips from the experts.

Warm up before working out. Your child can avoid

most stitches by taking time to warm up, says Eli Glick, a physical therapist at PhyCare Physical Therapy in Bala Cynwyd and Flourtown, Pennsylvania. "Before running or other active exercise, have your child do calisthenics like touching his toes and doing sit-ups. He should do this for about 10 to 15 minutes to increase blood flow and respiration," says Glick.

Stretch to stop stitches. The child should also stretch his arms and rib cage, says Glick. To stretch his arms, he should reach for the sky with his arms stretched over his head and slowly bend to each side. Lower the arms, then push forward with the arms, rounding out the back and shoulders. For rib cage expansion, have the child do a slow, gentle, large yawn. Repeat each stretch several times.

Encourage fitness. Side stitches are usually related to a lack of training. "The more fit your child is, the less likely

---

MEDICAL ALERT

When to See the Doctor

That pain in your child's side isn't *always* a side stitch. If the pain continues and is very severe, your doctor should check out the possibility of appendicitis or a bowel disorder, cautions John F. Duff, M.D., an orthopedic surgeon, founder and director of the North Shore Sports Medical Center in Danvers, Massachusetts, and author of *Youth Sports Injuries*. Seek medical care if any of the following symptoms exist.

- The pain remains after a bowel movement
- The child has a slight fever
- The pain lasts longer than three hours
- The stitches continue to occur even after several weeks of training

And never give a laxative to a child with a side pain, hoping to urge a bowel movement. If the problem is appendicitis and not a gas pain, the laxative could cause the appendix to burst.

she'll be to get frequent stitches," says Gregory Landry, M.D., staff pediatrician at the University of Wisconsin Hospital Sports Medicine Clinic in Madison and associate professor in the Department of Pediatrics at the University of Wisconsin–Madison Medical School. Be sure your child exercises regularly, not just occasionally. If she has just started a running program, she should gradually increase distances and speed, says Dr. Landry. A ten-year-old, for instance, should not run more than one to two miles per day or five to seven miles per week when she begins running for distance, according to Dr. Landry. After she runs that distance without any pain or stitches, she can gradually increase the distance an additional one to two miles per week.

Avoid big meals. Gulping a pizza and a giant slush drink just before a soccer game could give just about anyone a side stitch. A full belly increases the likelihood that the diaphragm and abdominal muscles will spasm, says John F. Duff, M.D., an orthopedic surgeon, founder and director of the North Shore Sports Medical Center in Danvers, Massachusetts, and author of *Youth Sports Injuries*. Your child doesn't have to avoid eating completely, but it's best if he only nibbles lightly before the big game.

Slow down. "If your child is running and gets a stitch, he should slow down and walk," says Dr. Landry. If the pain doesn't disappear, he should sit down and rest until it does. A stitch can also be a sign the youngster is pushing too hard and should cut back his workouts.

Take tiny breaths. Deep breaths will likely only make the stitch hurt more, says Janet Perry, a physical therapist with Rehabilitation Network in Portland, Oregon. She recommends that the child take small, shallow breaths for about ten breaths and then try to return to normal breathing.

Go slack—then massage. When the stitch hits, have your child slump over for a few seconds by bending at the hips and knees with their hands on the knees, suggests Perry. This makes the pained muscles go slack and your child may feel better in just a minute or two. Meanwhile, he may also want to massage the area that hurts, to provide relief, suggests Dr. Duff.

Ice the stitch. It helps to have an "instant icer" handy in case your child gets a stitch. Freeze some water in a paper cup, and take the cup along in a cooler when you go to your child's sporting event. "Tear a half inch of paper off the top of the cup, and you have what we call an ice stick," says Dr. Duff. Have your child rub the ice over the painful area for one or two minutes, he suggests. The first touch of cold ice is a shocker—but if he rubs it around, the ice stick really can help. Just be sure he keeps it moving so the skin doesn't get frostbitten.

Find a bathroom. If a side stitch persists for more than a few minutes, there's a good possibility the pain is caused by gas pain rather than muscle spasm, says Dr. Duff. There's a quick way to find out. Ask your child if she needs to have a bowel movement. If so, the problem may be gas pain, and it will subside soon after she moves her bowels.

SLEEP PROBLEMS

Getting In a Good Night's Rest

Babies, so the saying goes, are nature's way of showing you what the world looks like at 3:00 A.M. They just don't respect the difference between night and day. Whenever they have a crying need for something—which usually means food—they announce it by crying.

Things do get better. "By the time most babies are three to four months old, they're sleeping for longer stretches—even up to six hours," says Dena Hofkosh, M.D., assistant professor of pediatrics at the University of Pittsburgh School of Medicine and coordinator of the Infant Development Program at Children's Hospital of Pittsburgh. But most infants need some help learning to fall asleep by themselves—and to put themselves back to sleep after night wakings. Babies who don't learn this valuable skill may grow up to be children with sleep problems, says Dr. Hofkosh.

Because so many parents lose that precious opportunity to teach good sleep habits early on, some of the techniques that follow are also aimed at older children who have trouble falling or staying asleep.

Put your baby to bed awake, but tired. "Parents should try to put babies into their cribs while still awake," says Dr. Hofkosh. At bedtime, she says, get the baby into her sleeper and feed her. But don't let her fall asleep nursing or taking her bottle. "You want the child to be tired, but still awake, so she can have the experience of falling asleep on her own. Hopefully, she'll learn to do that when she wakes up in the middle of the night, too."

Encourage self-comforting behavior. Babies learn to associate certain rituals with the process of going to sleep, according to Ronald Dahl, M.D., director of the Children's Sleep Evaluation Center at Western Psychiatric Institute and Clinic in Pittsburgh, and associate professor of psychiatry and pediatrics at the University of Pittsburgh Medical Center. Often those rituals involve a parent's cuddling, rocking or singing.

"In fact, we're genetically wired to fall asleep only when we feel safe," he says. "For a lot of kids, safety means being in close contact with a parent." That's why babies and toddlers who wake in the middle of the night often cry out.

"The child goes into his deep sleep for one to three hours, and has a normal waking-up period after the first sleep cycle," Dr. Dahl explains. "But then the rocking isn't there anymore. So he starts to scream and cry." According to Dr. Dahl, the problem is that the child learns to rely on rocking as a comfort—and, of course, no parent can rock a child all night.

Children need to latch on to something that *is* available, like a thumb or a teddy bear, says Dr. Dahl. "If the child can begin to associate sucking his thumb or twirling his hair or having his teddy bear with feeling safe, then he's learning self-comforting behavior. Feeling safe, he can go back to sleep."

Plan daytime practice sessions. You want to teach your baby self-quieting skills—the ability to quiet herself when she gets upset, says Edward Christophersen, Ph.D., clinical psychologist at Children's Mercy Hospital, professor of pediatrics at the University of Missouri–Kansas City School of Medicine and author of *Beyond Discipline: Parenting That Lasts a Lifetime.*

"If she's fussing, but it's a situation that you know she can deal with, ignore her or leave her alone until she's quiet for a few seconds," notes Dr. Christophersen. "Or if she gets frustrated with a toy or activity, wait until she self-quiets before you redirect her to something else. In a study, we found that half the children who were taught self-quieting skills during the day no longer needed help with night-time sleep problems."

Set a regular bedtime. "Establishing a regular bedtime is really valuable," says Dr. Dahl. "By following a routine, infants and children are much more likely to fall asleep easily.

"That's because there's a biological clock inside each of us that controls when we get drowsy, when we secrete hormones, when body temperature rises and falls—a whole symphony of physiologic regulation. As anyone who has had jet lag knows, if you stretch the normal 24-hour pattern one way or the other, unsettling things occur—including sleep disturbance."

It's important, though, that in living by the clock you distinguish between bedtime and sleep time. "You can tell your child to go to bed—and enforce it—but there's nothing you can do to make him sleep," says John Herman, Ph.D., director of the Sleep Disorders Center at Children's Medical Center in Dallas, Texas. "At my house, we have only two rules for bedtime: Don't get out of the bed unless you have to go to the bathroom, and don't make any noise. That seems to work. I'm not saying the child has to sleep; I'm asserting this is bedtime."

Wean your baby from parental hovering. Most parents find the "cold turkey approach" to making their baby sleep through the night is just too painful. The more you try to ignore the crying, the louder it seems to get. "What's usually more helpful is a gradual weaning from parental assurances," says Dr. Hofkosh.

"Choose a period of time when you feel you can stand to listen to the baby cry for a while," she advises. "Start by waiting five minutes. Then you can go in and assure yourself and the baby that everything is okay, maybe give her a pat on the back, and then leave the room. Next time let her cry for ten minutes before going back in. Make the visits less and less frequent.

"The point is, you are reassuring yourself that the baby is okay, and you're letting her know that this is not punishment. In essence, you're saying, 'I'm still here. I still love you, but this is bedtime.' It may take several nights of crying before the baby realizes that she is not going to get picked up or get her bottle, just because she cries."

Tell yourself you're doing the right thing. That's often hard to remember when you're listening to your baby wail at 2:00 A.M. "It's akin to the mother bird pushing the baby bird out of the nest," says Dr. Herman, "It looks cruel, but it's actually for the baby bird's own good."

You need to keep this in mind, so you don't weaken and rush in. Says Dr. Hofkosh: "Try to remember that rather than punishing your child, you're teaching her something, helping her to develop a skill she's going to need."

Give early wakers a second chance. If you have an early riser, you might want to let her stay in bed—even if she's crying—until you're ready to get up. In many cases, says Dr. Herman, kids who wake up early fall back to sleep again.

Decide on bedtime etiquette—and stick to it. "Each family has its own notion of what sleeping arrangements should be," says Dr. Herman. "But whether you believe that everyone should sleep in his or her own bed, or that a child can pile into your bed, make the policy clear and be consistent."

If you decide that your child must sleep in his own bed—and stay there through the night—you can't give in when he cries and pleads for help getting back to sleep, says Dr. Herman. "No in-between techniques will work. Letting your child sleep with you sometimes and not other times will just prolong the misery indefinitely. If you decide your child is going to sleep by himself, this is a permanent decision, not a temporary one."

Have a bedtime ritual. Following a winding-down routine helps a child feel safe in the place where he's going to sleep, says Dr. Dahl. "The kind of things many families do—reading a bedtime story, having a special time with the child to talk about things in a supportive way, saying prayers, listing all the people who love the child—make sense in helping him feel secure and ready for sleep."

Don't punish a child by sending him to bed. "If a child begins to associate going to bed with fighting or being yelled at, that's going to interfere with sleep," says Dr. Dahl.

Don't overdo caffeinated beverages. A child who chugs down several caffeine-containing sodas in the course of a day can get a significant dose of this stimulant, says Dr. Dahl. "That may cause sleep difficulties the same way coffee does for adults."

SNORING

Measures to Silence the Sawing

That sawing you hear coming from your child's room may sound like a carpenter hard at work. But woodworking isn't the sort of activity that occurs in tykeland in the middle of the night. Snoring is.

"Many children snore occasionally," says David N. F. Fairbanks, M.D., clinical professor of otolaryngology at George Washington University School of Medicine in

Washington, D.C., a spokesperson for the American Academy of Otolaryngology/Head and Neck Surgery and author of *Snoring and Obstructive Sleep Apnea*. "Often it's because they have a cold, an allergy or an infection like tonsillitis."

Any one of those conditions can cause the tissues of the throat to swell. "The sawing sound you hear is caused by the tonsils, adenoids and palate partially blocking the airway and flapping in the breeze," explains William Potsic, M.D., director of otolaryngology at Children's Hospital of Philadelphia and a leading expert on sleep apnea in children.

When your child recovers from his allergy attack, cold or tonsillitis, the snoring should stop, says Dr. Fairbanks. "Snoring is not normal," says Dr. Fairbanks. "Any time there's snoring, there's airway obstruction. And the heavier the snoring, the more obstruction there is. There's nothing good about having obstructed breathing." Also, Dr. Fairbanks warns, snoring could be a sign of sleep apnea. So children should see a doctor whenever their snoring continues night after night.

However, if your child's snoring is the milder, temporary sort brought on by allergy or illness, the experts say you can treat it at home in much the same way you treat a cold.

Let salt water open things up. "If mucus is contributing to the blockage problem, you can flush it out with salt water," says Dr. Fairbanks. Saltwater nasal drops are available in drugstores. But you can make your own by dissolving ¼ teaspoon of salt in eight ounces of water, he says. Be sure to boil the water first to sterilize it—letting it cool down to body temperature before you put it in the nose dropper.

Try a decongestant. "Try an over-the-counter oral decongestant medication made especially for children," says Dr. Potsic. "A decongestant doesn't really cure a cold or allergy, but it does treat the symptoms," he says. "It helps kids breathe a little better so they feel a little better. And it may cut down on the snoring." If you do use a decongestant, be sure to read the package directions—or check with your physician—for the correct dosage for your child.

MEDICAL ALERT

When to See the Doctor

He's a restless sleeper, maybe a bed wetter. He snores loudly and irregularly—his growling snores sometimes interrupted by 5, 10, even 30 seconds of silence after which he rouses and turns over. After a little time passes, he begins snoring again and the pattern resumes.

These are the signs of obstructive sleep apnea, a potentially life-threatening disorder that needs to be treated by a doctor, says David N. F. Fairbanks, M.D., clinical professor of otolaryngology at George Washington University School of Medicine in Washington, D.C., a spokesperson for the American Academy of Otolaryngology/Head and Neck Surgery and author of *Snoring and Obstructive Sleep Apnea*. The problem is often caused by severely enlarged tonsils and adenoids.

At night, when the throat muscles relax, the enlarged tissues simply collapse on each other, completely blocking the airway. "So the child has multiple awakenings during the night to restart his breathing," Dr. Fairbanks explains. But sleep apnea also produces some signs that you should be alert for in the daytime, including:

- **Hyperactivity.** When children who don't get enough sleep start feeling drowsy the next day, they may jack up their activity to a frantic level in an effort to stay awake, says Dr. Fairbanks.

- **Reduced rate of growth.** "Some kids with apnea tend to be rather small because they fail to thrive," says William Potsic, M.D., director of otolaryngology at Children's Hospital of Philadelphia and a leading expert on sleep apnea in children. "They find it difficult to eat and breathe at the same time, so they're poor eaters—picky and slow. They also use a lot of energy to breathe, especially at night. The net result is they tend to be below average in weight."

- **Poor speech habits.** "Sometimes they talk like they have a mouthful of hot potato," says Dr. Potsic. "Doctors actually refer to it as 'hot potato voice.'"

continued

continued

- **Poor performance in school.** It's hard for kids with apnea to concentrate and be their best because they're not getting adequate rest.

  If you observe these symptoms, be sure to consult a doctor, suggests Lucinda Halstead, M.D., assistant professor in the Department of Otolaryngology and Communicative Sciences and the Department of Pediatrics at the Medical University of South Carolina in Charleston. "Most children outgrow the condition as they get older, usually around seven to nine years of age," she adds.

Steer clear of snore-triggers. You should avoid products containing antihistamines, which can be sedating and may actually *cause* snoring, says Dr. Potsic. "Sedating medicines relax nerves and muscles," he notes. "This reduces the muscle tone in the tissues of the throat, making them more likely to collapse and trigger snoring."

Find a better sleep position. "See if there's a position that allows your child to keep his airway open and to breathe more comfortably," suggests Lucinda Halstead, M.D., assistant professor in the Department of Otolaryngology and Communicative Sciences and the Department of Pediatrics at the Medical University of South Carolina in Charleston. "For example, some children do better lying on their sides with their heads propped up a little bit on the pillow."

Turn on a tape recorder. If your child's snoring is not responding to these measures or seems to be growing worse, there's something else you can do at home that will assist the doctor. "Parents can help the specialist by tape recording their snoring child as he sleeps at night," says Dr. Potsic.

Diagnosis of sleep apnea is sometimes difficult, he says, so this tape recording is a good reference. "During an office visit, your child is awake, smiling and happy. The doctor isn't able to observe the child struggling in his sleep. That's why it would be really helpful to play a recording of the noisy breathing."

SORE THROAT

Soothe the Scratchiness

Rare is the child who manages to get through the cold and flu season without at least one sore throat. So when your child comes to you complaining of scratchiness or hurting when he swallows, don't be alarmed. Because many sore throats are the result of viral infections, they typically last just a few days and then disappear on their own, says Lucinda Halstead, M.D., assistant professor in the Department of Otolaryngology and Communicative Sciences and the Department of Pediatrics at the Medical University of South Carolina in Charleston.

"Remedies for these viral sore throats are simply aimed at relieving the temporary symptoms," says Dr. Halstead. "But if your child's sore throat is caused by a bacterial infection, antibiotics will need to be prescribed."

That's why a call to the doctor is in order when a sore throat appears. There is always the risk that it is caused by streptococcus bacteria, the germ responsible for strep throat and tonsillitis. Your doctor will need to take a throat culture to rule out this more serious ailment.

If it turns out that your child's sore throat is just the result of a run-of-the-mill viral infection, you can try these home remedies to bring soothing relief.

Try a mouth-watering remedy. "You want to induce salivation, which can be done with cough drops, Life Savers or—for older children—medicated lozenges," says Russell Steele, M.D., professor and vice chairman of the Department of Pediatrics at the Louisiana State University School of Medicine in New Orleans. This will help reduce pain and also wash away waste material generated by the inflammation process, he says.

Serve a long, cool drink. "Offer your child something cool to drink," suggests Dr. Halstead. "Ginger ale or some other soda is often best, but let it go flat before serving. If it's too bubbly, it can 'burn' the child's throat. Carbonation can be very irritating."

Hold the O.J. "You don't want to give a child with a sore throat beverages that are too acidic—they can feel like sandpaper," says Dr. Halstead. So don't offer orange, pineapple, grapefruit or tomato juices until your child is feeling better. "On the other hand, apple juice is excellent," she says.

Spoon out some cold comfort. Here's some "medicine" your child certainly won't mind taking. "Ice cream works better than anything to soothe a sore throat," says Dr. Steele.

MEDICAL ALERT

When to See the Doctor

Though most sore throats in children turn out to be minor pain that soon gets better, the experts recommend that you call your physician as soon as your child starts complaining about it. "Your doctor can determine if there's something serious, like a strep infection, causing the symptoms," says Russell Steele, M.D., professor and vice chairman of the Department of Pediatrics at the Louisiana State University School of Medicine in New Orleans. "Once that's ruled out, he may recommend home treatments."

Even then, however, you should monitor your child's condition closely and call your doctor back if:

- The pain lasts more than two to three days.
- The child refuses to drink.
- The child is running a fever higher than 101°.
- You notice white patches in the back of the child's throat.
- The child's voice is affected.
- The child is experiencing breathing or swallowing difficulties.

But you might want to let it sit at room temperature for a few minutes before serving. "Anything that's *too* cold can be uncomfortable going down," says Dr. Halstead. However, if your child asks for something icy and can tolerate it, go ahead and give it to him. "Some kids love icy cold things like Popsicles when they have a sore throat," she says. "It all depends on the child."

Go back to the bottle. Even if your baby is old enough to be drinking from a cup, you might want to go back to a bottle for the duration of the sore throat. "A bottle is ideal because it washes the back of the throat and keeps it wet," says Dr. Steele. "You can fill it with anything the child will drink."

Moisten up the dry air. "Some sore throats can be caused by mouth breathing, especially while sleeping," says David N. F. Fairbanks, M.D., clinical professor of otolaryngology at George Washington University School of Medicine in Washington, D.C., and spokesperson for the American Academy of Otolaryngology/Head and Neck Surgery. Often the problem is compounded by excessively dry indoor air.

Placing a humidifier or small mist vaporizer in your child's room may help. "Just be sure it's close enough that the child is actually breathing in the mist," says Dr. Fairbanks. "Otherwise you really are not raising the humidity significantly." (But be sure to clean the humidifier or vaporizer frequently, following the manufacturer's instructions.)

Put a painkiller to work. "Acetaminophen (Children's Tylenol) can help soothe a mild sore throat," says Dr. Halstead. Check the package directions for the correct dosage for your child's age and weight. If your child is under age two, consult a physician. Dr. Steele says older kids might also benefit from an over-the-counter throat spray formulated to deaden sore throat pain, such as Vicks Children's Chloraseptic Spray.

SPLINTERS

Tips for Easy Extraction

Your nine-year-old has come back from day camp with a few unwanted splinters from the rough-hewn dock.

It looks like you'll have a marathon tweezer session ahead, and neither one of you is looking forward to it.

Don't despair! Splinter removal doesn't have to be major torture if you follow the tips of our splinter-removal experts.

Pull out the easy ones. Any splinter that can be easily grasped with tweezers, or even your fingers, should come out at once. "Removal of a splinter is a very good idea if it is easily gotten to," says Patience Williamson, R.N., a

---

MEDICAL ALERT

When to See the Doctor

"If your child has a splinter that is really deep and totally trapped under the skin, leave it alone and take your child to a physician," says Ann DiMaio, M.D., director of the pediatric emergency room at the New York Hospital–Cornell Medical Center and assistant professor of pediatrics at Cornell University Medical College, both in New York City. "You'll cause your child a lot of unnecessary pain if you attempt to dig the splinter out. That kind of delicate, invasive work should really be done under sterile conditions."

Splinters are usually minor medical problems, but bacteria can penetrate the skin with the splinter and cause an infection. "A small amount of redness and swelling is nothing to get excited about, but if the affected area is getting increasingly red, swollen and hot, and if your child has a fever, that indicates a more serious infection, which must be seen by a doctor and treated with antibiotics," says Dr. DiMaio.

certified school nurse at the Rand Family School in Montclair, New Jersey.

Ignore the tiny tough ones. Tiny splinters that are not easily removed can probably be left alone, according to Williamson. "For little splinters, do nothing for a day or two," she says. "The body will naturally try to reject the splinter without your intervention."

Williamson recommends that during the time that you are waiting for the splinter to work itself out, make sure that your child washes the area well and keeps it covered with a dab of antibacterial ointment to help ward off infection.

Soak 'em out. A lot of splinters will surface on their own if you give them a good soak, says Luisa Castiglia, M.D., a pediatrician in private practice in Mineola, New York. "Have your child take a nice, warm bath. Then, with a washcloth, rub the skin outward along the line of the splinter to see if it will surface." If the procedure doesn't work, try again another day, recommends Dr. Castiglia.

Make like Sherlock Holmes. Take Williamson's advice and use a magnifying glass if the splinter is hard to see. Or throw more light on the subject with a well-placed light.

Ply a sterile needle. If the skin around the splinter looks irritated or red, the splinter should be removed with a sterilized, extra-fine needle and tweezers, advises Dr. Castiglia. "The best way to sterilize your splinter-removal equipment is to hold it in a flame for a few seconds and then let it cool down naturally," she says. "Make sure that the needle and tweezers are really cool before you get to work."

Then use a gentle touch. "If the splinter is completely underneath the skin, soak the area for about ten minutes—the soaking softens the skin and makes removal easier. Then pat the area dry and cover with Betadine Solution," advises Dr. Castiglia.

"Using the very tip of your sterile needle, gently scrape the skin above the splinter. Don't gouge! Just open enough of the skin so that you can pull the splinter out with tweezers."

This may be easier said than done, admits Dr. Castiglia, because some kids start screaming at the first touch of a needle or if you simply lack confidence in attempting this procedure. (If they do, you may need to go to the doctor.)

Reward the sufferer. Once the splinter's out, you can do more than just breathe a sigh of relief. "Little ones up to the age of six or seven will love it if you draw a little smiley face on their Band-Aids, or give them a little sticker for their pains," says Williamson. "If they get a little treat, it makes the hurt go away faster."

SPRAINS AND STRAINS

A Line-Up to Halt the Pain

You're trying to fly a kite with your son, but you're having trouble getting it airborne. To get some extra lift, your son decides to take a running start down the hill. As the kite climbs upward, your son suddenly hits the turf, tripped by a treacherous rock.

You look at his swollen ankle and figure that he's probably gotten a sprain or a strain. And whichever it is, you probably wonder whether the injury needs a doctor's attention.

A strain is different from a sprain, though both may be treated in similar ways. A strain can occur when you overwork or overstretch a muscle. The pain and tenderness that results is a sign that muscle fibers have been torn. If you tear or overstretch a ligament (the tough, fibrous band that connects bones at a joint), the injury is called a sprain.

Though children's bodies are flexible, they do at times suffer a sprain or strain, according to Morey S. Moreland, M.D., professor of orthopedic surgery and vice chairman of the Department of Orthopaedic Surgery at the University of Pittsburgh and chief of orthopaedic surgery at the Children's Hospital of Pittsburgh. Both injuries involve pain,

AN OUNCE OF PREVENTION

It is impossible to prevent your child from ever getting a sprain or a strain when he participates in sports, but you can try to minimize his chances, says Brian Halpern, M.D., clinical instructor of sports medicine at the Hospital for Special Surgery in New York City and fellowship director of Sports Medicine at the University of Medicine and Dentistry of New Jersey, Robert Wood Johnson Medical School in New Brunswick.

"It's worthwhile to make sure that the playing field and equipment is in good condition, that your child stretches and warms up before the game and that everyone understands and plays by the rules. In addition, your child should avoid participating in contact sports until he is physically mature and in good shape."

swelling and tenderness, and both may cause some black-and-blue discoloration because capillaries (tiny blood vessels) in the injured area bleed underneath the skin. To make life more complicated, says Dr. Moreland, if your young child has *all* of these symptoms, there is a greater likelihood that she may have a fracture.

Anytime an injury causes swelling and pain, you should take your child to the doctor, says Dr. Moreland. But there are also some things you can do yourself if you suspect your child has suffered a sprain or a strain.

Take a load off. At the first sign of an injury, make sure that your child stops using the affected limb, says Lewis E. Zionts, M.D., assistant professor of orthopedic surgery at the University of Southern California in Los Angeles. "If your child has an injury, attempting to walk on the affected foot, for example, or trying to flex an injured wrist will only aggravate the condition," Dr. Zionts says.

Ice it down. The rule of thumb for all sprains and strains is to apply ice—immediately. "Ice eases the pain and limits the swelling," says Brian Halpern, M.D., clinical instructor of sports medicine at the Hospital for Special Surgery in

New York City and fellowship director of Sports Medicine at the University of Medicine and Dentistry of New Jersey, Robert Wood Johnson Medical School in New Brunswick. "Place a towel or cloth over the injured area, and apply ice in whatever form you have handy," says Dr. Halpern. Keep the injury iced for 20 minutes, and then let the area rest for a while. Reapply as needed.

"Commercial ice-packs do a good job, but so does a bag filled with ice cubes—or even a bag of frozen peas, if that's all that is available," says Dr. Halpern.

Immobilize the injury site. Splint a finger, keep an injured arm or wrist in a sling, wrap the ankle or knee with an elastic bandage to give it some support, suggests Dr. Moreland. "The less you move the damaged tissue, the less you damage it further," he says.

Elevate it. To help keep the swelling down, try to keep the injured area above your child's heart level if possible, suggests Dr. Zionts. For an injury involving the hand or wrist, elevate the area by using a sling. For an injured ankle, foot, knee or leg, prop it up on a pile of pillows.

Be alert to limping. "The injury may seem minor if you see very little swelling and no discoloration, but take the child to the doctor if she starts to limp," says Dr. Zionts. "Children don't usually limp unless they have a fair amount of pain, and if your child avoids using the injured body part in anyway, it could be a more serious problem."

STOMACHACHE

Comfort for a Tender Tummy

It's 6:00 A.M. and the weak voice from the bunk bed is apologetic. "Mommy, my tummy hurts."

And suddenly you're thinking—"All the things I have to *do* today"—as you try to figure out how a small person's tummyache will affect your commute, your career, your life. But foremost among your concerns is the almost shamefaced thought: "Does his tummy *really* hurt?"

If your child is under age 12, the answer is almost certainly *yes*, says pediatrician Catherine Dundon, M.D., of Goodlettsville, Tennessee, who is the mother of two children aged 6 and 9. "Children under 12 do not have the ability to malinger," she says. If your child says it hurts, you can assume it hurts.

Many times, stomachache in children is the result of indigestion, constipation or nervous upset, says Dr. Dundon. If the symptoms are severe, you'll want to give the doctor a call soon. If not, there are many things you can do to treat tummyache yourself. Here's what doctors recommend.

Apply warmth. Most children find heat a big comfort when their tummies hurt, says Bruce Taubman, M.D., a pediatrician in Cherry Hill, New Jersey, clinical associate professor of pediatrics at the University of Pennsylvania School of Medicine in Philadelphia and author of *Your Child's Symptoms*. An infant may find comfort if you place a hot-water bottle on your knees and then let the child lie tummy-down on the bottle. Older children can use a heating pad, but it should be turned on low, and an adult needs to be present. (A child should not lie on top of a heating pad, but on his back with the pad on his stomach, according to Dr. Taubman.)

Reduce the stomach's workload. "It's also a good idea to rest the gut," says Dr. Taubman. Hold off on food for 24 hours. "Give your child lots of clear liquids such as flat soda, water, Gatorade and chicken broth," he says. But keep everything else in the cupboard.

Relieve pain with medication. "Acetaminophen (Children's Tylenol) will take the edge off your child's pain," says Dr. Taubman. Check the package directions for the correct dosage for your child's age and weight. If your child is under age two, consult a physician.

MEDICAL ALERT

When to See the Doctor

"Most parents fear appendicitis whenever a child complains of stomach pain," says Bruce Taubman, M.D., a pediatrician in Cherry Hill, New Jersey, clinical associate professor of pediatrics at the University of Pennsylvania School of Medicine in Philadelphia and author of *Your Child's Symptoms*. "But a child with appendicitis will not be walking around saying, 'I have a tummyache.' He will be in severe pain."

"A child who can't get up or who is writhing in pain, needs to be seen by a doctor immediately," says Don Shifrin, M.D., a pediatrician in Bellevue, Washington, and president of the Washington State chapter of the American Academy of Pediatrics. "So does a child who—in addition to pain— has fever with nausea or vomiting not associated with meals. A child who develops pain, significant discomfort or vomiting after falling or being hit in the stomach area should also be checked." You should call your doctor for an immediate appointment if these symptoms begin, or take the child to an emergency room as soon as possible if your physician is unavailable.

Never mask the problem with codeine. One thing you *shouldn't* do for a tummyache is give your child a codeine-based medication left over from a previous illness, cautions Don Shifrin, M.D., a pediatrician in Bellevue, Washington, and president of the Washington chapter of the American Academy of Pediatrics. It may temporarily relieve the pain, but it can also mask the progression of something serious such as appendicitis or a blockage or infection.

Make time for bowel movements. "As our lives speed up, one of the things we're not giving our children is the time they need on the toilet," says Dr. Dundon. In fact, the way we're rushing our children around both at home and at school can cause major constipation, she says.

TOUCH THERAPY FOR A TENDER TUMMY

When a child has a mild tummyache rather than severe pain, massage is a good way to relieve it, says Ann Linguiti Pron, a certified registered nurse practitioner in private practice in Willow Grove, Pennsylvania. Especially if it's caused by excess gas, constipation or colic.

Even if the child is an infant, Pron suggests, you should tell her you're going to massage her tummy to make her feel better. Then start to gently massage in a clockwise, circular direction that mimics the movement of food and gas through the digestive system, says Pron. If you do it right, she says, you may not only relieve your child's pain, you may also encourage what's *causing* that pain to move toward the exit.

Here are some ways to help relieve that ache.

- Have your child lie down on his back and rub a quarter-size dab of vegetable or massage oil between your palms to warm it up. Using your oiled hand, massage the abdomen clockwise in a circular motion starting just below the rib cage, circling around to the groin and up across the belly, says Pron. Circle the abdomen for several minutes, then change your stroke.

- With your child still on his back, place one hand horizontally just under the rib cage and slide it straight down to the groin as though you were sweeping grains of sand off the abdomen. Alternate hands, in a rhythmic way, to massage the abdomen with steady sweeping strokes. Repeat several times, then massage the tummy again with a gentle, circling hand motion.

- If your child hasn't eaten within the last hour, you can also try lifting his legs as you do the sweeping motion, says Pron. Hold his feet with one hand and lift them to almost a 90-degree angle as you continue to sweep with the other hand. It's easy to raise the feet of an infant or younger child. If the child is older, you can ask him to lie down and bend his legs with his feet on the ground.

- For an infant to get additional relief from gas or colic, help the child bend his knees instead of raising his legs all the way in the air, suggests Pron. Lift one leg and gently bend the knee toward the belly, then quickly release it. Do the same with the other leg. Then bend and release both legs together. Repeat the exercise, then return to massaging your child's tummy.

"I see at least one kid a week in my office who's been holding back so long and so often that his bowel is dilated and he's lost a lot of the ability to move waste through," says Dr. Dundon. As a result, stool becomes impacted in the bowel, and liquid from higher up in the gut leaks past the impaction and out onto the child's clothes. "A child with an impaction may frequently have belly pain after eating," she says.

The way to prevent both the problem and the pain is to give your child five to ten minutes of *uninterrupted* time on the toilet every morning, suggests Dr. Dundon. "Most houses are a total zoo in the morning, but make this a regular part of the routine—just like brushing teeth," she says. Have your child sit on the toilet and read a book or listen to a story. Don't let anyone else come in and don't pressure him. Just give him the opportunity, and let nature take its course.

Cuddle to scuttle stress. "If your child's not vomiting or constipated, belly pain could be caused by stress," says Dr. Dundon. "Pain from stress is something we adults tend to get in our heads; kids get it in their bellies." Some causes of stress might be a family move or a death in the family.

How can you help? "What the child with stress-related stomachache needs is loving," says Ann Linguiti Pron, a certified registered nurse practitioner in private practice in Willow Grove, Pennsylvania. Hugs, kisses and cuddles are often enough to untighten an uptight tummy and relieve the pain, she says.

Ask about school. "If a child continues to complain of a tummyache throughout the week, however, there may be a problem at school that he has not been able to verbalize," says Pron. "He needs to talk—to you and maybe to a teacher or guidance counselor as well."

So put whatever you're doing to one side, and sit down and talk to your child. The problem may be as simple as a bully at the bus stop, a teacher who loses his temper or a seat assignment that forces your child to sit next to someone of the (horrors!) opposite sex.

Any of these situations can make your child want to

avoid school, says Dr. Dundon. "But even if 'school phobia' is the culprit, when a child says his belly hurts, it does. And he doesn't need you to tell him it doesn't. That just hurts him a second time."

Instead, says Dr. Dundon, when your child complains of tummyaches before school, offer hugs and gentle praise when he manages to get himself moving. Then, once he's off to school, pick up the phone and call his teacher. If the teacher knows that he's getting before-school tummyaches, she may be able to reduce the stress load at school by not calling on him in class, by moving Billy the Bully to the other side of the room or by offering more praise and support than she might normally give in a busy classroom.

STRESS

Helping Your Child Cope

S tress in *kids*? Isn't childhood supposed to be *carefree*? Unfortunately, for most kids it's not.

Far from being an adults-only problem, stress is part of the human condition right from the start. It probably begins the moment we make that perilous journey through the birth canal into the cold, bright and noisy world. Stress may accompany the first step, the first day of school, spelling tests, soccer tryouts and puberty.

"As it is for adults, stress in children is idiosyncratic and individual," says Jeanne Murrone, Ph.D., clinical psychologist and staff psychologist at the New York Foundling Hospital, a foster care agency in New York City. "Not everyone is stressed by the same thing." One child may breeze through his school days easily making A's, while another may find the competition so daunting he develops a stomachache or headache just at the sight of a school bus.

And children who feel a lot of stress react in different ways. Some young children may regress to babyish behavior, such as thumb-sucking and bed-wetting. Older children may show symptoms of depression, growing quiet and withdrawn, avoiding friends. Still others become behavior problems—having tantrums or temper outbursts that signal they feel out of control. It's not uncommon for stressed children to develop nervous tics and mannerisms, such as blinking, twitching, hair twirling or frequent swallowing.

Helping your child learn effective ways to cope with stress takes time and patience. Here are a few techniques that may help.

Remember what kid stress feels like. To a 2-year-old who is struggling with separation anxiety, the fact that you're going away for the weekend may be as stressful as a hospital stay. Your 11-year-old daughter who is going to her first dance may have sky-high stress because she's worried she's about to become a middle-school wallflower.

"What parents perceive as nonstressful may in fact be very stressful for a child," says Dr. Murrone. You can help your child through these rough times if you recognize what's happening. If you've forgotten your own childhood struggles, figure that anything kids do for the first time may make them anxious. Try to see the situation from their perspective, so you can understand their stress better, she advises.

Give her time to explain. Like adults, children under stress may need to talk it out. "Take a few minutes at bedtime and give your child the opportunity to talk about what's bothering him," says psychologist Peter Behrens, Ph.D., of the Pennsylvania State University, Allentown campus. "And don't feel you need to keep up the conversation yourself. Being quiet and simply listening is a prerequisite for getting a child to express his feelings."

Prepare your child for surprises. "The less we know about a new situation, the more afraid we are, which is why you need to familiarize children with what's coming," says Byron Egeland, Ph.D., professor of child development at the Institute of Child Development at the University of Minnesota in Minneapolis.

For example, a child who is going to have his tonsils

out can benefit by visiting the hospital beforehand and learning exactly what is going to happen to him. A child who is moving to a new neighborhood or starting at a new school should be given a chance to see his new home or visit his new classroom in advance.

"The more you communicate beforehand, the less you're going to stress the child," says Dr. Murrone. "If you start springing surprises on children, their anxiety level goes up."

Explain the time frame. Remember, very young children don't tell time the same way as adults. A child who is afraid she'll never see her mother again may not understand what you mean when you tell her that "Mommy will be back in three days from her business trip." "Explain things in a way the child can comprehend," says Dr. Murrone. "Tell her 'Mommy will be back in three sleeps.' " That way she knows how long she'll have to wait.

Don't demand all A's. One of the major stressors in a child's life can be the expectations of his parents, says Thomas Olkowski, Ph.D., a clinical psychologist in private practice in Denver. Often, those expectations need to be lowered to give the child a break.

"One mother I saw was worried that her 6-year-old hadn't chosen an interest she could enjoy for life," says Dr. Olkowski. "Her concern was that when her daughter applied to the best colleges, she would need to list some unique interests to impress the college recruiter. Here the child was only 6 and the mom was already worried about a decision to be faced at age 18. That kind of thing can be very stressful for a child."

Let your kid be a kid. "Today, parents are busier and they're expecting kids to do things to take care of themselves," says Dr. Olkowski. "What often happens is that children are expected to act like little adults. When they can't do that, kids aren't wise enough to question their parents' assumptions, they look to themselves and say, 'I can't do it; what's wrong with me?' They start to feel they aren't capable and life starts to feel out of control for them."

Children should only be expected to do what they're

HOW TO NIX NERVOUS TICS

In the two months before six-year-old Jason and his family moved to a new house, he developed a tic. Even at play, Jason would blink his eyes almost into a squint and swallow hard, sometimes making a noisy gulp. Although this behavior was obvious to everyone around him, Jason seemed unaware of what was rapidly becoming a nervous habit. Jason's parents—on the advice of a counselor—talked to Jason about the upcoming move and encouraged him to express his feelings, but they made no mention of his blinking and swallowing.

According to most experts, the best way to help a child overcome a nervous tic is to ignore it. "Pointing it out simply escalates the anxiety," says Jeanne Murrone, Ph.D., clinical psychologist and staff psychologist at the New York Foundling Hospital, a foster care agency in New York City. "A tic is simply a child's way of cueing you about his internal feelings. Once those feelings are addressed, the tic will often disappear."

What if it doesn't? Professional help may be needed, says Byron Egeland, Ph.D., professor of child development at the Institute of Child Development at the University of Minnesota in Minneapolis. "You want to keep an eye out for other symptoms that may accompany the tic. Mood changes, concentration problems, more fearfulness, a change in activity level—all of these can be signs of depression and anxiety." Check with your pediatrician or a school guidance counselor for a referral if these symptoms begin to show.

developmentally able to do, says Dr. Olkowski. "Kids really need to be kids."

Hold out your hand. "Whether it's your toddler struggling with controlling her temper or your preteen concerned about whether he'll fit in at junior high, your children need to know that you're the safe base they can return to if things go wrong," says Dr. Egeland. "Our research has found that the kid who has confidence that his parents will be there if the going gets tough will be the kid who best learns to master his environment. The more supportive the environment, the easier it is for a child to make the transition from dependence to functioning in a more independent fashion."

How can you "be there?" With toddlers and preschoolers, you may want to literally lend a hand. For example, a child who is afraid of the dark or of the strange new nursery school may need to hold on to you for a while until his fear subsides.

"Say, 'I know you're afraid, but I'll help you,' and the child will quickly realize, 'Hey, there's no reason to be afraid,' " says Dr. Egeland. "With older children, let them know you have confidence in them, but that you're available to help. Say, 'I know you're frustrated because you're fighting with your friends, but I know you can work it out. If you need me, I'll be here.' "

Tell what you remember. Share your ups and downs with your kids, and explain how you handled the stresses. "Tell your child stories from your own childhood about what hurt and embarrassed you," suggests Dr. Murrone. "It will normalize their own experiences."

Show some stress control. Nothing works better than showing kids the healthy ways you handle stress. When someone cuts in front of you on the crowded highway or when you have too much to do around the house, you can demonstrate that stress doesn't have to ruin your day, or your life.

"Try to balance sources of stress with points of calm and renewal—go for walks, eat good meals, talk with good friends and keep on a schedule," says Dr. Murrone. "When we have balanced lives, we're all able to tolerate stress better. And when we handle stress this way, our children will follow."

Set reasonable limits on after-school activities. A child who is overenrolled in sports and other extra-curricular activities is a prime candidate for stress. Frequently, there's no fun involved, for either the child or the parent.

"Parents need to step back, put limits on activities and

help the child do some things that are fun," says Dr. Olkowski. Don't get caught in the trap of "We paid a lot of money for that clarinet, so you have to stick with the lessons" if your child would be much happier spending that hour reading in her room.

Try imagery. School-age children can be trained to use imagery to relax. Have the child sit or lie down in a comfortable place. Then ask her to close her eyes and breathe deeply and rhythmically while she imagines a calm, peaceful place.

"When I do this with kids, I frequently have them come up with a 'secret cue' that they can use later on when they're feeling stressed," says Dr. Olkowski. One eight-year-old used the carefree cartoon cat Garfield as his relaxation cue. He put Garfield stickers on the brim of his baseball cap. He could look up whenever he wanted to relax, and the cue would remind him to feel calm.

Build their self-esteem. "People with good self-esteem look at stressful events as a challenge, not a problem," says Dr. Murrone. Help your child find something about herself that makes her feel good. Encourage her to pursue activities where she can experience success.

"With some kids, especially those who may be uncoordinated or learning-disabled, you may really have to search for activities that she does well. But the activity itself can be simple—as long as it's valued and praised by the parent.

"You're so reliable, I can count on you every night to help me set the table," are words that build self-esteem. Praising the child's accomplishments will help make up for things she can't do so well.

Show your love. Feeling unconditional love from his parents can inoculate a child from some of life's worst stresses. For example, a child who knows he is loved doesn't worry so much about competition, that big school-age stressor. "After about third grade, kids experience this creeping specter of competitive ranking, which says to them, 'You have to do this to be good, liked or accepted.' Tests or games are sometimes considered matters of life or death, which is simply not the case," says Dr. Behrens.

Children need to know they are loved by their parents, no matter how well they do in school or on the playing field. "Parents can reduce their children's anxiety enormously just by saying, 'You're okay, no matter what,'" says Dr. Behrens.

STUFFY NOSE

How to Break Up Nasal Gridlock

Your four-year-old is throwing another foot-stomping tantrum. This time, however, her defiant "no" comes out like "doe."

At one time or another, it seems, every kid gets a stuffed-up nose that makes her sound like Snuffle-upagus, Sesame Street's elephantine character with the nasally voice. Most often, it's because a cold virus has moved into the nose, says Bob Lanier, M.D., a pediatric allergist and immunologist in private practice in Fort Worth, Texas, and host of the nationally syndicated radio and TV program "60 Second House Call." The intruding virus irritates the delicate mucous membranes lining the nasal passages, causing blood vessels to swell. Fluid pools in the surrounding tissue. This triggers more mucus production until, finally, the result is nasal gridlock. Air can't move in and air can't move out.

For kids who are allergy prone, other irritants besides viruses may have the same effect. Feather pillows, dust or pollen can also swell nasal membranes. But whatever the cause, a child with jammed nasal passages is likely to be cranky, uncomfortable and unable to sleep. That means Mom and Dad don't get much sleep either.

And a baby's grouchiness can lead to all-night wakenings. "A stuffy nose can make a baby feel like she's suffocating," says Dr. Lanier. If her nose is blocked, she can't nurse, so she'll be even more frantic.

Here's what experts recommend to get mucus moving and breathing passages open again, no matter what your child's age.

MEDICAL ALERT

When to See the Doctor

"If your baby is stuffy and has a fever or is unable to nurse, you should let your doctor know immediately," says Michael Macknin, M.D., head of the Section of General Pediatrics at the Cleveland Clinic Foundation in Ohio, clinical professor at Pennsylvania State University Medical School in Hershey and associate professor of pediatrics at Ohio State University Medical School in Columbus.

For an older child, it's time to call the doctor if there's no improvement after about ten days or there's a fever of 103° or higher.

Parents should also be aware of any strong odor that accompanies the discharge from one nostril. The odor "may indicate that a tiny toy or some other foreign object is stuck up the nose," Dr. Macknin says.

If your child is a chronic mouth breather, the doctor may test for specific allergies and then prescribe treatment. Some mouth breathers, however, may have enlarged adenoids. These tonsil-like tissues at the back of the nasal passages can swell for unknown reasons and interfere with air flow. Adenoids can be surgically removed, according to Dr. Macknin.

For moister air, turn on the shower. "In Seattle, where we have misty weather, I often tell parents who have porches to rock their stuffy babies to sleep out in the moist air," says Helen Baker, M.D., clinical professor of pediatrics at the University of Washington in Seattle. But Dr. Baker also recommends an even better remedy that's available to anyone year-round: "First, run the shower tap on hot for several minutes to steam up your bathroom. Then go in and sit with your child for 15 to 20 minutes. That should help loosen nasal secretions," she says.

Try a mist machine at night. If your child often wakes up stuffy, it may be because the air in your house is too dry. If so, you can use a cool-mist vaporizer or ultrasonic humidifier. These are safer in kids' rooms than the old-fashioned steam-type vaporizers, according to Michael Macknin, M.D., head of the Section of General Pediatrics at the Cleveland Clinic Foundation in Ohio, clinical professor at Pennsylvania State University Medical School in Hershey and associate professor of pediatrics at Ohio State University Medical School in Columbus. But you have to clean them often to avoid fungus and bacteria buildup (follow manufacturer's instructions).

"These misters spew minute particles that can end up deep inside the airways. If there's contamination, it may trigger bronchitis or other breathing problems," says Dr. Macknin. He recommends rinsing the machine daily with hot water. Every third day, scrub the tank with a diluted bleach solution and rinse thoroughly.

Keep filling her favorite cup. When your child has to breathe through her mouth for long periods, it can have a dehydrating effect, says Dr. Lanier. Drinking lots of water, juice or other liquids helps guard against that, and also promotes mucus flow and drainage, he says. Milk is fine, too. "It's a myth that milk thickens mucus," says Dr. Lanier.

Try a tender touch. "For children who panic when they get stuffy, reassurance is important," says Dr. Baker. "A calming rock in a rocking chair, for example, may help settle your child so she can fall asleep."

Dr. Baker doesn't advise rubbing your child's chest with a strong-smelling over-the-counter ointment containing menthol, oil of wintergreen or eucalyptus. "These give parents something to do, but they really don't improve air flow," she says. And in babies and very young children, these ingredients can be absorbed into the bloodstream, where they might have toxic effects.

Suction out the stuffiness. If you have an infant with a stuffy nose, a handy suction device called an ear bulb can be a great help. Available at drugstores, the ear bulb makes a great mucus extractor, says Dr. Baker. (She prefers it to a nasal aspirator because it has a longer, easier-to-use tip.)

To use one, hold your baby's head still with one hand. With the other hand, squeeze the bulb, then insert the tip in one nostril. Quickly release the bulb to suction up secretions. Remove the tip and squirt the contents in a tissue. Repeat with the other nostril. "After use, be sure to sterilize the bulb by boiling it," adds Dr. Lanier.

Try homemade saltwater nose drops. "I've been recommending these drops for 30 years to loosen stubborn secretions in infants," says Dr. Baker. Her recipe: Mix ¼ teaspoon of salt in a ½ cup of warm water, and store it in a clean jar—but not for more than a few days. Make up a new jar if needed.

To get the drops to baby's upper nasal passages, you'll need gravity's help, she says. Sit on the edge of a chair, with your legs straight out and your feet flat on the floor. Position your baby's head down the incline of your legs so her nose points to the sky. Hold her still with one arm. Using an eyedropper, place one drop of saltwater in each nostril. Wait a few minutes. (If necessary, you can sing to her to calm her.) Then, using an ear bulb, suction out the secretions. Both the eyedropper and the ear bulb should be boiled, to sterilize them, before you use them again.

To insert drops in an older child's nose, have him lie face up on the bed with his head over the edge. Place two drops in each nostril. Let them seep in for about two minutes. Then have him gently blow his nose.

Or buy the ready-made kind. Saline (saltwater) drops are available at drugstores. But you'll need to administer them with a steady hand. If the tip should touch your child's nose, the dropper could become contaminated, cautions Steven D. Handler, M.D., associate director of otolaryngology at Children's Hospital of Philadelphia. "If contact is made, don't replace the dropper in the bottle," he cautions. Sterilize the dropper before you use it again.

Be cautious with medicated syrups. Over-the-counter decongestant syrups shrink swollen blood vessels and open up the airways, says Dr. Handler. Different children react in different ways to the individual products. Some kids get jittery, says Dr. Handler, while for other kids, the same product puts them out like a light. "It's a matter of trial and error," he says.

These products aren't meant for kids under one year old, cautions Dr. Baker. For older children, carefully follow the directions on the bottle or consult your physician for the correct dosage for your child.

STUTTERING

Smoothing the Way to Surer Speech

British statesman Sir Winston Churchill was a stutterer, as were scientist Sir Isaac Newton and writer W. Somerset Maugham. So are singer Carly Simon and actors Bruce Willis and James Earl Jones. That your child is in such distinguished company may be small consolation, though. Stuttering is a problem that can affect your child's social life, his school performance and his self-esteem.

There are many theories on why people stutter, but none is conclusive. One thing that is clear is that stuttering—or disfluency, as the experts call it—is a problem of childhood. "Ninety percent of the people who are going to stutter start to do so by the time they're seven," says Edward Conture, Ph.D., a professor of speech-language pathology and chairperson of the Department of Communication Sciences and Disorders at Syracuse University and one of the nation's leading experts on childhood stuttering.

There is good news: Most children who begin to stutter gradually stop. Therapy with a trained speech and language pathologist tends to be quite successful, says Barry Guitar, Ph.D, professor of communication sciences and disorders at the Eleanor M. Luse Center for Communication Disorders at the University of Vermont College of Arts and Sciences in Burlington.

However, intervention needs to be undertaken early,

FALSE STARTS CAN BE NORMAL

Your three-year-old can't seem to get out a thought without countless false starts. Each sentence he utters seems to double back on itself as he edits and re-edits every phrase. Occasionally, he trips over a word. Is your child a stutterer?

There's a good chance he's just experiencing the normal period of disfluency many children go through sometime between the ages of 18 months and six years, says Barry Guitar, Ph.D., professor of communication sciences and disorders at the Eleanor M. Luse Center for Communication Disorders at the University of Vermont College of Arts and Sciences in Burlington. "Children with normal disfluency problems will repeat words or syllables once or twice, li-li-like this," he says.

When is there cause for worry? "We get concerned when kids repeat parts of words more than once or twice," says Dr. Guitar. "There's also some cause for concern if a child gets stuck on a word and it just won't come out, or if the child appears to be struggling, showing physical tension as he speaks."

If you suspect your child could be a stutterer, contact a trained speech and language pathologist who specializes in stuttering. Both the American Speech, Language and Hearing Association, 10801 Rockville Pike, Rockville, Maryland 20852, and the Stuttering Foundation of America, P.O. Box 11749, Memphis, Tennessee 38111-0749, can make referrals.

says Dr. Guitar, himself a stutterer. "With the majority of kids under five, treatment helps so much they will either overcome their problem or have only a minor disfluency. If the stuttering is severe, treatment is usually successful in helping the child learn to deal with it so it doesn't interfere with communication."

Though stuttering generally requires professional help, there are many supplemental things parents can do at home to help their child overcome this relatively common problem. Here are some simple techniques suggested by the experts.

Talk like Mister Rogers. That means slow down and speak clearly. Although many parents find this television personality's delivery annoying, his rate of speech does closely match kids' speech-processing abilities, according to Dr. Guitar. "On the other hand, if a child is listening to an adult speaking at a very rapid rate, the child will also try to speak rapidly and may become discoordinated," says Dr. Guitar.

By slowing down, you're modeling a way of speaking that your child is realistically able to achieve, adds Dr. Conture. "It also provides the child with sufficient time to smoothly and easily generate his own speech. Initially, in a conversation with your child, you may only need to do this for about five minutes. Then you can probably go back to a more typical speaking rate, provided you don't talk *too* rapidly."

Take the pause that encourages. Don't be too hasty in responding to a child's comment or question, says Dr. Conture. "Pause for one or two seconds before you respond," he says. This will underscore the calm, slow pace of conversation and make it easier for the stuttering child to keep up his end of the conversation.

Set aside a special time to chat. Life is busy for everyone these days, and parents can't always drop everything and engage in slow, measured conversation. "But it helps if a child knows that he has a certain time each day when the parent is going to listen to him. Even if you can only set aside five or ten minutes, that can compensate for the fact that life is too busy and rushed," says Dr. Guitar.

Let the child talk about his feelings. When you set aside some time to be with your child, let the child direct the conversation, says Dr. Guitar. Children who are going through a tough period may have a lot of feelings and thoughts that have gone unexpressed, he notes. These quiet times with you, when the child is in charge, may give him the sense of security he needs to express himself. "It can really be magical if you create an environment where the child feels free to talk about feelings and where all feelings are considered okay and normal."

Use the salt shaker trick. A child who stutters may get shut out of fast-paced dinner conversations. One way to make things easier is to give dinner-table talk a special structure, says Dr. Guitar. "One family used a salt shaker that was passed around the table. If you had the salt shaker, it was your turn to talk and no one could interrupt you. This kind of structure is good for the stutterer because he doesn't feel he always has to struggle to get a word in."

Avoid "simultalk." "Try not to talk over the end of your child's utterance," says Dr. Conture. Though you sometimes may be tempted to finish your child's long, labored sentences, complete his thoughts or interrupt him in a rush to get the conversation moving, let him finish. Otherwise you could possibly make his stuttering worse.

Don't be so picky. Kids who stutter need to know that they don't have to be perfect, that they can make mistakes and still be okay. Many of these children worry more about how they talk than what they say. "They worry about being perfect in talking, rather than just talking," says Dr. Conture. "Parents can help though, by not being so picky about everything—the child's room, his fingernails, his homework, his chores. Give the kid some slack," says Dr. Conture, "so he can learn he can screw up and make mistakes and the world doesn't end."

Let speaking skills come naturally. Parents who are constantly correcting speech mistakes or stressing verbal skills can worsen their child's stuttering problems. "Take away any pressures," says Dr. Guitar. "Kids will develop language and speech skills on their own just by hearing conversation. They don't need to grow up in households where there's a lot of time spent learning vocabulary and the names of all the dinosaurs."

Make the teacher your ally. It's important that your child's teacher understand how to handle speech problems.

"Giving oral reports, volunteering answers in class and reading aloud are all difficult things for the stuttering child. Don't ask the teacher to excuse your child from these activities," says Dr. Guitar, "but open up communication so the child feels comfortable talking to the teacher about it. Kids who stutter will have good days and bad days. Your child may want to strike a deal with the teacher that he's only called on when his hand is up, so his good days can be taken advantage of and his bad days forgiven."

SUNBURN

Ways to Counter Risky Rays

You're probably well aware that too much sun can increase your child's skin cancer risk later in life— as well as make him pretty miserable *now*—so you probably take care to spread sunscreen on that vulnerable young skin before he goes outdoors.

But sometimes you miss a patch. Or a bike ride in the blazing sun causes your child to sweat away the first coating of sunscreen. Or the sunscreen washes off from constant dips in the neighbor's pool. Whatever the reason, your child comes home with a classic case of red-hot sunburn. And he's exquisitely uncomfortable.

Here's what you can do to help your sunburned child get through the healing process as comfortably as possible—and some tips on how to protect your child's skin from future sun damage.

Treatment

Soak in cool water. Put your child in a cool—but not icy cold—bath. That can help draw the heat out and give quite a bit of comfort to hot, burning skin, says Richard Wagner, Jr., M.D., professor of dermatology at the University of Texas Medical Branch in Galveston.

MEDICAL ALERT

When to See the Doctor

Almost anyone will get burned skin if she stays out in the sun too long without protection. But severe sunburn in very young children—particularly if it appears in a short period of time—could indicate another problem, says Frances Storrs, M.D., professor of dermatology at the Oregon Health Sciences University in Portland.

"If your child exhibits such a sensitivity, it should be discussed with his or her doctor or dermatologist immediately. There are a number of serious illnesses that are associated with extreme sensitivity to the sun," says Dr. Storrs.

Children with normal skin, however, only need medical attention if there is blistering over a large area of the body or if the sunburn is accompanied by headache, chills or fever, says John E. Wolf, Jr., M.D., chairman of the Department of Dermatology at Baylor College of Medicine in Houston. These are all signs that infection or heatstroke could have occurred. For that, you need prompt professional help.

Add oatmeal to the bath. Aveeno colloidal oatmeal, added to a body-temperature bath, is very soothing to sunburned skin, says John E. Wolf, Jr., M.D., chairman of the Department of Dermatology at Baylor College of Medicine in Houston. You can find Aveeno at most drugstores, with directions for use on the box.

Or put on a wet wrap. If a cool bath isn't practical, just wrap a burned child in a wet shirt or wet towel, suggests Frances Storrs, M.D., professor of dermatology at the Oregon Health Sciences University in Portland. This is a particularly helpful tactic if you're camping or at the beach, she notes.

Apply a moisturizer. "After giving your child the Aveeno bath or wet towel wrap, apply a moisturizer to soften the skin and help trap some of the water," says Dr. Wolf. It's not a good idea to apply a moisturizer until you've cooled the skin off, however, as the moisturizer could trap heat.

Powder up. Calamine lotion can be comforting because the powder suspended in the lotion helps the skin lose heat, explains Dr. Storrs. "Even plain talcum powder can be quite soothing," she says.

Give acetaminophen. Acetaminophen (Children's Tylenol) can provide pain relief to a cranky child with a painful burn, says Dr. Wolf. The pain is worst the first two days after exposure, and then subsides. Check the package directions for the correct dosage for your child's age and weight. If your child is under age two, consult a physician.

Try an antihistamine. Once the burn is not as painful, it may begin to itch unbearably. "If your child can't stand the itching, you can give an over-the-counter antihistamine such as Benadryl," says Dr. Wolf. Be sure to read package directions to make certain the product is recommended for your child's age. For the correct dosage, follow package directions or consult your physician. Some doctors don't advise Benadryl cream or spray because it could cause a reaction.

Preventive Care

Apply sunscreen frequently. Apply the sunscreen about 30 minutes before you send your child outdoors, says Dr. Wagner. And remember, even waterproof sunscreens don't last forever, especially if your child is playing hard and sweating or swimming. "It's important to reapply sunscreen periodically, and make sure you apply a uniform coat over your child's skin," he says. "That usually requires quite a bit of the product."

Think 15. "For kids older than two, you should always use a sunscreen with an SPF (sun protection factor) of at least 15, regardless of skin type," says Dr. Wagner. "Otherwise your child is simply not getting enough protection."

Bring in the new. Sunscreens don't last forever. "Throw away the sunscreens left over from a year ago," advises Dr. Wagner. "The active ingredient becomes less effective as the sunscreen ages."

Apply sunscreen under clothing. Yes, it's a good idea to put a protective T-shirt on your tyke playing in the water, but clothing doesn't *completely* protect against sunburn, says Dr. Wagner. "Cotton shirts give about an SPF of 8, and when a shirt gets wet, the sun protection is even less. So you should apply sunscreen *under* your child's T-shirt, too. Thinner fabrics let in even more damaging rays," he says.

Take special care with infants. Babies have fragile, vulnerable skin, so limit their time in the sun. "When you do go out, make sure your baby is covered with light clothing—or place a fabric screening over the carriage," suggests Dr. Wolf.

You should also use sunscreen on your infant, no matter how young the child is. "There has been some concern about how much of the chemical in sunscreens was being absorbed into the baby's skin," says Dr. Storrs. "But, in my view, as long as you use a sunscreen with an SPF between 8 and 15, there should be no hazard from the sunscreen for infants."

Avoid peak burning hours. The time of greatest sun damage is usually from 10:00 A.M. to 3:00 P.M., so it's best for your child to avoid being out on the playground, beach or playing field during those hours. But the peak hours can vary depending on where you live, says Dr. Wagner. "In Texas, for example, studies have shown that there is substantial sun damage between 8:00 A.M. and 6:00 P.M. during the summer," he says. The solution? Avoid what seem to be the hottest parts of the day and take precautions at all times.

Provide a head covering. It doesn't take much convincing to get a young boy to wear a baseball cap—but try to get him to wear it with the bill in front, instead of backwards. Supply hats for all children, with sun bonnets for babies, says Dr. Wagner. "Safari-type hats that have a drape over the neck are particularly good," he says. Longer hair styles give the ears some sun protection, too, adds Dr. Wagner—and ears are a common site for skin cancer.

Watch out for freckles. Freckles may be cute, but they're an early warning sign that your child is getting too much sun, says Dr. Wagner. If freckles appear, enforce the always-wear-a-hat rule and take special care with sunscreen.

Remember the winter sun. Many parents don't think about too many rays in the wintertime, but January sun can be just as harmful as August's. "If your child likes winter sports or you're in a high-altitude region, the sun can be damaging even in the dead of winter," says Dr. Wagner. "Be sure to apply sunscreen, especially when snow is involved, since snow reflects the sunlight."

Feel free to use PABA. At one time, there was some concern that the active ingredient in many sunscreens—called para-aminobenzoic-acid (PABA)—could cause an allergic reaction in people, says Dr. Storrs. "Allergy to sunscreens does occur but is *extremely* rare," she says. "If your child is allergic to anything in the sunscreen, it is more likely to be the preservatives or perfumes, not the PABA." Look for brands labeled hypo-allergenic and fragrance-free.

SWIMMER'S EAR

Safeguards against a Perennial Problem

Your child has taken to his swimming lessons like a duck to water. Now you can hardly get him out of the pool. But a duck's feathers have built-in waterproofing. Your child's ears don't.

All that exposure to moisture can take its toll on the delicate lining of the ear canal, making it angry, red and itchy. Doctors call the problem otitis externa, or swimmer's ear. Left untreated, the irritation can develop into a painful infection.

Full-blown swimmer's ear infection in children isn't hard for a doctor to diagnose, says Jeffrey Fogel, M.D., a pediatrician in Fort Washington, Pennsylvania, and staff physician at Chestnut Hill Hospital in Philadelphia. To check, a doctor gently jiggles the child's earlobe. "If the child has extreme pain, there's a good chance it's swimmer's ear," he says.

Once infection and pain set in, a visit to the pediatrician or family physician is essential, says Dr. Fogel, because you'll need a prescription for antibiotics and cortisone eardrops. But experts say you can treat the condition *before* it becomes infected—while it is still just an itchy irritation—or even prevent it with these simple measures.

Try over-the-counter eardrops. Most drugstores carry eardrops labeled specifically for swimmer's ear to ease the pain and itching and head off infection, says Russell Steele, M.D., professor and vice chairman of the Department of Pediatrics at Louisiana State University School of Medicine in New Orleans. "The fluid in the drops is acidic, so it helps prevent bacteria from growing," he explains.

Give it a shake. Since swimmer's ear is often caused by the irritation of water still trapped inside the ear canal, getting it out can help head off problems. "After the child has been swimming, he should shake his head, tip it to each side and pull on each earlobe a couple of times while shaking to try to get all the water out," says Dr. Fogel.

Make your own eardrops. If you don't have a commercial preparation handy, your medicine chest may contain the makings of swimmer's eardrops, says Dr. Fogel. "Put some hydrogen peroxide or rubbing alcohol in a dropper," he says. "After your child swims, place two or three drops in each ear and leave it in. This will help displace any water that might be trapped inside." (The drops combine with the water in the ear and aid rapid evaporation, he explains.)

Another method is to use vinegar in a dropper, says Kevin Ferentz, M.D., assistant professor of family medicine at the University of Maryland School of Medicine and a family physician in Baltimore. "Vinegar contains acetic acid, which is the same ingredient in some over-the-counter eardrops. Just use a couple of drops in each ear." Gently jiggle your child's ear to get the vinegar to the bottom of the canal, he advises. Then tilt the child's head to let it drain out.

Ban underwater adventures. "A child is more likely to get swimmer's ear if he's diving underwater," says Dr. Fogel. That's because at greater depths there is more pressure pushing against the ears and water is more likely to get in. So try to have your child stay on the surface as much as possible.

Don't depend on ear plugs. Plugs can help keep water out of the ear, but they're not foolproof. "One problem with store-bought ear plugs is that they can irritate the ear canal," says Dr. Fogel. Instead, he recommends moistening some cotton with petroleum jelly and placing it at the edge of the ear opening. "Just remember that no plug is 100 percent watertight," he cautions.

Use your hair dryer for hair, not ears. Many experts recommend that adults use a hair dryer on low setting to dry out their ears after swimming. But Dr. Fogel doesn't recommend this for kids. "The appliance is simply too noisy and can potentially impair a child's hearing," he says.

SWOLLEN GLANDS

When Infection Sends Signals

L ymph glands are like little crisis-management centers located throughout the body. Ordinarily, these pea-size glands are filled with cells called lymphocytes, which produce the antibodies needed to fight off invading organisms like bacteria or viruses. When your child gets a viral infection such as a cold, or a bacterial infection such as impetigo, the lymphocytes multiply rapidly in the lymph gland nearest to the source of the infection, which makes the gland somewhat swollen.

The fact that your child has swollen glands doesn't mean that he has an illness. Rather, it's a sign that your child's immune system is at work. When your child's glands are swollen, you may actually be able to feel and see the swelling, and the glands may be tender to the touch. If you examine your child carefully, you may even be able to discover the infection or injury that has caused the gland to swell, says Jack H. Hutto, Jr., M.D., chief of pediatric infectious disease at All Children's Hospital in St. Petersburg, Florida.

For instance, says Dr. Hutto, a swollen gland in the groin may be due to an ingrown toenail or an infected knee, while a swollen gland in the front of the neck may indicate a cold or tonsillitis. A swollen gland under the armpit could be due to the immune system's reaction to an infected finger.

You can expect your child to have many swollen glands as she confronts the numerous cuts and colds of childhood, and for the most part, it shouldn't worry you, especially if you keep in mind the following tips.

Leave it alone. Unless the gland has a bacterial infection within it, leave it alone, says Lorry Rubin, M.D., chief of the Division of Pediatric Infectious Diseases at Schneider Children's Hospital of the Long Island Jewish Medical Center in New Hyde Park, New York, and associate professor of Pediatrics at the Albert Einstein School of Medicine in New York City. With swollen glands, it is more important to diagnose and treat the source of infection. The glands themselves need no treatment.

See if it moves. A lymph gland at work on a minor infection should feel relatively soft, may be tender and should be somewhat mobile, says Blair M. Eig, M.D., a pediatrician in private practice in Silver Spring, Maryland. To make sure the infection is minor, you should try moving the gland with your fingers, he suggests.

Be alert to warmth and pain. On occasion, the glands can become overwhelmed with bacteria, causing the infection to spread and grow in the lymph gland. If the gland itself becomes infected, the skin overlying the lymph node gets red and hot, and it will be very tender and very sore, says Dr. Rubin. For pain relief, you can give your child

MEDICAL ALERT

When to See the Doctor

If your child has a swollen gland that is red and painful or is larger than two inches, or if your child feels ill or feverish, consult your pediatrician, says Blair M. Eig, M.D., a pediatrician in private practice in Silver Spring, Maryland. The swollen glands may be responding to a bacterial infection that needs to be treated with antibiotics.

Lorry Rubin, M.D., chief of the Division of Pediatric Infectious Diseases at Schneider Children's Hospital of the Long Island Jewish Medical Center in New Hyde Park, New York, and associate professor of Pediatrics at the Albert Einstein School of Medicine in New York City, says his rule of thumb is: If the gland is big enough to see, take your child to the physician. Also, if your child has a gland that is persistently enlarged but is not tender or mobile, have it evaluated by a physician. In rare instances, it could indicate a more serious medical condition.

a dose of acetaminophen (Children's Tylenol). Check the package directions for the correct dosage for your child's age and weight. If your child is under age two, consult a physician. This type of infection may require antibiotic therapy and perhaps surgical drainage, Dr. Rubin says.

TEETHING

Relief for Sensitive Gums

When your baby begins to chew on everything in sight and starts drooling like Niagara Falls, it's a good guess the difficult teething months have officially begun.

Teeth begin to push through the gums when your baby is about six months old. This process can make the gums red and sensitive, and some babies will be fussy and irritable with every tooth that erupts. (Other babies, however, sail through the process with scarcely a whimper.)

The process continues until all 20 teeth come through, at about age 2½. Here's how to help your child deal with the discomfort from those emerging teeth.

Rub the gums. Just rubbing your baby's gums with your finger may make her feel better. And if you rub gently with a small gauze pad, you'll not only help relieve teething pain, but also clean your baby's mouth and get her used to the sensation of having her teeth cleaned, says John Bogert, D.D.S., pediatric dentist and executive director of the American Academy of Pediatric Dentistry in Chicago.

Offer soothing comfort. Sometimes a little tender care can ease the discomfort of a teething baby, says James F. Steiner, D.D.S., professor of clinical pediatrics and associate director of the Division of Pediatric Dentistry at Children's Hospital Medical Center in Cincinnati. Cuddling your baby, rocking him or walking with him can often make him feel better.

Supply a washcloth to chomp on. Give your baby a clean, wet washcloth to chew on, suggests Linda Jonides, R.N., a certified pediatric nurse practitioner in Ann Arbor, Michigan. If you chill the cloth in the refrigerator beforehand, it provides even more relief, by cooling those tender gums.

Ice is nice. Wrap a piece of ice in a bit of cotton cloth, says William Kuttler, D.D.S., a dentist in Dubuque, Iowa. "Rubbing this gently on the gums helps to numb them, and the pressure seems to feel good, too," he says. Be sure that the ice itself doesn't touch the gum, however, and that you keep the wrapped ice moving rather than holding it in one place.

Supply a teething ring. Teething rings with liquid centers intended for freezing are great for gum relief, says Dr. Steiner. But instead of freezing the ring, chill it in the refrigerator. "A child who holds a frozen teething ring against

MEDICAL ALERT

When to See the Doctor

Teething can cause your child to be uncomfortable, but it usually doesn't require medical care. Normal symptoms of teething include:

- Chewing.
- Fussing.
- Drooling.
- Crying.
- Red, swollen gums.

Teething does *not* normally cause fever, vomiting, diarrhea or loss of appetite, says John Bogert, D.D.S., pediatric dentist and executive director of the American Academy of Pediatric Dentistry in Chicago. If your child has any of these symptoms, they're likely caused by some other condition. Check with your pediatrician.

his gums can actually get frostbitten gums," explains Dr. Steiner. "Refrigerating them gets the rings cool enough to comfort the baby's gums without the potential harm from direct ice."

And although it may be tempting to attach the ring to the baby's clothing with a bit of string so you don't have to keep retrieving it, don't, warns Jonides. You don't want to risk your baby choking on the string.

Consider an OTC pain reliever. If your baby is in serious discomfort or having trouble sleeping because of pain, call your doctor and ask about giving an over-the-counter pain reliever. Acetaminophen (Children's Tylenol) can help a baby who seems to be very uncomfortable, says F. T. Fitzpatrick, M.D., a pediatrician in private practice in Doylestown, Pennsylvania. Be sure to get a pain reliever that's specifically for infants, and check with your doctor for the correct dosage.

Try a gum preparation. Products that numb the gums,

such as Orajel or Anbesol Baby Teething Gel can help ease gum pain, says Dr. Kuttler. Just follow directions on the package for use.

Mop up the drool. Drooling goes with teething. And clothing that has become wet from drooling can cause a rash, particularly on the neck and upper chest, says Dr. Fitzpatrick. To prevent this, change your child's clothing often, or keep a soft cloth or bib around your baby's neck to soak up the drool.

Protect your baby's face. Your child may need a bit of extra protection to keep from getting a rash on her face. "If your baby is drooling a great deal, put a coating of petroleum jelly around her mouth and chin, avoiding the lips," says Jonides.

TEMPER TANTRUMS

Techniques to Tame the Rage

It may happen at any time from about 14 months on. Your sweet cuddly baby suddenly becomes a raging monster, throwing a temper tantrum that reminds you of demonic possession. So you may be surprised to learn that temper tantrums are perfectly normal in humans of *all* ages, according to William Sobesky, Ph.D., assistant clinical professor of psychiatry at the University of Colorado Health Sciences Center and research psychologist at Children's Hospital, both in Denver.

"Everybody has tantrums. We don't ever outgrow them completely. As adults, we just get more subtle about expressing our displeasure," says Dr. Sobesky. "Two-year-olds, on the other hand, are more direct and challenging. They just let it all hang out."

Your role as parent of a child in his "terrible twos" is to teach him to control his rages, to learn some of that subtlety and restraint at which adults are so practiced.

WHEN TANTRUMS TAKE THE BREATH AWAY

If you're one of those unlucky parents whose child, in the throes of a tantrum, holds her breath, take a deep breath yourself—and then remember this: "Breath-holding is almost always harmless," says Francis J. DiMario, Jr., M.D., assistant professor of pediatrics and neurology at the University of Connecticut in Farmington.

While breath-holding can seem like a form of manipulation, children usually don't do it on purpose, Dr. DiMario explains. "It's actually a reflex, triggered when the crying child forcefully exhales the majority of air in her lungs. At that point she becomes silent—her mouth is open but nothing comes out." Most of the time, these breath-holding incidents are resolved in 30 to 60 seconds, when the child catches her breath and begins yelling again.

There's not very much you can do about this unpredictable sequence of events, says Dr. DiMario.

While the wild-eyed flailing and screaming that characterizes toddler tantrums usually diminishes—with help—by age three, some children have a more difficult time than others handling their tempers, Dr. Sobesky says.

But here are some techniques that can help you prevent the terrible twos from stretching into the terrible twelves.

Recognize and avoid flash points. Kids are more likely to lash out if they're tired, hungry or feeling rushed. "If you can predict those times when there will be problems, often you can work around them," says Dr. Sobesky.

You may be able to eliminate the dreaded checkout-line tantrums, for example, by not shopping when your child is hungry. A child who throws a fit during the morning "rush hour" around the house—when parents are headed for work and older siblings for school—may need to get up a half-hour earlier. "Know your child's bad times so you can prevent tantrums," says Dr. Sobesky.

Intervene early. It's a lot easier to stop a tantrum that's just starting than one in full bloom, says Dr. Sobesky. With young children, distraction often works. "Get them interested in something else, such as a toy or a game," he says. "Even getting silly or tickling them sometimes works."

Switch from "stop" to "go." Young children are more likely to respond to parental requests to do something—so-called go instructions—than to heed stop requests, says Mark Roberts, Ph.D., professor of psychology at Idaho State University in Pocatello. "So if your child is yelling and screaming, ask him to come to you instead of asking him to stop screaming. He's more likely to obey," says Dr. Roberts.

MEDICAL ALERT

When to See the Doctor

In very rare instances, a child who becomes emotionally upset and holds her breath may have a true seizure. "She may lose consciousness, get stiff, make a few jerking movements and then resume breathing," he says. "The first time anything like this happens, it can be really scary," says Francis J. DiMario, Jr., M.D., assistant professor of pediatrics and neurology at the University of Connecticut in Farmington.

Though it may only happen once, you should report the episode to your doctor, says Dr. DiMario. Some neurological problems can also cause seizures, so your doctor may want to evaluate your child to make sure she is in good health. Dr. DiMario, who has studied the phenomenon and published his findings in the *American Journal of Diseases of Children*, offers these suggestions for coping with breath-holding episodes.

- Treat the event the same way you would if your child fainted. Lay her flat on the ground with her head tipped to the side to avoid choking in case she vomits.
- Be as reassuring as possible to the child, who may be disoriented afterward.
- After the episode, once again set limits on bad behavior. Don't back off just to avoid breath-holding spells.

Name that emotion. A two-year-old may not be able to express in words—or even understand—his feelings of rage. To give him some control over his emotions, you have to give them a name, says Lewis P. Lipsitt, Ph.D., professor of psychology and medical science and founding director of the Child Study Center at Brown University in Providence, Rhode Island.

"Without making a judgment about his emotions, try reflecting back to the child what he is feeling, such as 'Maybe you're angry because you can't have a cookie,' " says Dr. Lipsitt. "Then make it clear that despite his feelings, there are boundaries to his behavior. Tell him, 'Even though you are angry, you must not yell and scream in the store.' " This helps to teach the child that there are certain situations where such behavior is not permitted.

Tell the truth about consequences. "With younger children, it's often helpful to explain the consequences of their bad behavior," says Dr. Lipsitt. "Explain things very simply: 'You are acting out of control and we don't allow that here. If you continue, you will have to go to your room.' "

Call time-out. "Chair time-outs are the discipline of choice for preschool children," says Dr. Roberts. He explains that a child who is having a tantrum should be required to sit on a chair that's next to a wall (away from all entertaining or dangerous objects) for a certain minimum period of time.

"From our research we know that less than one minute is not effective," says Dr. Roberts. Usually it takes between two and five minutes for the child to calm down, he says. You should not speak to the child during that time.

When the time is up and the child is calm, explain that his tantrums will not be tolerated. Then give a few suggestions for alternative behavior and allow things to return to normal, says Dr. Roberts.

Send the child to a time-out room. As many parents discover, an out-of-control toddler may not stay in a time-out chair. "In these situations, a brief, solitary time-out in a separate room can be helpful," says Dr. Roberts.

"If the child refuses to stay on the time-out chair, take the child by the arm and put him in his room," he suggests. "Close the door, hold it shut and wait for 60 seconds, listening carefully for 'dangerous' sounds—such as bouncing on the bed—that would require intervention. What usually happens is the child continues his tantrum at the door. After 60 seconds, carefully open the door, march the child back to the time-out chair and tell him to stay there and be quiet." You may have to do this three times or more before the child stays on the time-out chair, Dr. Roberts says. If a child aggressively and repeatedly refuses to stay on the chair during time-out, it's time to seek professional counsel, he adds.

Follow through on your warning. Once you tell a child that he'll have to take time-out in his room or in a chair, you must follow through consistently, adds Dr. Roberts. "Otherwise, it's like the story of the boy who cried wolf. Empty warnings don't accomplish anything. Children tune them out like background music."

Count to ten (or higher). It's not just the child who needs a time-out. *You* may need a break, too, especially if you are on the verge of losing control yourself after your child's temper outburst. "Just tell the child, 'I'm too upset with you right now. I need to settle down before we talk,'" suggests Dr. Sobesky.

"It's okay to be angry, but not okay to lose your temper," he says. "When parents yell and scream, they're not being good role models for their kids. If you do lose your temper, apologize. Say, 'I'm sorry. That was my anger talking, not me.' Kids are very forgiving."

Counter fear with love. A child who is having a temper outburst is likely to be frightened by the intensity of his own out-of-control emotions. "Rage reactions scare the person who is angry," says Dr. Lipsitt. "In the midst of anger, children often feel like hitting—which is a particularly upsetting feeling for an older child."

The best way to bring these feelings under control is to express your love and concern. "Tell the child that everything is going to be all right soon," says Dr. Lipsitt, "and that his feelings are natural although not to be desired."

Conjure up a calm image. A useful tip to try with your child to keep his temper under control is to ask him to imagine something calming or actually, physically cool, says Thomas Olkowski, Ph.D., a clinical psychologist in private practice in Denver.

"When the parents of one child I worked with tried this approach, the boy came up with a number of images to help him remember to 'keep cool.' Initially, he pictured himself sitting on a block of ice or going outside in a snowstorm. But he finally settled on a stuffed penguin as his imaginary reminder, because penguins always keep their cool."

If they can't cut it out, help them cut it back. A child who is temperamentally a hothead isn't going to change overnight, but she can make small changes daily, says Dr. Olkowski. "Let's say your child blows her stack three times a day. Pick a day and work with her to cut those outbursts down from three to two, just to give her a feeling of control. At that point she may think, 'Hey, I've done it once. Maybe I can do it again.' That gives her a sense of accomplishment."

THUMB-SUCKING

Helpful Hints to Break the Habit

At 11, Brian was still sucking his thumb. Not all the time, and never at school or at friends' houses. But whenever he was lost in thought at home—whether studying the contents of the refrigerator or watching TV—his thumb would rise toward his mouth. And at night he'd fall asleep with that comforting thumb wedged firmly in place.

"I had visions of him going off to college sucking his

thumb," says his mother. But as it turned out, he stopped before sixth grade. Brian made the decision himself—and he succeeded with help from his parents.

Experts agree that sometimes thumb-sucking isn't a problem at all. "It's *not* a sign of insecurity—it's simply a habit," says Susan Heitler, Ph.D., a clinical psychologist in Denver. "It's a coping skill, much like pacing or cigarette smoking is to an adult," says Dr. Heitler. "If a child is agitated, it calms him down; if he's bored, it stimulates him."

If the child is under five, the best policy might be to ignore it. "If the child thumb-sucks only occasionally and it doesn't appear to be harming teeth or fingers, there's no need to do anything," says Stephen Goepferd, D.D.S., professor of pediatric dentistry and director of dentistry in the Division of Developmental Disabilities at the University Hospital School at the University of Iowa in Iowa City.

Problems can occur, however, if a child is vigorously thumb-sucking after age five, says Patrick Friman, Ph.D., associate professor of psychology at Creighton University Medical School and the director of clinical research at Father Flanagan's Boys' Town, in Boys' Town, Nebraska. "The child may be at risk for buck teeth, malformation of the sucked fingers or thumbs and fungal infections under the nails," he says.

And frequent thumb-sucking can take a social toll once a child starts school or preschool. A child who sucks his thumb in school will probably have to put up with the jokes and teasing of classmates, according to Dr. Friman.

So if your youngster still has a thing for his thumb as school age approaches, you might want to take some positive action. Here are some steps that can help.

Can the nagging. No matter what your child's age, don't scold him about his habit. "If you've been nagging your child about his thumb-sucking, now is the time to call it quits," says Dr. Friman. Don't mention thumb-sucking unless the child brings it up. Particularly don't pull your child's thumb out of his mouth, he says. Sometimes just making a nonissue of thumb-sucking can help to cut back on it. If not, at least you've stopped making your child miserable about the habit.

Tune in to your child's signals. If you want to gently steer your child away from thumb-sucking, take note of what's going on whenever your child's thumb goes in her mouth, says Dr. Heitler. "If your child automatically sucks her thumb when she's tired, hungry or bored, help her verbalize those feelings and look for other solutions," she suggests. "For instance, you can say to her, 'You must be feeling bored,' and then get her interested in a book or toy to take the place of her thumb."

Abandon cuddly props. Sometimes thumb-sucking and hugging a blanket or teddy bear are habits that are linked together, and your child automatically does one while doing the other. "Dragging around a blanket or teddy bear may trigger unnecessary daytime sucking," points out Dr. Heitler. If you make a rule that the blanket or teddy must stay in the child's bedroom, you'll likely cut down on thumb-sucking *outside* the bedroom.

Consider your timing. If you believe it's time for your child to actively try to break the thumb-sucking habit, pick a time when life is relatively calm, advises Dr. Goepferd. You probably won't get anywhere if there's been a death in the family or a serious illness, or if a divorce is in progress, he notes. "Postpone any program until later, when things are calm again."

Give a reason to quit. If you want your child to quit because you think other children will make fun of him when he starts kindergarten, explain this. "It's easy for a child to see that he probably doesn't want to be sucking his thumb in front of all those other kids at school," says Dr. Heitler.

You can also explain that the pressure from the thumb could harm his teeth—and it helps if your pediatrician or dentist also mentions this. "It may take a heart-to-heart talk to convince your child that ending the habit is important," says Dr. Heitler.

Team up to stop the habit. Once your child is interested in quitting, discuss possible solutions together, says Dr. Friman. "That way, it's not something the parent is doing *to* the child, but rather something that the child is doing for himself." Parents can help with reminders, he says, but the child feels more in charge this way.

Pick a milestone for stopping. "It's often a good idea to tie the time for your child to stop sucking his thumb to a milestone or special event in her life, such as starting kindergarten, by New Year's or before summer vacation begins," says Dr. Heitler.

Once you've chosen the "stop" date, sit down with your child and design a colorful chart where you can record the hours or days he goes without sucking his thumb, suggests Dr. Heitler. This gives your child a sense of control, she says, and lets him see the progress he has made.

Reward success. "Build into your charting system little treats or rewards—something for your child to work toward in her endeavor to quit the habit," says William Kuttler, D.D.S., a dentist in Dubuque, Iowa, who has been treating children for more than 20 years. "It's very motivating."

He suggests giving a child a star for each day she gets through without sucking her thumb. You and the child can determine ahead of time how many stars she needs to collect before she earns a particular treat, such as a new toy.

Or make a dot-to-dot game. A personalized dot-to-dot game can give the child not only an incentive, but a sense of control, says Dr. Friman. First, find a picture in a magazine of a treat the child would like, and then put a sheet of white paper over the picture and draw dots along the outline of the treat. Post the dot-to-dot game in a prominent place in your child's room.

"A child who doesn't suck his thumb all day gets to connect two dots. When all the dots are connected, the child gets the thing he's drawn," explains Dr. Friman. "If there are days when the child feels he must suck his thumb, then no dots are connected, but the child still hasn't *lost* anything. He's still the one in control."

Develop a warning system. "The hardest part of quitting is for the child to realize that his thumb is in his mouth, since it goes in by automatic pilot," says Dr. Heitler. You need a way to warn your child that the thumb is moving toward his mouth. Discuss it with your child, and pick something that will remind him what he's doing. A small adhesive bandage around the thumb may do the trick.

"If the plain bandage isn't enough, try putting a bit of vinegar on it," suggests Stuart Fountain, D.D.S., a dentist in Greensboro, North Carolina, and associate professor of endodontics at the University of North Carolina's Chapel Hill School of Dentistry. "The taste of the vinegar will remind your child that he's trying to quit."

Put a sock on it. If your child sucks her thumb when she's sleeping, even a bandage on the thumb may not stop it from going in the mouth. Instead, your child may want to put some gloves or socks over her hands while she sleeps, suggests Dr. Heitler.

Try thumb-painting. For the child who is trying to quit with little success, try Stopzit or a similar over-the-counter product, suggests Dr. Friman. These pharmacy products are safe for children, but contain bad-tasting ingredients that jolt the child's taste buds.

But be sure your child doesn't think of this as a punishment, warns Dr. Friman. "You can say to your child, 'Here's some medicine that can really help you when you forget and put your thumb in your mouth,' " he suggests. "The child gets the message that his parents aren't *making* him quit, they're *helping* him quit."

Offer an encouraging word. "Don't underestimate how difficult breaking this habit is for your child," says Dr. Heitler. "Thumb-sucking is a very rewarding habit, and doing without it creates a feeling of loss or emptiness. Much like what an adult feels when he gives up smoking." So be patient with your child, and offer frequent encouragement.

And even if your child quits, it will be easy for him to relapse during the first few weeks, points out Dr. Heitler. "Your child will have to work extra hard to guard against slipping back. It usually takes at least 30 days for the sucking impulse to subside."

TICK BITES

Tactics to Stop the Tiny Attacks

These tiny little critters always were a nuisance, but since the discovery of Lyme disease in 1975, they've become even more ominous.

The common tick is about an eighth of an inch long and easy to spot, while the deer tick—which can carry the bacteria that causes Lyme disease—is smaller and harder to see.

If you live in tick territory, it's important to keep a sharp eye out for these tiny animals and remove them from your children as soon as possible. Here are some tips from the experts.

Perform a tick search. "After the child comes in from a tick-infested area, especially the woods, do a tick check," says Gary Wasserman, D.O., a pediatric emergency medicine specialist, chief of the section of clinical toxicology and director of the Poison Control Center at The Children's Mercy Hospital in Kansas City, Missouri. Check your child carefully from head to toe, including the groin area. Look carefully through her hair, paying particular attention to the scalp border, where ticks like to latch on.

Tweezer that tick off. If a tick is still crawling, you can pluck it off with tweezers without pulling at the skin. But if the tick has already latched on, care is required. First, explain to your child that you need to pull off the tick, but it won't hurt. (Even when a bit of skin is pulled away along with the tick, there's very little pain involved.)

MEDICAL ALERT

When to See the Doctor

Two of the most common tick-related ailments are Lyme disease, which causes joint pain and other complications, and Rocky Mountain spotted fever, which can cause serious illness from high fever.

Fortunately, both usually have distinctive rashes that should alert you to seek immediate medical attention, says Gary Wasserman, D.O., a pediatric emergency medicine specialist, chief of the section of clinical toxicology and director of the Poison Control Center at The Children's Mercy Hospital in Kansas City, Missouri.

The telltale sign of Lyme disease is a rash shaped something like a bull's-eye. It can appear anywhere on the body. Look for a red dot that expands into a large, roughly circular red area. Other symptoms may include fever, headache, muscle pains and lethargy.

A child infected with Rocky Mountain spotted fever will develop small pink spots on the wrists and ankles that then spread to the rest of the body. Other possible symptoms are mild fever, loss of appetite, headache, nausea and vomiting.

Now grip the tick as close to the skin with the tweezers as possible and gently pull it away, but not too fast, cautions Herbert Luscombe, M.D., professor emeritus of dermatology at Jefferson Medical College of Thomas Jefferson University in Philadelphia and senior attending dermatologist at Thomas Jefferson University Hospital.

Caution: Jerking the tick out can leave mouth parts behind that can infect the skin. And never use your fingers to remove a tick since bacteria from the tick can penetrate even unbroken skin.

Avoid scary remedies. Some people advocate trying to get a tick to loosen its grip by applying a lighted cigarette or sizzling match tip. That's just too frightening for children, says Dr. Wasserman, and it's less effective than using tweezers.

Also, don't try nail polish. "This will likely suffocate a tick," he says, "but it may take as long as four hours and by then the tick may have already infected the child."

Dispose of the tick. Ticks will drown in a mixture of water and electric-dishwasher detergent. Stir about one teaspoonful of detergent in a cup of water, then drop the tick in the solution, says Dr. Wasserman.

Disinfect the area. Wash the bitten area thoroughly with soap and water, says Claude Frazier, M.D., an allergist in Asheville, North Carolina, and the author of *Insects and Allergy: And What to Do about Them*. Then apply an antiseptic ointment.

Cover up. To avoid bringing in ticks from woods and fields, help your child dress properly. He should wear long pants and a long-sleeved shirt. Clothes should be light-colored, so you can see ticks more easily, suggests Dr. Wasserman. To fend off ticks falling from tree branches, your child should also wear a hat or cap.

TOILET TRAINING PROBLEMS

Try a Worry-Free Approach

Though successful toilet training is often regarded as a milestone in a child's life, experts say parents spend far too much time worrying about it. And that can cause unnecessary problems.

"I always tell parents, 'I've never heard of a kid who went off to college carrying a diaper bag,'" says Jeffrey Fogel, M.D., a pediatrician in Fort Washington, Pennsylvania, and staff physician at Chestnut Hill Hospital in Philadelphia. "The point is: Even if you did nothing, your child would eventually learn how to use the toilet."

Most kids are toilet trained by the time they're three, but it's not unusual—or abnormal—for a child of 3½ or 4 to still be untrained, notes George Sterne, M.D., clinical professor of pediatrics at Tulane University Medical School and a pediatrician in New Orleans. Boys seem to train later than girls, he adds.

If there's one word you should keep in mind about toilet training, say the experts, it's *relax*. "Toileting isn't something you can force," says Dr. Fogel.

But experts also say you can make toilet training easier for both you and your child if you follow these suggestions.

Buy a potty chair. "A potty chair can serve the same way as those little plastic lawn mowers parents buy for their kids. It's something that helps Junior act like Daddy," says Thomas Bartholomew, M.D., pediatric urologist and assistant professor of surgery and urology at the University of Texas Health Science Center in San Antonio.

"Put the child's name on the chair and have him sit on it during a favorite activity—when he's hearing a story or watching a video, for example," adds Barton D. Schmitt, M.D., professor of pediatrics at The University of Colorado School of Medicine, director of consultative services at the Ambulatory Care Center at Children's Hospital of Denver and author of *Your Child's Health*. "You really ought to have the chair in place and the child enjoying it *before* you bring up the idea that this is also the place where he should go."

Step up to a potty seat. If your child is willing, you might start him on a potty seat that goes on top of the regular toilet seat, suggests Lottie Mendelson, R.N., a pediatric nurse practitioner in Portland, Oregon, and coauthor of *The Complete Book of Parenting*. "Provide the child with a stool to help him get on and off," she suggests.

Or maybe he's ready for the big time. "Children who are strong enough can learn to go directly on the toilet by sitting backward—facing the water tank—to steady themselves," says Mendelson. Most kids want to try out the adult seat as soon as they're able, she points out.

Be a role model. Tell your child what you want him to do, but better yet, show him, suggests Dr. Bartholomew. For obvious reasons, it's best if the same-sex parent performs this particular duty. "It's like anything else—kids like to imitate their parents," says Dr. Bartholomew. "When they see you use the bathroom, they're going to want to use the bathroom."

Skip the transition. Though it may be tempting to use the diaperlike transition pants, Dr. Fogel doesn't advise it. "That sends a mixed message to kids," he says. "We're saying to them: 'You don't like those big bulky diapers? Fine, here's something that's thin, it's light, it looks just like underwear but you can pee and poop in it.' That takes away the big incentive of graduating from a diaper into the big-boy or big-girl pants." If protecting clothing and furniture is a high priority, and your child stays dry 95 percent of the time, you can buy training pants that are simply underwear with a padded crotch. They don't eliminate leaking, but they do reduce it, says Dr. Fogel.

Make a fuss over success. "Provide extra attention or play a special game if your child has a successful elimination in the toilet," says Cathleen Piazza, Ph.D., assistant professor of psychiatry at Johns Hopkins University School of Medicine and chief psychologist of the neurobehavioral unit at Kennedy Krieger Institute in Baltimore. She suggests that you give your child a particular toy, stickers or a favorite food item as a toilet training reward.

Find out what motivates your child. "You can give children reasons to use the potty, but they have to be reasons that matter to them," says Dr. Fogel. He suggests that you listen to your child's cues. "For example, if your kid sees the big-boy underwear in the store and says, 'Oh, look at that, the Ninja Turtles,' you can say, 'Well, when you're fully dry during the day, you can have them, too.' That way, the motivation is coming from him," says Dr. Fogel.

Don't let the bathroom become a battleground. Don't ever fight with your child about using the toilet. "Fighting

WAIT FOR SIGNS OF READINESS

The biggest mistake parents make in toilet training is to start too soon, experts say. "All that does is set kids up for failure," says Jeffrey Fogel, M.D., a pediatrician in Fort Washington, Pennsylvania, and staff physician at Chestnut Hill Hospital in Philadelphia. "They know you want them to be dry, but they know they're still wetting. So they feel like a failure, and it lowers their self-esteem.

"You wouldn't push someone who wasn't prepared out of an airplane and say, 'When you feel like it, pull the chute.' It's the same with toilet training, if introduced prematurely," says Dr. Fogel. "You can't expect a child to handle a process he isn't yet capable of mastering."

Instead, be patient and look for these signs that your child may be ready to start using the toilet.

- Your child is talking well enough to communicate his needs. "Although this usually occurs in the 1½- to 2-year age range (when a child is also walking), don't go by your child's age," cautions George Sterne, M.D., clinical professor of pediatrics at Tulane University Medical School and a pediatrician in New Orleans, Louisiana.
- Your child is obvious about having a full bladder or needing to defecate. "You can usually tell this if the child suddenly stops what he is doing and runs behind the couch or into a corner," says Robert Mendelson, M.D., a pediatrician and clinical professor of pediatrics at Oregon Health Sciences University in Portland.

   "Some children may grab their genitals, others may do 'the pee-pee dance,' as some parents call it, or do a lot of squatting and grunting," adds Barton D. Schmitt, M.D., professor of pediatrics at the University of Colorado School of Medicine and director of consultative services at the Ambulatory Care Center at the Children's Hospital of Denver.
- Your child wakes up dry fairly regularly. According to Dr. Fogel, "You can say to your child, 'You've been dry now for a few days, and we're very proud of you. Would you like to wear your big-boy pants?' If he says yes, put him in the pants and get on with life."

is counterproductive," says Dr. Fogel. Instead, think of toileting as a skill that will come naturally, given some time and patience. "It's like any other developmental milestone," notes Dr. Fogel. "A child has to want to do it and be able to do it. Just as you can't force a child to walk, to crawl or to roll over, you can't make him use the toilet."

Parents who try to force the issue risk getting locked into a "battle of the bowels" that could, if unresolved, require the help of a professional therapist, says Dr. Sterne.

If he starts withholding, back off. It's a clear sign that a child is not ready to use the toilet if he begins to withhold stools, says Dr. Sterne.

"If that happens, back off," he says. "Say, 'You don't want to use the potty? Okay. If you want to wear your diaper, wear your diaper. I can see you're uncomfortable about letting go.'"

Withholding can also occur because of fear. "Some children are afraid of falling into the toilet," says Dr. Sterne. "Others may get scared if you flush the toilet while they're still sitting on it. You may need to give your child more time to get used to the whole idea."

TOOTHACHE

Making Molar Misery Milder

Your child approaches you holding the side of his face. His tooth aches, and he wants you to make it better. This is one hurt, however, that a loving kiss won't cure. You call the dentist immediately and make an appointment, but the earliest appointment isn't until tomorrow afternoon. Now what?

"A toothache can be caused by any number of problems," says Edward Grace, D.D.S., director of behavioral sciences at the University of Maryland Dental School in Baltimore. "While it could be a cavity, there could also be a crack in the enamel, a permanent tooth trying to break through, an irritated gum or just a loose baby tooth causing discomfort."

Because you probably don't know for sure what's causing your child's tooth to hurt, the experts suggest that you try as many of the following remedies as necessary to help ease the pain during the hours you must wait before seeing the dentist.

Look for the obvious. "Sometimes a piece of food can get jammed between two teeth and cause soreness," says William Kuttler, D.D.S., a dentist in Dubuque, Iowa, who has been treating children for more than 20 years. Look carefully in the area where your child has pain, using a penlight if necessary, to see if anything is stuck there. Then carefully try to remove any material with dental floss, or have your child try to do it himself if he's old enough. (Children aged seven or eight can usually manage the floss themselves.)

Try a saltwater rinse. If you can see that the gum is a bit swollen or irritated, a saltwater rinse may be the ticket to relief. "Mix a teaspoon of salt in an eight-ounce glass of warm water," advises Luke Matranga, D.D.S., president of the Academy of General Dentistry and chairman of the Department of Comprehensive Dental Care at Creighton University Dental School in Omaha. "Have your child swish the warm saltwater around and spit it out." Repeat this every few hours.

Test a warm water swish. If you can't see any gum irritation, plain warm water may help. "If your child has eroding or cracked tooth enamel, then bathing the sensitive tooth in a warm water rinse may help soothe the pain," says Dr. Matranga. Give your child a glassful of warm water to swish around his mouth, and repeat as required if the tooth starts hurting again. (He can swallow unsalted water—but he may want to spit it out.)

Or serve up cold water. If the warm water doesn't help, try cold. "There are some causes of tooth pain that feel better with a cold water rinse," says Dr. Grace. "You can even take a cup of cold water with you on the drive to the dentist, so your child can swish it around and swallow it on the way."

Apply an ice-pack. If the pain is severe, a cold pack may provide relief. Wrap a bag of crushed ice in a towel and hold it against the painful jaw, suggests Dr. Kuttler.

Choose soft, lukewarm foods or liquids. A painful tooth can feel even worse if your child chomps down on it while eating, says Dr. Matranga. Opt for soup, broth or anything soft—but avoid very hot foods. If cold irritates the tooth, avoid cold drinks and ice cream as well.

Select bland foods. If the problem appears to be an irritated gum, spicy foods could make it more painful, says Dr. Matranga. "Stay away from vinegar, mustard and salt, for example, because they could irritate the area," he says. You should also skip sugary foods or juice, because if the problem's a cavity, sugar will make the pain even worse.

Keep the lips zipped. "Tell your child to keep her lips together and the jaw relaxed so the upper and lower teeth don't touch," says Dr. Grace. "That will keep her from placing any pressure on a sore tooth—or sucking in air that may hurt a tooth that's sensitive to cold."

Give an OTC painkiller. Over-the-counter products such as acetaminophen (Children's Tylenol) may help relieve the pain of a toothache, says Steven Vincent, D.D.S., associate professor at the University of Iowa College of Dentistry in Iowa City. Check the package directions for the correct dosage for your child's age and weight. If your child is under age two, consult a physician. Children should not be given aspirin because of the risk of Reye's syndrome, a life-threatening neurological disease.

Use a little eugenol. Some over-the-counter oral pain-relief products such as Dentemp contain eugenol, which is made from oil of cloves. That's the same spice used on holiday hams. "Or you may want to try one of the other over-the-counter oral pain medications, such as Num-Zit or Anbesol," says Dr. Kuttler. Some of these contain clove oil. For amounts and application, follow the instructions on the package.

Distract your child. There are many ways you can help take your child's mind off the pain while waiting for the dental appointment, says Dr. Kuttler. Let your child curl up in a comfortable chair and read to him, or turn on a favorite video or television show. Playing games or listening to some favorite music can also provide distraction until it's time to leave for the dentist's.

TOOTH GRINDING

Ways to Halt the Gnashing

The first hint that your child is a tooth grinder may be audible in the middle of the night. If you hear a mysterious sort of *gritting* noise coming from your child's room, you'd better investigate.

About 50 percent of kids grind their teeth at some time, says Jed Best, D.D.S., a pediatric dentist and assistant clinical professor of pediatric dentistry at Columbia University School of Dentistry in New York City. For most kids, occasional grinding—also called bruxism—causes no problems, and many children outgrow the habit.

But during acute episodes, a child may wake up in the morning with a headache, a toothache or even an aching face. This can be serious business. "If tooth grinding persists for months and years, the teeth can actually wear down," says Luke Matranga, D.D.S., president of the Academy of General Dentistry and chairman of the Department of Comprehensive Dental Care at Creighton University Dental School in Omaha. There can also be damage to the temporomandibular joint, which is the joint where the jawbone is "hinged" to the side of the head.

Experts say if your child's grinding is persistent, you should consult with your dentist, who may make your child a special mouth splint to keep the teeth apart. If your child grinds his teeth only occasionally, however, you can try these remedies from the experts, or you may want to try them in addition to the mouth splint.

Give the jaw a rest. Any time your child is not chewing, swallowing or speaking, the upper and lower teeth should not meet, says Steven Vincent, D.D.S., associate professor at the University of Iowa College of Dentistry in Iowa City. If the teeth are meeting, this is clenching, and it's just one step away from grinding. Explain this to your child, and ask him to try to keep his teeth just slightly apart when relaxed.

Encourage exercise. Regular exercise may help your child relieve stress and muscular tension, which in susceptible individuals could be the cause of nighttime tooth grinding, says Bernadette Jaeger, D.D.S., adjunct associate professor in the Section of Orofacial Pain and Occlusion in the School of Dentistry at the University of California, Los Angeles.

Slow down just before bedtime. No more wrestling, tag or other rowdy activities just before bedtime. "Tight muscles need time to relax before your child goes to sleep," says Edward Grace, D.D.S., director of behavioral sciences at the University of Maryland Dental School in Baltimore. "Make the hour before bedtime reasonably quiet." This is a good time to read a story to your child or encourage him to read or look at a picture book.

Try an early-to-bed treatment. "Your child may be overtired—and that can trigger tooth grinding during sleep," says Dr. Grace. An earlier bedtime may help. "If your child usually goes to bed at 9:00 P.M., try having him go to bed at 8:00 P.M."

Skip the bedtime snack. If digestive juices are working the midnight shift, they could be making your child more tense during sleep. "Don't let your child eat or drink anything except water within an hour before bedtime," advises Dr. Grace.

Talk out your child's problems. If your child is worried about a troublesome homework assignment or an upcoming school play, that may be causing her to grind her teeth during the night. "If something is bothering your child, don't let her take it to bed with her," says Dr. Grace. "Simply talking it out often helps reduce the worry." As a part of the tucking-in routine, have a five- or ten-minute chat with your child before she goes to sleep.

Apply warm, wet compresses. If your child's jaw aches in the morning, dip a washcloth in warm water, wring it out and apply it to her jaw until she feels better, says John Bogert, D.D.S., pediatric dentist and executive director of the American Academy of Pediatric Dentistry in Chicago. This may help soothe the pain.

TOOTH KNOCKED OUT

Fast Action to Save a Smile

Kids play hard—sometimes too hard. After unexpected contact with a ball, bat, jungle gym or a fist, your child can come home with a gap in his smile where one or two teeth used to be. Usually, it's the upper front two that take the brunt of the blow.

If it's a baby tooth, of course, you don't think twice about saving the tooth. It's best to alert your dentist, however, because if the permanent tooth is years away from making its appearance, your child may need a spacer to keep the rest of the teeth from shifting out of place.

But if the tooth that gets knocked out is a permanent one, you *do* want to take quick action to try to preserve the tooth. And you need to get to the dentist quickly so it can be replaced. If you act fast and take the recommended steps, there's a good chance that knocked-out tooth can be saved.

Here's what you need to do.

MEDICAL	ALERT

When to See the Doctor

For the best chance of saving a permanent tooth that's been knocked out, it's imperative to get your child and his tooth to the dentist as soon as possible, says Steven Vincent, D.D.S., associate professor at the University of Iowa College of Dentistry in Iowa City.

"If the tooth can be replanted within 30 minutes after being knocked out, the chances of success are 80 to 90 percent," he says. The odds drop after that, but don't give up even if it takes you an hour or more to find the tooth—there's still a chance of successfully replanting it.

Once you've retrieved the tooth, head for the *nearest* dentist. "If your child's dentist is way across town, go to one who's closer," says Luke Matranga, D.D.S., president of the Academy of General Dentistry and chairman of the Department of Comprehensive Dental Care at Creighton University Dental School in Omaha. "I don't know of any dentist who would turn you away in this kind of emergency," he adds. If no dentist's office is open, head to the nearest emergency room.

If a tooth isn't knocked out completely, but loosened significantly, leave it in place. It's still urgent to get to the nearest dentist or emergency room, however. The loose tooth can probably be "splinted" to the adjacent teeth until it heals, but that needs to be done quickly.

Handle with care. Once you've found that precious tooth, hold it by the crown, not the root. "The root is covered by a delicate tissue, called the periodontal ligament, that needs to be protected if the tooth is to be successfully replanted," says Steven Vincent, D.D.S., associate professor at the University of Iowa College of Dentistry in Iowa City. For the same reason, don't scrub the tooth.

Replace the tooth. The safest place to store that tooth is where it came from—back in the socket. Rinse the tooth quickly with milk or saline contact lens solution. (Use tap water as a last resort because it usually contains chlorine, which can also damage the important periodontal ligament.) If your child is calm—and willing to cooperate—gently put the tooth back into place.

"Even if you insert it facing the wrong direction, that can be corrected later," says Luke Matranga, D.D.S., president of the Academy of General Dentistry and chairman of the Department of Comprehensive Dental Care at Creighton University Dental School in Omaha. "The important thing is that it's in the best location possible, its own natural home." Once it's in, have your child bite down gently on a gauze pad or tissue to hold it in place and get to your dentist as quickly as possible.

Reach for the moo-juice. If reinserting the tooth isn't possible, put it in a jar or cup of milk. According to dentists, milk has the right kind of chemical makeup—measured in terms of alkalinity (pH)—to help keep that tooth in good shape for a while. "Milk is an excellent transport medium because it has a pH compatible with the periodontal ligament tissues," says Dr. Vincent. "But that doesn't mean you can dawdle; milk won't preserve the tooth for an extended period of time."

Or put the tooth in *your* mouth. No milk on hand? "If the only moisture available is inside your own mouth, then put the tooth there, between your teeth and cheek," advises Stuart Fountain, D.D.S., a dentist in Greensboro, North Carolina, and associate professor of endodontics at the University of North Carolina's Chapel Hill School of Dentistry. You can also put it inside your child's mouth if you're sure he's old enough and calm enough not to swallow it.

Wrap it up. A final option is to wrap the tooth in a moist tissue or cloth, says John Bogert, D.D.S., pediatric dentist and executive director of the American Academy of Pediatric Dentistry in Chicago. Another option is putting the tooth in a plastic bag with a little water or milk. That will help prevent the tooth from drying out and also help protect it.

HELPING THE TOOTH FAIRY

If your child has a loose, wobbly baby tooth, usually all you need to do is wait until it comes out on its own. But if the soon-to-exit baby tooth is dangling, you may want to give it a helping hand so it doesn't come out during the night and possibly cause your child to choke.

Here are some ways you can help remove the tooth.

- Chill the gum with ice so your child won't feel the tooth coming out, suggests Stuart Fountain, D.D.S., a dentist in Greensboro, North Carolina, and associate professor of endodontics at the University of North Carolina's Chapel Hill School of Dentistry. "Hold an ice cube on the gum beside the loose tooth for three to four minutes," he says.
- Give your child a tissue so he can grasp the tooth and pull it out, says John Bogert, D.D.S., executive director of the American Academy of Pediatric Dentistry in Chicago.
- If your child prefers that *you* pull the tooth, remove it by twisting it quickly, Dr. Bogert advises.

The only time to consult the dentist about losing baby teeth, doctors agree, is if a permanent tooth starts coming in *before* the baby tooth has loosened. In that case, the baby tooth may need to be removed so the permanent tooth can come in straight.

Conversely, if a baby tooth is lost prematurely, a dentist may recommend a space-maintaining device so there will be room for the permanent tooth.

Supply a handkerchief to bite down on. This will help stem bleeding and ease the pain, says Dr. Vincent. "Actually a sterile gauze pad is better, if you have one handy. But a towel or handkerchief will do."

Avoid future losses. If you know your child is going to be active in sports, particularly skating, outfit her with a protective mouth guard, says Dr. Fountain. You can find these at sporting goods stores.

TV ADDICTION

Getting Tube Time to a Minimum

Six-year-old Alex's family was planning an extra-special cross-country trip in a camper. When Alex found out there would be no television for the entire three weeks, he couldn't believe it. "But what will I *do?*" he squawked.

Whenever ten-year-old Tracy enters her room, she turns on her TV set. It's as automatic as flipping on the light switch. Whether she is doing homework, playing with friends or talking on the phone, her TV is always on.

Both Alex and Tracy are TV addicts. In some ways, they are as dependent on the flickering screen images as many grown-ups are on cigarettes or alcohol. And the consequences can be serious.

As many studies have shown, children who watch a lot of television are fatter and less fit and have higher cholesterol levels than kids who watch less. Some experts think excessive tube-watching may even foster a more accepting attitude toward violence and promote aggressive behavior.

If you're concerned that your child is watching too much television, here are some tips for cutting back.

Log in those viewing hours. "Keep a record of how much television your child actually watches," suggests Nicholas A. Roes, president of the Education Guild and author of *Helping Children Watch TV.* You may be quite surprised at how many hours per week are spent that way. Once you know the extent of the problem, you'll be in a better position to institute needed changes, says Roes.

Short-circuit the electronic babysitter. "Don't get in the habit of using television as a babysitter, no matter how busy you are," says Marie Winn, author of *Unplugging the Plug-In Drug.* Instead, come up with some *active* pastimes your child can pursue when you're not available to supervise.

You might provide a wide variety of drawing materials,

for instance, or purchase some simple musical instruments for your child to play with on his own. If you read to your child—and do a lot of reading yourself—you'll encourage your child to be entertained by books as well as television.

Map out a week's worth of watching. "Go through the channel listings with your child each weekend and select programs for the coming week that you would feel comfortable having her watch," says Carole Lieberman, M.D., a Beverly Hills psychiatrist, media consultant and assistant clinical professor of psychiatry at the University of California, Los Angeles. "Choose programs that are educational and nonviolent, that espouse the kinds of values you want your child to have."

If the show is part of a series, she suggests you watch at least one episode with your child to make sure it's really suitable. Important: As soon as the chosen program is over, and before your child can get hooked on the one that happens to follow, turn the set off, Dr. Lieberman says.

Take a day off. "Designate a single day every week as No-TV Day," suggests Winn. "Some families do this on Saturday or Sunday as part of their Sabbath observance." Explain that everyone—Mom and Dad included—will just have to find more creative ways to fill their free time on that day.

Make time for homework. Try the "no TV on school nights" rule, which is the easiest one to enforce, according to Winn. Discuss the rule first in a family meeting, so your child knows why you feel it's so important.

"Children won't necessarily watch TV all weekend to make up for what they've missed on week nights," says Winn. In fact, because they haven't fallen into the viewing habit during the week, they'll be more likely to look to other leisure activities once Saturday rolls around.

Try a TV Turn-Off Week. Occasionally, you can present your children with the challenge of keeping the set turned off for a whole week, suggests Winn, who has organized TV Turn-offs around the country. "That's when you'll see

HOW TO TURN THE ENEMY INTO AN ALLY

Used intelligently, television can be a positive, educational force in your child's life, says Nicholas A. Roes, president of the Education Guild and author of *Helping Children Watch TV*. Here are a few of his suggestions.

- If your child enjoys watching game shows, make it a whole-family activity. Pick some topics that come up regularly on the shows, and spend time together with an almanac or encyclopedia preparing for next week. Then tune in and let your child field each question and keep his own score.

- To encourage critical viewing, assign "TV show reports" to your child in the same way book reports are assigned in school. Depending on your child's age, each report might contain comments on factors including plot, pacing, character development, clichés, setting, music and special effects.

- If violence crops up on a show you're watching, discuss alternative, nonviolent means the characters might have used to solve their problems.

- Suggest that your child write letters to producers, advertisers and networks to express his feelings about various programs.

how dependent your family is on television." The insight may be sobering, but it could help you to set limits in the future, she points out.

Expect withdrawal symptoms: Your kids may beg to watch "just one" favorite show. But hold firm.

"Just be sure you present it as a scientific experiment or an adventure—absolutely not as a punishment," says Winn. "As additional motivation, think up a reward for the end of the week. You might decide to take a special family trip or purchase a new game or other play equipment."

Enlist the aid of your VCR. "By making more use of videotaping, you can gain more control over what your children watch, and when," says Dr. Lieberman. Also, if a troubling or confusing issue arises in a taped program you're viewing, you can hit the pause button and talk things over with your child.

"You can also fast-forward through offensive commercials," she adds. Or you can choose to watch some of the commercials with your child, then pause the tape to teach some healthy skepticism. "You might discuss how the ad suggests that if your child gets this toy, she'll be the most popular child on the block," says Dr. Lieberman. "You can point out just how unrealistic that is."

Don't let TV intrude on sleep time. Set a regular bedtime for your child that doesn't change from night to night depending on when certain television programs end, advises Bobbi Vogel, Ph.D., a family counselor in Woodland Hills, California, and director of the Adolescent Outpatient Program at Tarzana Treatment Center in Tarzana. And don't put a TV set in your child's bedroom, unless you want to completely lose control of how and when she uses it.

Switch off background temptation. Discourage your child from leaving the television on as background noise, advises Dr. Vogel. "It's too visually stimulating," she says. Before you know it, she could be watching instead of just listening. If she likes to hear something while she's drawing or doing other things, she can play a record or listen to the radio instead.

VIDEO GAME ADDICTION

Tips to Tame the Kid Who's Hooked

E very afternoon at 3:00, Chad rushes home from fifth grade and goes straight to his room. There he sits, shoulder muscles tensed, jaw clenched, eyes staring straight ahead at a monitor screen. His fingers are poised over a set of buttons. When he is called to dinner, he doesn't answer. His homework sits untouched.

Chad is a video game addict.

Chad's behavior is not unusual. Some youngsters, particularly preteen boys, would rather spend their time playing video games than doing almost anything else. Their parents worry about the violence in the games, the lack of social contact in their children's lives and the fact that family activities are becoming only a memory.

But where do experts draw the line between enthusiastic involvement and true dependency?

"Notice if your child is going into a trancelike state while playing," suggests Carole Lieberman, M.D., a Beverly Hills psychiatrist, media consultant and assistant clinical professor of psychiatry at the University of California, Los Angeles. "That signals an addiction."

MEDICAL ALERT

When to See the Doctor

Sometimes a child's video game addiction can be a symptom of a more serious underlying problem, points out Carla Perez, M.D., a psychiatrist in San Francisco who specializes in addictive behavior and author of *Getting Off the Merry-Go-Round: How to Control Your Destructive Habits in Relationships, Work, Food, Money.* "For example, a child may be playing video games as an escape because of major difficulties at school or tremendous tension between family members at home."

"Serious addiction stemming from relationship problems requires professional intervention from a family therapist to help with the whole family system," says Steven Silvern, Ph.D., professor of early childhood education at Auburn University in Auburn, Alabama. "The family may be out of control, and it's not just the kid's responsibility to get things straightened out."

If your family is going through a time of stressful change or transition and your child is spending a lot of time in front of the video monitor, ask your physician to refer you to a family counselor or therapist, he suggests.

Steven Silvern, Ph.D., professor of early childhood education at Auburn University in Auburn, Alabama, uses another benchmark. "If you've tried limiting your child's video game playing, and he stubbornly resists, causing a power struggle, it's an addiction," says Dr. Silvern. "As in adult addictions, the addicted child finds all kinds of ways to circumvent the rules and do what he's not supposed to be doing."

Video game addicts need help. If you suspect you have one in your house, try the following suggestions from the experts to get your child's habit under control.

Develop an incentive system. Work out a system in which children must earn video game play privileges, suggests Donald Jackson, Jr., Psy.D., director of The Psychological Services Center of Widener University in Chester, Pennsylvania. Don't let the child believe she's automatically entitled to these privileges.

"Use video games as a reward for doing chores, completing homework or accomplishing something special around the house," says Dr. Jackson. "If the child can prove she's responsible in such ways, *then* she can have the freedom to deal with the special appeal of video games."

Set limits on playing time. You can buy a TV metering device, called TV Allowance, to help control playing time, says Dr. Jackson. You can program the device to permit a certain number of playing hours per week—and no more. It's available from the TV Allowance Company, 5605 S.W. 74th Street, Number 21, South Miami, Florida 33143.

Schedule "reality breaks." "After one hour of video game play, the child should be required to take a 'reality break' to discuss briefly with a family member or friend what else is going on in the house," suggests Dr. Jackson. "It's a way of focusing attention away from the fantasy world of the games for a few minutes."

Rest tired eyes and muscles. Between reality breaks, it's a good idea to have your child take a brief eye-focusing break every 20 minutes to prevent eyestrain, says Dr. Jackson. Have her look up from the game and focus on something in the distance for several seconds.

While you're at it, encourage her to get up and move around for a minute or two to relieve muscle tension. These posture breaks will also help remind your child there's a world beyond the video monitor, says Dr. Jackson.

Change the cues. Changing the context in which your child is used to playing video games may make it easier to enforce limits on the amount of play, says Dr. Silvern. "For instance, you could shift the time your child plays. Instead of allowing him to always sit down the minute he comes home from school, don't permit him to play until after dinner. Or only allow him to play on weekends."

Make it a social occasion. "Invite friends over for your child to play video games with, so he isn't always playing by himself," says Dr. Silvern. "Whenever possible, choose games that allow two kids to play. Even with solo games, two kids can play in parallel with each other, by taking turns and commenting on each other's performance."

Don't beat 'em, join 'em. "Play the games yourself so you understand what's at stake in each game and what your child is talking about," suggests Marsha Kinder, Ph.D., professor of critical studies at the University of Southern California School of Cinema–Television in Los Angeles and author of *Playing with Power in Movies, Television and Video Games*. Ask him what he likes, so you can help him develop better taste in choosing more positive, less violent games.

"By playing video games *with* your children, it becomes a shared experience," adds Dr. Silvern. "As you watch him play, raise some questions. When he's completed a level of play, have him pause the game and ask him something, such as, 'I noticed that you picked up that sword. Why did you do that?' This gives the child an opportunity to teach you more about the game."

Push for computer games instead. "Encourage your child to switch over to playing educational-type games on computers," suggests Dr. Lieberman. "Even it hand-eye coordination is what he values most in video games, there are computer games that provide this and are more worthwhile than most of the video games." She suggests that parents check out "Concentration," "Jeopardy," "Sesame Street," "ABC and 123" and other challenging computer games.

Change the power source. Kids get a sense of power from playing and mastering video games, but there are many more positive ways to help give your child a sense of powerfulness. "Look for interactive activities that give your child power through participation and learning, rather than through zapping little men or cars on a video screen," says Dr. Lieberman. If your child excels athletically, she'll get that kind of empowerment through participation in her favorite sport. For a child who gets a lot of gratification from games, mastering a challenging board game like chess can be very satisfying, according to Dr. Lieberman.

Look for the school connection. Is your child turning to video game escapism because of slumping grades at school? "In the long run," says Dr. Lieberman, "getting him a tutor may be less expensive than buying lots of games." And the results will do more for his self-esteem. "The important thing is to attack the problem at its source instead of condoning substitute ways of dealing with the frustration," she says.

Go for the real thing. "Instead of purchasing a video game based on a sport like baseball or hockey, take him to a real game," suggests Dr. Lieberman. That not only gets him away from the screen, it also gives you and your child the camaraderie of spending time together, she says.

VOMITING

How to Quell the Queasiness

Was it too much cake and ice cream at your first-grader's birthday party? Something in the sausage pizza? Or that third ride on the merry-go-round? What prompted that colorful return of lunch may keep you guessing. But one thing you know for sure: You hope it doesn't happen again.

And in most cases, it won't. "Most vomiting is caused by gastroenteritis," says pediatrician Marjorie Hogan, M.D., an instructor of pediatrics at the University of Minnesota and pediatrician at the Hennepin County Medical Center in Minneapolis. "That's a viral infection of the gastrointestinal tract which is simple and self-limiting." In other words, it probably won't last long.

On the other hand, if vomiting does continue, it could lead to dehydration. "Vomiting a few times is usually no big deal," says Dr. Hogan. "Kids usually have enough fluid on board. It's when vomiting persists, when it's accompanied by diarrhea or when the child is a baby or toddler that you need to be careful."

Older children are more able to tell you when they're parched and thirsty. "With infants," says Dr. Hogan, "it's hard to know when they've crossed that line. That's why you need to contact a doctor immediately."

Most children need some parental comfort, since vomiting can be pretty scary. And while you're nursing your child back to a state of settled stomach, try these tactics.

Give that tummy a rest. "The first thing to do is to stop putting things in the child's stomach. Give it a rest," says Loraine Stern, M.D., associate clinical professor of pediatrics at the University of California, Los Angeles, and author of *When Do I Call the Doctor?* That also goes for babies who are still breastfeeding or bottlefeeding, says Dr. Stern. "Just skip a regular feeding until the stomach seems to settle." Offer oral rehydration fluids such as Pedialyte, instead, in small, frequent sips. You can ask your pharmacist

MEDICAL ALERT

When to See the Doctor

If your child has been vomiting, you need to be alert to signals that he is becoming dehydrated. If the child refuses fluids, stops urinating, cries without tears, has dry mucous membranes or appears lethargic, listless, drowsy or confused, he may need to be taken to the hospital and given fluids intravenously or put on a special oral rehydration program, says Marjorie Hogan, M.D., instructor of pediatrics at the University of Minnesota and pediatrician at the Hennepin County Medical Center in Minneapolis. In any case, call the doctor if the vomiting persists for more than two to three days, which increases the likelihood of dehydration.

You should also be on the lookout for symptoms of more serious illnesses or injuries. These include:

- Projectile vomiting in a baby, especially under four months of age. This forceful vomiting may be a symptom of pyloric stenosis, an obstruction at the end of the stomach that prevents food from passing through.
- Vomiting accompanied by fever. This can be a symptom of meningitis, bowel infection or some other serious condition.
- The stomach is hard and bloated in between episodes of vomiting. This could indicate an intestinal or stomach obstruction that could lead to life-threatening problems—so immediate attention is a must.
- Vomiting after recovering from a viral infection. This could be a symptom of Reye's syndrome, an inflammation of the brain and liver that can be fatal.
- Vomiting after a head injury. This may signal a concussion or bleeding in the brain.
- Vomiting yellow or green liquid (bile) repeatedly. This sometimes means there's an obstruction in the stomach.
- Vomit that resembles coffee grounds. This usually means there is blood in the stomach, a sign of internal bleeding.
- Vomiting after an accident involving the stomach, especially a bicycle handlebar injury. Even if the vomiting occurs a week or two later, you should call the doctor, says Loraine Stern, M.D., associate clinical professor of pediatrics at the University of California, Los Angeles, and author of *When Do I Call the Doctor?* This kind of vomiting may mean there's a bruise in the intestines.

WHY BABIES SPIT UP

If you're the first-time parent of a newborn, there's one very important thing to remember: Spit happens.

Many babies have a condition known as gastroesophageal reflux, says Marjorie Hogan, M.D., instructor of pediatrics at the University of Minnesota and pediatrician at the Hennepin County Medical Center in Minneapolis. That means the sphincter muscle at the bottom of the esophagus isn't working well yet, so breast milk or formula sloshes back up, creating that foolproof identifying mark of a new parent, the shoulder splotch.

There are a few ways to minimize spitting up until the baby's esophageal sphincter tightens up.

Handle gently. Don't jostle the baby during or after a feeding. Don't automatically fling him to your shoulder and start to burp him, says Loraine Stern, M.D., associate clinical professor of pediatrics at the University of California, Los Angeles, and author of When Do I Call the Doctor?

Follow baby's cues. "Pay close attention to the baby's feeding cues," says Dr. Hogan. "Feed at his tempo, stop when he seems to want to stop, and when he wants to take a rest, take a rest. Don't try to feed past fullness."

When in doubt, call the doctor. "Babies who spit up a lot can sometimes absorb fluid in their lungs, which can lead to lung disease," says Dr. Hogan. "Your doctor can also tell you if your baby is growing well and if the spitting up is caused by an obstruction. If a baby is vomiting a lot, don't deal with it at home. See a doctor right away."

for these drinks, which basically contain sugar, salt and a few other nutrients and are available at most drugstores.

Offer reassurance. "Vomiting can be very scary to a child," says Dr. Hogan. "Assure her that she's going to be all right." A young child may want you to hold her and stay with her for a while. For older children, it's comforting to be tucked into bed until they feel better.

Start foods slowly. Wait for your child to express an

interest in eating, then start with clear liquids, says Dr. Stern. Your main objective is to avoid dehydration. Many children can't tolerate water after vomiting but will suck on ice chips or even a cold, wet washcloth. Offer juices (unless there's also diarrhea), ice pops, oral rehydration liquids and gelatin, suggests Dr. Hogan.

If the clear liquids stay down, you can offer dry toast or crackers. "Avoid milk and milk products, though, which aren't well-tolerated."

Pour a cola. Things do go better with Coke. This is an old home remedy that has stood the test of time. "There's something about lukewarm Coca-Cola Classic that makes it stay down better than most things," says Dr. Stern. "Serve it lukewarm and a little bit flat. Stir it a little to make the bubbles disappear."

Ask about this OTC remedy. "If, after waiting a few hours, you've given the child sips of liquids and those don't stay down, an over-the-counter antinausea medicine called Emetrol may help," says Dr. Stern. However, consult your doctor first—and ask for the proper dose for your child's weight and age.

Trust your child. Whether she says she wants tea and toast or a pepperoni pizza, serve it up. When children are ready to eat again, it's best to go with what they feel they can eat, says Dr. Hogan.

With younger, less verbal children, says Dr. Hogan, stick to bland foods such as toast, crackers, rice or potatoes at first. If the child's stomach tolerates those foods, you can gradually introduce others.

WARTS

Causes, Quirks and Cures

They spring up like forest mushrooms after a spring rain—knobby little growths on knee or elbow or finger.

But even though they look peculiar, warts are harmless. They are actually nothing more than little growths caused by a virus, says Richard Johnson, M.D., instructor of dermatology at Deaconess Medicine, Harvard Medical School in Boston. They're relatively common in kids, particularly on areas prone to minor injury, such as hands, elbows and knees, where it's easy for the virus to enter through a break in the skin.

Warts can be annoying to your child if they're on the hands and interfere with day-to-day activities or with nail growth. And some kids get self-conscious about them, which is natural enough, since they can be unsightly. But the only warts that cause outright pain (usually) are the kind that appear on the feet, called plantar warts. It doesn't

---

MEDICAL ALERT

When to See the Doctor

Every wart should be checked out by your pediatrician to make sure it *is* a wart before you take active measures to remove it. Your pediatrician should also check out any unusual or wartlike growth anywhere on your child's body to ensure that it is not a cancerous growth.

Because of the possibility of scarring, you should also never try to treat or remove any wart on the face, lips or eyelids yourself, says Richard Johnson, M.D., instructor of dermatology at Deaconess Medicine, Harvard Medical School in Boston. "It's often difficult to remove a wart and not leave some sort of scar behind," he says. For these warts, consult your child's pediatrician or dermatologist.

take long for a plantar wart to become flattened and painful from the pressure of walking.

Before deciding to actively treat a wart yourself, check with your doctor to be sure that what's growing on your child is indeed a harmless wart. If the doctor says yes, you can try these tips from the experts to cope with these growths.

Treatment

Wait it out. Warts will eventually go away all by themselves, although it could take months or even years. "If your child can stand them, just leave them alone," advises Moise Levy, M.D., a pediatric dermatologist and an assistant professor in the departments of dermatology and pediatrics at Baylor College of Medicine in Houston. But if your child is being taunted about his warts or they get in the way, you may want to help them along.

Wish them away. The first thing to try is—wishing the warts away. No kidding. Studies have found that some people who imagine their warts dissolving *do* lose their warts. "With young kids, suggestion sometimes actually works," says Dr. Levy. "Simply have your child think about getting rid of his warts for several minutes every day, and it could happen." Be sure to explain to your child that this is an experiment, however, so she doesn't feel that she has failed if the warts don't magically disappear.

Consider an OTC. If your doctor has confirmed that these growths *are* warts and are candidates for home treatment, you may decide it's time for more drastic action. Enter the over-the-counter wart removal products. There are many choices, including Wart-Off, Compound W and Trans-Plantar, says Kenneth R. Keefner, Ph.D., a pharmacist and associate professor of pharmacy in the School of Pharmacy and Allied Health Professions at Creighton University in Omaha.

It's important to remember, however, that most of these products are mild acids and work by burning the skin. For this reason, you should not use an over-the-counter product on children under six years old. If you do decide to use one, you should read directions carefully and follow them to the letter, says Dr. Keefner. It's also a good idea to coat the area around the wart with petroleum jelly to avoid getting the acid on healthy skin.

Try a liquid remover. A wide array of wart removers come in liquid form. All you do is drip the remover onto the wart. Look for products that list salicylic acid as the active ingredient, suggests Dr. Keefner. "They all come in various strengths—up to 40 percent salicylic acid," he explains. "For younger children, it's best to select a lower concentration, such as 17 percent, because their skin is more delicate."

Or choose a pad remover. Another option is wart remover pads or disks that may be easier to use on squirming children than liquids, says Dr. Keefner. "These can be cut to the size of the wart and then placed directly on top of it," he says. The pad is treated with salicylic acid, so be sure to cut the pad no larger than the wart itself.

Wait a bit . . . but not forever. No matter what over-the-counter product you choose, you may have to use it for a couple of weeks before the wart begins to vanish. But you shouldn't apply a nonprescription treatment indefinitely, says Michael L. Ramsey, M.D., a dermatologist in group practice in Wharton, Texas, and clinical instructor of dermatology at Baylor College of Medicine in Houston. "If I didn't see some results from an over-the-counter treatment in two weeks," he says, "I'd scoot in and see my family doctor or dermatologist." A plantar wart in particular may be a painful problem that needs further attention, he says.

Preventive Care

Stop the spread. Warts are contagious and picking at them can spread them to other parts of the body. To prevent that, be sure to explain to your child that warts shouldn't be touched or scratched. "Warts on the hands can easily wind up on the face, nose and mouth from scratching and biting the fingernails," says Dr. Johnson.

Furnish shower footwear. It's a simple matter for a barefoot child to pick up the wart virus in the shower or in the locker room at the pool or gym. You can help your child avoid plantar warts by buying flip-flops to wear in the shower, suggests Suzanne Levine, D.P.M., a podiatric surgeon, clinical assistant professor at the New York College of Podiatric Medicine in New York City and author of *My Feet Are Killing Me.* And because you probably don't have time to constantly disinfect the shower stall at home after a child with warts has used it, encourage your children to wear them when showering at home as well.

Assign personal laundry. Because warts are contagious, children with warts shouldn't share towels with anyone else, says Dr. Levine. To avoid singling out the child with warts, assign each child his own matching towel and washcloth. Pick bright colors or designs that are easily distinguishable or, better yet, let your children pick out the towels themselves. And remind your children not to share shoes or slippers—or any clothing for that matter, unless they have been freshly laundered.

Attack the virus. If you're battling warts in your house, you'll want to vanquish the wart virus when it's time to clean the bathroom. Household disinfectants such as Lysol or chlorine bleach will do the job on bathroom floors or showers, says Dr. Levine. Normal laundering in warm water with detergent will take care of the virus on towels and clothing, she says.

Slow down the pace. People tend to get warts when they're under a lot of stress or eating poorly, says Dr. Levine. If your child has a tendency to get warts and is leading a hectic lifestyle crammed with piano lessons and soccer practice and Girl Scout meetings, it can't hurt to slow down the pace a bit and make sure she's eating well.

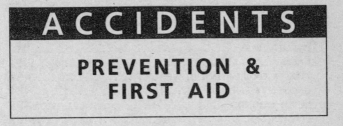

ACCIDENTS
PREVENTION &
FIRST AID

TIPS ON SAFETY

Parents always *hope* their children will somehow be accident-free their whole lives long.

Never possible, of course. But there are ways to keep accidents to a minimum in those early years—and ways to take care of emergencies in a hurry when they do occur. Take a few moments to read through this section. Under "Prevention," beginning below, you'll find hundreds of tips about how to accident-proof your home to avoid common childhood injuries, plus a few tips on things you should have on hand, just in case emergencies do happen.

Under "First Aid," beginning on page 475, you'll find step-by-step first-aid procedures.

We suggest that you review this information when the house is quiet and the kids are asleep, because real-life emergencies can occur without warning, and you may not have time to look up what to do. Be prepared, so you know what to do . . . just in case.

As you read through this section, you'll notice that true emergencies need medical attention—fast. While we do suggest some first-aid procedures, skills such as cardiopulmonary resuscitation (CPR), artificial respiration and the Heimlich maneuver can't be learned from a book alone. The best way to master these techniques is to take a course through the American Heart Association, the American Red Cross or your local hospital. The skills you learn may one day help save your child from harm.

PREVENTION

Bike Safety

Whizzing down the block may be your child's idea of freedom, but it is your responsibility to teach her how to do it safely. "Bicycles are vehicles, not toys, and any child who rides a bike without wearing a helmet is at serious risk," says Michael Macknin, M.D., head of the Section of General Pediatrics at the Cleveland Clinic Foundation in Ohio, clinical professor at Pennsylvania State University Medical School in Hershey and associate professor of pediatrics at Ohio State University Medical School in Columbus.

The vast majority of bicycle-related deaths and serious injuries are due to head injury. Eighty-five percent of head injuries and 88 percent of brain injuries could be prevented by wearing helmets, says Dr. Macknin.

Contrary to what you might think, the majority of accidents do not involve cars. "If your child can get his bike up to a speed of 20 miles per hour (and most kids can), taking a fall will generate the same amount of force as jumping off a three-story building," Dr. Macknin says.

Dr. Macknin offers the following tips.

Wearing Helmets

- Buy a crash-tested helmet. Be sure that the helmet meets the safety standards of the American National Standards Institute (ANSI) or the Snell Memorial Foundation. Look for a sticker on the helmet stating that it meets the standards of one of these organizations.

  Caution: Never let your child use a football helmet or hard hat instead of a bicycle helmet. They are not designed to protect your child in a crash or fall.

- Make helmet-wearing a rule. Any child who rides a two-wheel bicycle must wear a helmet. If your child has just started to ride—even a tricycle or a bike with training wheels—enforce this rule until it becomes a habit. Let him know if he doesn't wear a bike helmet, he can't go bike-riding.

- Have the helmet checked after a fall. If your child has taken a fall, the Styrofoam lining inside her helmet may be compressed, which means it might not provide enough protection if she takes another fall. Take the helmet to your bike store and ask an experienced salesperson if the helmet should be replaced.

Suggestion: Some helmet manufacturers will replace the helmet if you answer a questionnaire about your child's accident. Call the company to find out.

- Get together a helmet-buying group. Buying a helmet can be expensive, but you may get a discount if you buy as a group. To find out how to set up a group-discount program, check at bicycle shops in your area.

Safe Cycling

- Use "kiddy seats" with caution. Do not take your little one bike-riding in a bicycle seat until he is at least a year old and can sit well. Children younger than one year old may not have sufficient head control to ride safely.

  Caution: Any child riding in a bicycle seat should also wear a bicycle helmet.

- Buy a bicycle that fits your child. Riding an oversized bike is dangerous.
- When your child is skilled enough to ride on the street, teach him to ride on the right side, with traffic.
- Also, be sure to teach your child to use hand signals and to respect traffic signals.

Burn Prevention

Most accidents involving burns happen in the kitchen and bathroom, says Barbara Lewis, a burn technician and community burn educator at Saint Barnabas Burn Foundation in Livingston, New Jersey. To decrease the possibility of scalding your child (or yourself), she recommends setting the thermostat on your hot water heater to a maximum of 120°F. That's hot enough for normal washing, but not so hot that it will scald a child.

In addition, Lewis recommends that parents observe the following precautions in the kitchen and bathroom.

In the Kitchen

- Cook on the back burners and turn pot handles toward the back of the stove.

- Try to keep kids out of the kitchen while you are cooking. If they won't stay out, at least keep them away from the stove.
- Make sure that kids are at a safe distance away when you open the oven door.

    Suggestion: If kids want to help in the kitchen, let them mix dry ingredients like pancake batter or dried cereal (for "pretend") in a bowl—well away from the stove and other appliances.
- Test the temperature of food by touching it or tasting it yourself, especially if it has been cooked in a microwave oven. Microwaves heat some food unevenly, and your child can burn her mouth badly if she bites into a "hot spot."

    Caution: Don't heat a baby's bottle in the microwave.
- Keep all appliances on short electrical cords.
- Keep hot liquids away from the edges of countertops and tabletops.
- Don't drink hot beverages while holding a child.

In the Bathroom

- Before bathing a child, test the water with your elbow. Young kids have very sensitive skin, and what feels nice and comfortable to you may be very hot to the child. What you feel on the sensitive skin near your elbow is about what a child feels on his skin.
- Never leave a child unattended in the bathroom while bathing or at any time. It takes only a second for a child to turn on the hot water and get burned.
- Don't allow a young child to play with faucets, even if you're in the bathroom with her.
- Don't allow older kids to bathe younger ones.
- If you are building a new home or are renovating, install plumbing fixtures that automatically protect against scalding. Plumbing contractors and supply stores carry information.

Car Seat Safety

Good car safety starts the moment you strap your newborn securely into a car seat for her first ride home from the hospital. From then on, buckling up should be a habit.

"Your child should always be buckled up in an appropriate car safety seat, booster or seat belt, even for a trip around the block," says Elizabeth Orsay, M.D., assistant professor of emergency medicine and associate director of the Office of Research and Development at the University of Illinois at Chicago. "Most car collisions occur close to the home," she observes.

To make sure your child is as safe as possible, Dr. Orsay suggests the following:

- Use an appropriate car safety seat. For an infant who weighs less than 20 pounds, use a federally approved car seat that is designed so the child faces backward. When your child is more than 20 pounds, you can switch to a car seat that faces ahead—or, if you have a convertible seat, turn it around.

  Caution: If you do have a convertible car seat that can be turned from back-facing to front-facing, be sure to make the necessary adjustments in the shoulder straps and in the seat belt position. Follow the instructions in your owner's manual.

- Install your car seat in the rear middle seat, if possible. It will be the safest place in the car if there's ever an accident.

- Follow the manufacturer's instructions *to the letter* for your particular car seat. Be sure that the seat belt is threaded through the proper places and well-tightened.

- Use the car seat as long as possible—usually until a child weighs about 40 pounds.

- When your child weighs about 40 pounds, consider switching to a booster seat. A booster seat provides better protection in an accident than a seat belt, and makes the seat belt fit properly and more comfortably.

  Caution: Seat belts were really designed for adults, not children. When a child is fastened in a regular seat belt, the shoulder harness tends to cut across the neck, and the lap belt may ride up over the abdomen (which could cause abdominal injuries in a car crash). For this reason, booster seats are recommended for children weighing 40 to 60 pounds.

- If a booster seat isn't available, have your child sit as near as possible to the seat-belt buckle. That way, the lap strap will be low on his abdomen and the shoulder harness will be down off his neck.

    Suggestion: Don't put the shoulder harness behind your child. Even if the harness rides high, it provides much more protection than a lap belt alone. For increased comfort, buy a special belt cover, or fold a soft cloth over the part of the shoulder harness that crosses near your child's neck.

- If you have the kind of shoulder belt that stays slack when pulled, you can allow up to an inch of slack to keep the belt away from your child's neck. Don't exceed one inch of slack, though, because this decreases the effectiveness of the seat belt.

- A shoulder harness should always cross the chest: never put it under one arm. (If you have an accident, your child's spleen could be damaged by a seat belt in the underarm position.)

Choking

Children under the age of three are especially at risk for accidental choking. Infants and toddlers explore the world by putting objects in their mouths—so be on your guard and keep small items out of reach. Your child may choke on such common household items as coins, nails, tacks, screws, safety pins, crayon pieces, marbles, small parts of a toy, a broken or deflated balloon, jewelry or small batteries.

Round, hard food should never be given to a child because it can completely block your child's airway. That's why if your child is under four, you should usually avoid serving these foods: hot dogs, nuts, raisins, hard candies, raw carrots, grapes and popcorn. Some of these foods can be cut or chopped before serving, but you should ask the doctor whether your child is old enough to eat them without choking.

You can reduce the chance of having a choking accident in your home if you follow some prevention strategies, says Katherine Karlsrud, M.D., a clinical instructor in pediatrics at Cornell University Medical College in Ithaca, New York, pediatrician in New York City and a consultant with the Family Alert Program, a nonprofit consumer information program dealing with issues of child safety. Here are some of her suggestions.

- Take a first-aid and CPR course. The techniques used to rescue a choking victim need to be practiced first-hand, and this is the best way to learn them.
- Any food that has a diameter somewhere between a sour ball and a hot dog is the same size as your child's trachea. Cut the food into small pieces before serving it. A grape or a hot dog should be sliced lengthwise, then cut up into small chunks.
- Don't allow your child to run with food in her mouth.
- Be extra vigilant when visiting other people's houses during the holidays. Raw vegetables, hard candy, nuts and candy canes are often accessible. These hors d'oeuvres and treats can be dangerous to young children.
- If your child is in day care or going to camp, find out what kind of food she's eating. Insist that inappropriate foods be eliminated from the menu.
- Serve only tender meat to children under four. Most preschool kids don't chew well and may have trouble with tough food like steak. When your child is between the ages of four and seven, cut hard-to-chew foods into tiny pieces, just to stay on the safe side.
- Balloons or pieces of popped balloons are the most frequently choked-on toy. Keep them away from your children.
- Be sure that your baby or toddler doesn't have access to an older child's toys that could be chewed, swallowed or partially swallowed. Teach your older child to keep

toys with small pieces on a shelf out of reach. And he should play with them only when the baby is not around.

- Buy sturdy toys from a reliable manufacturer. More fragile, cheaply made toys may have small parts that break easily.
- Remove any detachable strings or ribbons from toys and clothing.

Drowning

In Florida, drowning is the number-one cause of death for children between the ages of one and four, according to Betti Hertzberg, M.D., a pediatrician and head of the Continuing Care Clinic at Miami Children's Hospital.

Most of these drowning deaths occur in the family pool or in a pool that belongs to a friend or relative. "It doesn't take long for a drowning accident to occur," says Dr. Hertzberg. "In 77 percent of these accidents, the children were missing for less than five minutes," she says.

But young children can be at risk of drowning in very little water—in a tub, a fish bowl, even a cleaning bucket. Dr. Hertzberg believes that adequate supervision can prevent the vast majority of drowning fatalities. Here's what she suggests.

Around the House
- While you are cleaning, keep your eye on your bucket of water or cleaning fluid. Empty it as soon as you are done.
- Keep the bathroom door closed. Toddlers have drowned in the toilet.
- Make sure any fish tank is out of reach of toddlers and babies.

General Water Safety
- Never leave a young child alone near the water.
- Enroll children over three years old in swimming lessons

taught by instructors who are certified by the American Red Cross. But keep in mind that lessons don't make your child water-safe or drown-proof.

- Take a CPR course, and keep your skills current.
- Even when your child knows how to swim, he should swim with a buddy, never alone.
- Do not allow horseplay in a pool or swimming area.

Home Pool and Spa Safety

- Spas and pools must be fully enclosed with a four-sided fence that is at least four feet high and is equipped with a self-closing and self-latching gate. The latch should be above the reach of your toddler.

  Caution: Even if you do have a fence around the pool, children should be supervised when they're in the area. Many children quickly figure out how to climb over a fence—and it's a temptation.
- Never leave tricycles and wheeled toys near a pool.
- Supervise children whenever they're in a wading pool. Empty the pool after the kids are through, and store it upside down.
- If you have a pool or spa indoors, keep the room locked.
- Never place chairs or tables near the pool fence. Children may climb on the furniture to get into the pool area.
- You should have a clear view of the pool or spa from the house. Keep flowers and hedges trimmed.
- If you use a cover for your pool or spa, remove it completely when the pool or spa is in use. Children have been known to drown when trapped under the cover.
- If you drain the pool for the winter, drain all of the standing water. One or two inches of standing water is all it takes to cause a fatal drowning accident.
- Don't allow a child to walk on a spa or pool cover.
- If your child is missing, look in the pool or any standing water first.
- Keep rescue equipment by the pool.
- Keep a cordless phone by the pool.

Electric Shock

There's a lot you can do to prevent electrical injuries in the home. Mary Ann Cooper, M.D., associate professor of emergency medicine and residency research director of the Program in Emergency Medicine at the University of Illinois College of Medicine in Chicago, suggests the following ways to reduce the chance of your child getting shocked.

- Take a complete survey of your home to determine where hazards exist. Open sockets are a particular hazard to small children who may insert pins or other metal devices in the holes.
- Teach kids not to touch cords and outlets.
- Install outlet covers over every electrical outlet. These must be tough enough to endure your child's ingenious attempts to remove them.
- Use plastic cord shorteners (available in most home centers and hardware stores) to shorten electrical cords. Or wind up excess cord and wrap it with duct tape.
- Keep electric and extension cords out of reach. A child can burn his mouth or face by chewing on the cord. If you must use an extension cord, put it in an inaccessible place such as behind the television, refrigerator or bookcase.
- Where an appliance is plugged into an extension cord, wrap electrical or duct tape around the connection so that the appliance plug can't be pulled out of the extension cord.
- Never leave an extension cord plugged in on one end and exposed at the other. If a child sucks on the exposed plug, he can get a severe, high-temperature burn that will cause permanent disfigurement.
- Never plug a three-pronged plug into a two-hole extension cord.
- Don't use an electric appliance near the tub, sink or any water. Electric extension cords should not be left near swimming pools.
- Have ground-fault interrupter (GFI) receptacles installed in areas of high risk such as the bathroom, work-

shop and patio. A GFI automatically cuts off the current if the receptacle gets wet or if it short-circuits. You can purchase a GFI at most home centers and hardware stores.

- Do not touch any downed electric power lines, even if they are insulated lines leading to your house.

  Caution: The insulation on high power lines protects against corrosion, not against electric shock.

- Teach your children not to touch electrical boxes on utility poles. And they should never try to climb telephone poles.

Fall-Proofing Your Home

From the moment a baby appears on the scene, parents realize how closely that new resident needs to be watched— and how much "child-proofing" needs to be done around the house. A baby can easily fall off a changing table or tumble out of a crib. And as for toddlers—it's amazing how *fast* those kids can move.

Even the safest-looking house may have a number of treacherous areas where your child might fall and get injured.

"Of all the childhood injuries, injuries resulting from falls are among the leading causes of emergency room visits," says Mark D. Widome, M.D., professor of pediatrics at the Pennsylvania State University Children's Hospital in Hershey and former chairman of the Committee of Injury and Poison Prevention of the American Academy of Pediatrics.

But with a little common sense and planning, you may be able to prevent some falls and reduce the chance of injury, Dr. Widome says. Here's what he suggests.

Precautions with Babies

- Before you change your baby's diaper, have your supplies ready so you won't have to run to the bathroom to get wipes or diaper cream.

- When your baby is on the changing table, never turn your back on her, even if a safety strap is fastened around her. (The strap might not protect her from a fall.) Keep one hand on her at all times.
- If the phone rings and the baby is on the changing table, pick up your baby when you go to answer it. (If you have an answering machine, let the machine take the call.)
- Don't leave your baby alone on a bed or sofa. A child may learn to roll over any time between the ages of two and five months—and he can easily roll off a bed if left alone for a minute.
- Place carpet under your baby's changing table and crib. If your child should ever fall to the floor, she'll hit a more forgiving surface than the hard floor.
- Keep an eye on the crib. If the crib rail is at the level of your child's nipples when your child is standing and the crib mattress is at its lowest setting, your child is too tall for the crib. Move her to a bed with a safety rail.
- Avoid using a baby walker. Too many babies are injured—approximately 20,000 children a year need medical treatment for injuries related to baby walkers. If you must use a walker, never leave your baby unattended.

Precautions with Toddlers

- Buy your toddler shoes that have good traction. Avoid shoes with shiny leather bottoms because they tend to be slippery.
- If you have bare-wood or vinyl floors, allow your toddler to walk barefooted around the house rather than walk around in socks. She'll get better traction in bare feet.
- Install gates at the top *and* the bottom of any stairway. Use the gates until your child can negotiate the stairs well.

    Caution: If you only have a gate at the top of the stairs, your toddler may crawl halfway up the stairs and then fall down.
- Be sure you have railings and banisters at child height installed everywhere a child might fall—on the stairs

inside your house, alongside the basement stairs and on the porch.

- Move chairs and other pieces of furniture away from windows so that your young climber won't be able to open windows or get up on windowsills.
- Install window guards to cover the bottom of any accessible window. An unguarded window that is opened only five inches can be a danger for kids under ten. Window guards are available at most hardware and home-supply stores.

  Caution: A window screen is not strong enough to keep a child from falling out.
- Use nonskid decals or a rubber mat in the tub for extra traction.
- Have a "no running" rule for all kids in the house. That rule should include friends.
- Cushion the corners of coffee tables and any sharp-cornered furniture. Even better, move this furniture out of the main "traffic lanes" until your toddler grows up a bit.

Firearms

If you own a firearm for sport or for protection, you should know that a gun in the home is more likely to kill a family member or friend than an intruder. The steady increase in gun-related injuries and deaths of children in our country has prompted the American Academy of Pediatrics to call firearm injuries an epidemic: about 11 children and teenagers now die daily as a result of firearm injuries.

To reduce that chance that your child will be hurt or killed by a firearm in the home, Susan P. Baker, M.P.H., professor and codirector of the Johns Hopkins Injury Prevention Center at the Johns Hopkins School of Public Health in Baltimore suggests the following tips.

- The best way to reduce firearm injuries is to remove handguns from the home.

- If you do keep a gun, store it in an inaccessible, locked cabinet or box. Be sure that the gun is stored unloaded.
- Keep ammunition in a separate, locked area.

Fire Safety

The following safety tips for fire prevention and emergencies are recommended by Bill Kamela, associate director of the National SAFE KIDS Campaign, a nonprofit organization devoted to preventing childhood injury.

- Make sure that every sleeping area has a working smoke detector. Check the smoke detector once a month to make sure the batteries are working.
   Suggestion: Change the smoke-detector batteries in the spring and fall when you reset the clocks for daylight saving time. That way, you'll always remember to put in new batteries twice a year.
- Keep fire extinguishers in the kitchen, garage and basement.
   Check their labels to make sure they're up to date.
- Keep lighters and matches out of children's reach.
- If you are building or renovating a home, install sprinklers. Sprinklers add two to three thousand dollars to the cost of a house, but an automatic system does save lives and reduce property damage.
- Practice fire escape routes with your children.
   Suggestion: Your children should learn how to leave the house by two different routes in case one is blocked by fire. Have a designated meeting place outside the house for your family, so you can make sure everyone got out safely.
- If your house needs an escape ladder, be sure to get one and leave it near a window where it's easily available. As soon as your child is old enough, she should learn how to use the ladder in an emergency.
- Teach kids to crawl *underneath* the smoke. (More people die from smoke inhalation than from fire.)

- Tell your children they should never hide under their beds or in closets if there's a fire in the house.

  Suggestion: Some children are afraid of firefighters. Take your child to your local fire station so they get familiar with firefighters and their uniforms. Remind your child he should never run away or try to hide if firefighters come in the house.

- Tell your child she should never re-enter a burning home.

- Don't allow children to play near wood stoves, radiant heaters or other heating sources.

Frostbite

Children run a greater risk of frostbite than adults, according to Charles Steiner, M.D., a family practitioner at the Tanana Valley Clinic in Fairbanks, Alaska, and chairman of the Disaster Preparedness Committee at Fairbanks Memorial Hospital. According to Dr. Steiner, children lose heat from their skin more rapidly than adults, and they may lack the judgment to come in from the cold in time to prevent injuries.

"Prevent frostbite injuries by respecting the elements, not by avoiding them," says Dr. Steiner. "Teach kids the right way to approach the cold by being prepared and staying close to home. Once kids are more experienced, the family can branch out into more winter sports and activities," Dr. Steiner says.

Here's what he suggests to reduce the chance of cold injury.

- Babies too young to run and play have to be superinsulated because they lose a lot of body heat. Add extra padding on the baby's bottom if you plan to pull him along in a sled or toboggan.

- Be on the lookout for frostnip (see page 219). It usually strikes the face, cheeks and ears and gives the skin a bleached, white look. At the first sign of frostnip, go indoors or warm the area.

- Have your children dress in loose, warm layers and choose synthetics over cotton. (Cotton conducts the cold when wet, so it's not a good insulator. The innermost layer should include long underwear, followed by pants or sweatpants, thick wool socks, a T-shirt and a sweatshirt. The outermost layers should be either a one- or two-piece snowsuit that sheds the snow. (Dr. Steiner says his own children—in Alaska—enjoy playing outside as long as they're bundled up like this and the temperature is warmer than $-10°F$.)

- For added protection, your child can wear a fleece or wool balaclava—a hat that covers the head and neck but leaves the face exposed. If your child is participating in winter sports in severe cold and wind, he should wear a wind-shedding face mask of nylon, fleece or neoprene in addition to the balaclava. Both the balaclava and face mask are available in outdoor specialty stores.

- Mittens are warmer than gloves, but the warmest combination is a pair of mittens *on top of* gloves or glove liners. Attach your child's mittens to the coat with clips.

- If you are out for extended periods of time, have extra warm clothing and mittens. Plan for the unexpected.

- If you're planning outdoor winter activities, carry along juice, water, hot cocoa or soup in a Thermos, and let your child drink as frequently as possible. A child who becomes dehydrated is more likely to get frostbite.

- Older kids should be given special warnings about the danger of drinking alcohol or smoking cigarettes in the cold. Alcohol increases heat loss, and smoking decreases circulation to the extremities.

- Avoid contact with metal on bare skin. It can produce a frost injury within seconds.

- Don't drink superchilled drinks. They can cause esophageal damage. (For example, when you're backpacking in cold conditions and you pull a drink from your backpack, it may be superchilled even though it's not frozen. Let the drink warm up a bit before your child takes a swallow.)

Playgrounds and Sports

To avoid injuries, inspect the playgrounds in your area before your child gets on the swings or climbs the jungle gym, suggests Mark D. Widome, M.D., professor of pediatrics at Pennsylvania State University Children's Hospital in Hershey and former chairman of the Committee of Injury and Poison Prevention of the American Academy of Pediatrics. Dr. Widome offers the following suggestions for parents of young playground-goers and sports enthusiasts.

- Soften playground surfaces. Many kids take a spill off playground equipment, so be sure that where your child plays, the surface underfoot is soft. It should be made of special padding or a thick layer of some kind of loose material such as gravel, shredded tires or wood chips.

  Caution: Grass, packed dirt and asphalt surfaces increase the chances of injury.

- Use proper sports equipment. Your young athlete needs to be protected with a helmet and extra padding for some sports. Football, skating, skateboarding and bicycling are among the sports in which injuries are high.

- Look for good coaching. A good coaching staff will make sure your child learns to fall properly and will match him with players of equal ability as well as size. Your child will also get the proper conditioning to insure that he's in good physical shape. These factors will make it less likely that your young athlete will sustain an injury during sports activities.

Poisons

A lovely bottle of perfume, a common houseplant, a handy spray bottle of window cleaner, some iron tablets—all these common household items can be poison to your child. If you have a child under five, he is especially at risk for accidental poisoning in the home. A child of that age is curious, has little understanding about what is dangerous to eat and drink, and he has a strong urge to imitate what you do.

"The best way to keep your child from being accidentally poisoned is to never leave a poison and your child alone together," says Jude McNally, R.Ph., a registered pharmacist and assistant director of the Arizona Poison and Drug Information Center in Tucson. Here's his advice on how to poison-proof your home—and how to be prepared for emergencies.

- Assume your child can get into anything. Go through your house room by room and put all poisons out of reach. Keep all dangerous substances on a high shelf, preferably in a locked box.
- Keep your eye on cleaning products and other dangerous substances while you are using them, and put them away as soon as you are finished. One study showed that as many as 40 percent of pediatric household poisonings occurred when parents were using the product. Assume that a child can always get his hands on the poison when your back is turned.
- Never coax your child to take medication by saying that it tastes like candy.
- Don't leave medication lying around where children can reach. Studies show that, given time, kids can figure out how to open up child-proof packaging.
- Do what pharmacists do: Always read the label before giving your child a dose of medication. Don't assume that you remember the proper dose.
- At night, always turn on the light before giving medication. Tragic mistakes have been made by giving medicine from the wrong bottle.
- Clean out your medicine cabinet. Flush outdated medication down the toilet or pour liquid medicines down the sink. Store other medications in a locked box.
    Caution: The medicine cabinet is the worst place to keep medication because children can easily climb up, open the cabinet door and help themselves.
- Be sure that all poisons are stored in locked cabinets or

well out of reach in your basement, gardening shed and garage as well as the house.

- Don't leave vitamins out on the kitchen counter. A child can eat a bóttle of iron tablets as though it were candy.
- When you have visitors in your home, ask them to keep their medication, perfume and make-up in a locked travel case or well out of the reach of toddlers.
- Be especially careful when you bring your children into other people's homes. Your friends may not be as careful about poisons as you are.
- Always keep your Poison Control Center's telephone number posted or taped on the phone.
- Keep ipecac syrup on hand for certain types of poisonings. (But only use it when instructed to do so by a Poison Control Center or physician.)
- Avoid the following plants in and around your home. Not all of the varieties of these plants are poisonous—but many varieties are hazardous. To be on the safe side, keep these plants out of the reach of children.

Bird of paradise	Mescal bean
Bull nettle	Mexicantes
Castor bean	Mistletoe
Chinaberry tree	Morning glory
Crocus	Mountain laurel
Daffodil	Night-blooming jasmine
Deadly nightshade	Nutmeg
Dieffenbachia (dumb cane)	Oleander
Foxglove	Philodendron
Glory lily	Poison ivy
Hemlock	Poison sumac
Holly berry	Pokeweed
Indian tobacco	Poppy
Iris	Potato
Jimsonweed	Privet
Lantana	Rhododendron
Larkspur	Rhubarb
Lily of the valley	Water hemlock
Marijuana	Wisteria

Snakebite

Though most snakes are nonpoisonous, snakebites are almost always painful, and they can cause infection. If your child does encounter a venomous snake, the consequences can be severe.

The best way to avoid snakes is by taking some simple precautions recommended by Kenneth W. Kizer, M.D., M.P.H., professor of emergency medicine and medical toxicology at the University of California, Davis, School of Medicine. Discuss these precautions with your child.

- Always look over logs before stepping over them. Snakes often nap on either side.
- Never put your hand into a hole unless you can see into it. A snake may be in there.
- Don't poke around hollow logs or reach into stumps of trees. These are the types of places where snakes like to hide.
- Never try to grab or touch a snake, even if you know it's not poisonous. (And some kids have been known to dare each other to kiss a snake. So warn your child, "Never!")
- When walking in the woods or fields, where snakes are likely to be, wear high-top boots or high-top leather sneakers that cover the ankles.
- Wear long pants. A heavy fabric such as denim is more likely to fend off a snake's fangs than thin cotton.
- Wear sturdy gloves if you go out to the woodpile. It's a favorite lurking place for snakes.
- If you meet a snake, stop in your tracks. Snakes usually strike when they feel threatened. If you stand still, there's a good chance the snake will retreat.

Suffocation

"Suffocation, the most extreme form of breathing difficulty, occurs when a child can't get air into his lungs," says Modena Wilson, M.D., M.P.H., a specialist in pediatric injury prevention and director of general pediatrics at Johns Hopkins Children's Center in Baltimore. "Suffocation results when the nose and mouth are covered so that no air can pass or when the neck is compressed," says Dr. Wilson.

"Most suffocation accidents can be eliminated if parents are attuned to the danger," Dr. Wilson adds. Here are some of her suggestions for preventing suffocation.

- Do not put an infant to sleep on soft surfaces that he can sink into such as a beanbag chair, a basket with soft sides, soft pillow or water bed. Babies have suffocated on these surfaces because they were not able to free their faces.
- Put your baby to sleep in a standard crib, cradle or bassinet with a snug-fitting, firm mattress. When visiting a friend or relative, don't put a baby to sleep on an adult bed. Children have been trapped between the headboard and the mattress.
- Avoid antique cribs with curlicues or high posts that can catch a child's clothing or trap the head or neck.
- Use a crib with slats that are no more than 2⅜ inches apart. The Consumer Product Safety Commission requires that all new cribs meet this standard, but old or antique cribs may not. If the slats are too far apart, the baby's body might slip through, trapping the baby's head.
- Keep all plastic bags away from a baby. If the baby's mouth or head is covered with plastic, air won't pass through.
- Remove the plastic covering from a new mattress, and don't cover a mattress with a plastic bag.
- Keep all pillows out of the crib.
- Don't have balloons on a string around the crib.
- Don't dangle toys from strings into the crib. Crib gyms can be a hazardous if the baby's clothing gets tangled in them. (A mobile that has a short cord and is high enough to be out of reach is fine.)
- Don't place cribs near blind or drapery cords. Cut drapery cords so they don't dangle near the floor. Buy draperies that are closed with rods.

- When your baby is in a playpen, keep the mesh sides up. Young children have become entangled in the folds when a side is collapsed and have suffocated.
- Don't put a pacifier on a string around the baby's neck.
- Avoid using the old accordion-style gates; children's heads have been trapped in them. More modern, safe designs are available in toy stores.
- Older kids should not play in the playground with a string, scarf or necklace around their neck. These could get caught on the equipment and cause strangulation.
- Toys should not be stored in a toy chest that has a lid that might fall down on a child's neck or trap him inside.
- If you're storing an old refrigerator or freezer, remove the door. (Most new appliances are built to open from the inside, but older appliances don't have this safety feature—and they are usually airtight when shut.)
- If you are visiting a farm, warn children to stay away from granaries and silos. Children have been suffocated by falling into silage.
- If you use an automatic garage door, it should automatically retract when it comes in contact with an obstruction. (You can test this with a block of wood. The garage door mechanism should stop and reverse itself when it encounters the block.)
- Be aware of bunk bed hazards. Children have been trapped and suffocated because of poorly constructed bunk beds. Children under six should be kept out of the top bunk, and there should be no openings that would allow children to be trapped and strangled in the openings between the mattress, bed ends or guard rail. The bed frames should be supported by strong cross pieces, and the mattresses should fit snugly. Allow no horseplay or jumping on the beds.

FIRST AID

Bleeding

If your child has punctured or severed an artery, bright red blood will spurt out with each beat of the heart. Arterial bleeding can be life-threatening.

Severe bleeding from a vein is usually less dangerous and is distinguished by flowing rather than spurting blood.

If your child is bleeding heavily—from either an artery or vein—you should take the following steps as soon as possible.

1. Calm and reassure the victim. The sight of blood can be very frightening.
2. Locate the source of the bleeding.
3. Wash your hands.
4. Put on sterile gloves if you have them. Remove any obvious loose debris from the wound.
5. Using a sterile dressing or clean cloth, apply direct pressure to the wound to stop the bleeding. Direct pressure is almost aways appropriate for brisk bleeding; however, do not use direct pressure on an eye injury, on a wound that contains an embedded object or on a head injury if there is a possibility of skull fracture.
6. Raise the bleeding part above the level of the victim's heart if you don't suspect a broken bone and if elevating the injury doesn't cause the victim more pain.
7. If the bleeding doesn't stop or if you need to free your hands, apply a pressure bandage. This is a roller bandage or long strip of cloth tied firmly over the wound. (The pressure bandage should be tight enough to keep pressure on the wound, but not so tight that it cuts off circulation.)
8. If the bleeding doesn't stop after 15 minutes of direct pressure, or if the wound is too extensive to cover effectively, use pressure point bleeding control—

applying pressure to a major artery—if you are trained in the procedure.

9. If the bleeding stops with direct pressure but then starts up again, reapply direct pressure.

10. If the bleeding is severe, take steps to prevent shock while you await medical help. Lay the victim flat, raise his or her feet 8 to 12 inches and cover the victim with a coat or blanket. Do not place the victim in the shock position if you suspect any head, neck, back or leg injury or if the position makes the victim uncomfortable.

11. If bleeding is not severe, wash the wound with soap and water. Rinse well and place a sterile dressing or a clean cloth over the wound. Then apply direct pressure for a few minutes to control any bleeding.

Breathing Problems and Suffocation

If your child is having severe breathing problems, it may be caused by a number of conditions that include injury, sudden illness or an underlying medical problem. Here's what to do.

- Call for emergency medical service.
- Loosen any tight clothing.
- While you wait for help to arrive, do not move your child or put him in any position that he finds uncomfortable.
- Do not put a pillow under your child's head since this can close his airway.
- Do not give him anything to eat or drink.
- Be as calm and reassuring as you can. Anxiety can worsen the problem.
- If your child becomes drowsy or stops wheezing, do not assume that his condition is improving. His condition may have taken a turn for the worse. But if you've already called the emergency medical service, help should arrive quickly.

Minor Burns

If a burn appears to be just superficial (red skin and perhaps a blister) and is smaller than a quarter, you can treat it as a minor burn. Take the following steps.

1. Cool the burn immediately by immersing it in cold water (not ice water) or under gently running cold water for at least ten minutes. A clean, cold, wet towel might also help reduce the pain. If a blister forms, leave it alone.
2. Pat the area dry with a clean (sterile, if possible) cloth and cover it with a nonadhesive sterile dressing. This will help prevent infection.

    Caution: Call for medical attention for any burn that involves your child's airway, eyes, face, hands or genitals. Additionally, if a minor burn doesn't heal normally, call your doctor. Even with a minor burn, you should make sure your child is up-to-date on his tetanus immunization.

Severe Burns

A severe burn can be caused by any prolonged exposure to intense heat, fire, electricity, chemicals or scalding liquids. It destroys all skin layers and may affect the underlying fat and muscle. The child needs immediate emergency medical treatment. Call an ambulance and take the following steps while you wait for medical help to arrive.

1. Check your child's ABCs: Make sure the airway is open, and check his breathing and circulation. Start rescue breathing, CPR or bleeding control as needed.

    Caution: Someone who is certified in CPR and first aid is best suited to do these techniques. You and every member of your family can easily learn them and become certified. First-aid and CPR courses are offered by local chapters of the American Red Cross. The American Heart Association also gives instructions in CPR.

2. Calm and reassure your child.
3. Treat your child for shock. Have the child lie down and elevate his feet 8 to 12 inches. If you think he has a head, neck, back or leg injury, just keep your child calm and comfortable.
4. Don't take any other steps to treat your child for a severe burn. Also, don't give him anything to eat or drink, and never apply cold compresses, creams, ointments, sprays or oils. Trying to remove blisters or dead skin may cause severe complications.

Choking

If your child gets food, liquid or an inedible object in his airway, he will automatically begin coughing to eject the obstruction. The choking sensation can be frightening to a child, but as long as he can speak, breath or cough forcefully, he will probably be able to expel the object by himself.

But you must intervene if your child seems to be in real trouble. Take action right away if your child has convulsions or loses consciousness. You should also take immediate action if he can't breathe, cry, speak or cough forcefully, or if his face looks pale and bluish. A correctly performed Heimlich maneuver could save his life.

You or someone else should call for emergency help as soon as possible. But don't wait for the ambulance to arrive before performing the Heimlich Maneuver.

Heimlich Maneuver for a Baby

For a baby who is newborn up to one year of age, use this method to restore breathing.

1. Place the baby face-down along your forearm, with his head toward the palm of your hand. Lower your arm slightly, so his head is lower than the rest of his body.
2. Support your baby's head with your hand. Hold the

baby's jaw between your thumb and finger. Rest your forearm on your thigh.

3. Deliver four forceful blows with the heel of your hand to the baby's back, between the shoulder blades.

4. Then turn the baby over, so he's lying on his back. Place him on your thigh or a firm surface, with his head lower than his chest.

5. Place your index and middle finger on the baby's breast bone just below the nipples and above the notch at the end of the breastplate.

6. Give four quick thrusts down, pressing the breast ½ to 1 inch each time. Each thrust is a separate attempt to clear the airway by forcing air out through the windpipe.

7. Continue the series of four back blows and four chest thrusts—turning the baby from stomach position to back position—until the object is dislodged. If the baby becomes unconscious, however, you should stop this maneuver. (You can provide first aid for an unconscious infant using techniques taught in a first-aid course.)

8. Seek medical attention even if your baby starts to breathe normally.

Heimlich Maneuver for a Child over One Year of Age

1. Stand or kneel behind your child and wrap your arms around his waist.

2. Make a fist with one hand. Place the thumb side of your fist in the middle of your child's abdomen. Place the fist above navel and well below the breastbone.

3. Grab your fist with your other hand.

4. Keeping your elbows out, give four quick, upward thrusts into the child's abdomen.

5. Repeat this procedure until the object pops out of his throat and the airway is cleared. But stop the procedure if the child loses consciousness. (You can provide first aid for an unconscious victim using techniques taught in a first-aid course.)

6. Seek medical attention even if your child starts to breathe normally.

Convulsions without Fever

During a convulsion (also known as a seizure), a child becomes unconscious for a brief period of time. The convulsion may be accompanied by falling; drooling or frothing at the mouth; vigorous, involuntary muscle spasms; loss of bladder or bowel control; and a temporary halt in breathing. In some cases, there are no convulsive movements, but the child becomes pale and limp.

Convulsions are associated with many medical conditions. But if your toddler has no previous history of convulsions and suddenly experiences multiple seizures, he may have swallowed poison. Call the Poison Control Center and get immediate emergency medical aid.

While seizures are frightening to parents, they are usually short-lived, generally lasting from 30 to 45 seconds. Once a seizure has begun, there is no way to stop it. The best thing you can do for your child is to get medical help while you take steps to prevent him from hurting himself. Here's what you should do to protect your child during a seizure.

• Place your child on the ground in a safe area. Clear away any sharp or hard objects.
• Protect his head by placing cushions around it.
• Loosen his collar, pants, belt or any other tight clothing.
• Roll your child onto his left side to keep his airway clear.
• Do not try to restrain your child during a seizure, and do not try to put anything between his teeth.
• When your child regains consciousness, he may fall into a deep sleep. This is typical: Do not try to wake him.
• Do not give him anything to eat or drink until is he fully awake and alert.

Drowning

If your child has been submerged in the water and is no longer breathing, you may still be able to save his life if you take immediate action. Here's how.

- Call for emergency medical help and rescue the drowning child.
- Check your child's ABCs—airway, breathing and circulation. If necessary, begin rescue breathing or CPR if you have been trained.
- Remove any cold, wet clothes. Cover your child with a blanket, coat or any other clothing to prevent hypothermia.
- As your child revives, he may cough and have trouble breathing. Try to be calm and reassuring while you wait for medical help to arrive.
- Near-drowning victims should always be checked by a physician because lung complications may develop as a result of the accident.

Electric Shock Injuries

Electrical injuries can be minor if your child has only brief contact with a low current, but a high-voltage shock from a generated electrical current or a lightning strike can cause devastating injuries: severe burns, internal and external damage, cardiac and respiratory arrest, neurological damage and sometimes death. If your child has sustained an electrical injury, take the following measures.

- Check to see if your child is still in contact with the electric current. If he is, don't touch him, even with a wooden branch, pole or broomstick. A high-voltage current may be able to travel through wood.
- Shut off the power at a wall switch or circuit box.
- Check the ABCs—airway, breathing and circulation. If necessary, begin CPR if you know how.
- Call for emergency medical service.

Eye Injuries

When your child gets an eye lash or a piece of dirt in her eye, she can probably remove it herself by blinking—or her tears may flush out the small object. But if your child has a more serious eye injury, it could jeopardize her sight.

Be very cautious, however, about touching your child's eye. Even if your child has chemicals or a foreign body in her eye, you may not be able to help her immediately—and if you try, you could make the eye injury worse. Also, your child will undoubtedly resist your attempts to help her.

Because an eye injury requires expert medical care, your main role is to ensure that the eye is protected as much as possible until help arrives. Take these steps.

Foreign Body in the Eye
If the eye seems seriously injured by the foreign body, call for emergency medical service.

- While you wait for help to arrive, tilt your child's head so that the injured eye is down. Flush the object out of the eye, from the inside corner of the eye outward, using a sterile saline solution if you have it. (If you have none, plain tap water will do.)
- Try to hold your child's eyelid open to make sure the eye is properly flushed. Keep flushing for 15 to 30 minutes, or until you have medical help.
- Do not press or rub the eye.
- Do not try to remove the object with your fingers, with a cotton swab or with anything else.

Foreign Body Embedded in the Eye
- Call for emergency medical service even if the object in the eye is small.
- Leave the object alone. Do not touch it or let anything press on it.
- If the object is large, place a cup or cone over the injured eye and tape it into place. Cover the uninjured eye with

an eye patch or sterile dressing. If the object is small, cover both eyes with eye patches or a sterile dressing.

- Try to calm and reassure your child.

Chemical Exposure

- Call for emergency medical service, then try to determine the type of chemical. Call the Poison Control Center in your area for specific advice.
- Do not press or rub the eye or allow the child to rub the eye.
- Tilt your child's head so the injured eye is down. Flush the eye with fresh water, pouring the water from the inside corner of the eye outward. Continue to do this for at least 15 to 30 minutes or until help arrives. (You may have to force the eye open to be effective.)
- If both eyes are affected, do this procedure in the shower.
- Even if only one eye is affected, cover both eyes with sterile dressings after the flushing procedure. Keep the eyes covered until help arrives.

Falls

If an infant or toddler doesn't start to use an injured arm or leg within hours of a fall or he or she continues to cry when the injured area is touched, assume the child has a broken bone. Take the following measures.

- Call for emergency medical help.
- Don't move the child unless the injured limb is immobilized. If you know first aid, splint the limb in the position you found it.
- Keep your child still while you wait for help to arrive.
- Do not try to straighten or test a misshapen bone or joint.
- Do not give your child anything to eat or drink.
- If the injury involves an open wound, do not blow on it, wash it or probe it. Cover the wound with sterile dressings.

- Take steps to prevent shock. If you can do so without moving the limb or causing pain, raise the child's feet 8 to 12 inches. Cover him with a blanket.

  Caution: Do not attempt to move a child whom you suspect to have a neck injury. Call for help. (You should cover the child with a blanket while you're waiting for help to arrive.)

Finger or Toe Injuries

An injured finger or toe may turn black and blue under the nail. Often there's swelling as well as some bleeding around the cuticle. When there's bleeding underneath the nail, the end of the toe or finger will turn black or dark blue. The pressure underneath the nail will be very painful.

If your child has a smashed finger or toe, take the following steps.

- Call your child's physician if there appears to be excessive swelling, a deep cut, blood under the fingernail, bleeding or if the finger or toe appears broken.

  Caution: Don't attempt to straighten the injured part.
- If the swelling and bleeding is less severe, wash the injured area with soap and water and cover with a soft, sterile cloth. Then apply an ice-pack or soak it in cold water to relieve pain and minimize swelling.
- Cover with a soft, sterile cloth.
- If you notice increased pain, swelling, redness, pus or fever within 24 to 72 hours of the injury, notify your child's physician at once. An infection has probably set in.

Frostbite

A frostbite injury, caused when bitter cold and wind freeze body tissue, can be severe enough to penetrate the skin and everything beneath it including blood and bones. Any part of the body can be affected by frostbite, but it commonly strikes the exposed areas of the face, the fingers, toes, ear lobes and nose. Frostbitten skin is frozen, waxy and numb;

when it thaws, the skin may blister, swell and turn red, blue or purple.

It is often hard to judge how serious the frostbite damage is, so you should play it safe by beginning first-aid treatment whenever you suspect your child *might* have a case of frostbite. Then get your child to a doctor as soon as possible. Here's what to do.

- Move your child out of the cold.
- Remove any constricting or wet clothing and replace with dry clothing.
- For frostbite, rewarm the frozen area for at least 30 minutes by using wet heat. Immerse the frozen limb in water that is slightly warmer than body temperature (100° to 105°F). Help the warming process by circulating the water with your hand. For areas that can't be immersed in water, such as the cheeks and nose, apply warm compresses.
- Expect that rewarming may be painful. Your child will experience a burning sensation, swelling and color changes on the skin. When the skin looks pink and is no longer numb, the area is thawed.
- After the skin has thawed, apply dry, sterile dressing to the area. If fingers have been affected, place the dressing between each finger, too. Use the same procedure if the toes are frostbitten.
- Move the thawed areas as little as possible.
- Prevent refreezing by wrapping the rewarmed areas.
- Don't thaw out a frostbitten area if it's not possible to keep it thawed.
- Do not use direct heat such as a radiator, car heater, campfire, or heating pad to thaw the frostbitten area.
- Do not massage or rub snow on the frostbitten area.
- Do not disturb the blisters on the frozen skin.

Head Injuries

Your active child may receive a good wallop on the head as she runs, climbs and plays, but as long she is up and running again after the injury, it is not likely that she has sustained serious damage. You should watch her for the next 24 hours, though, since the symptoms of a serious head injury may be delayed. Check with your doctor at least by telephone for any head injury that causes even momentary loss of consciousness. And, for infants, consult the doctor for all but minor head injuries.

Be alert for such symptoms as severe or repeated vomiting, dazed or confused behavior, increased irritability, restlessness, a personality change or drowsiness during the times when your child would ordinarily be alert. According to doctors, you should also watch out for headache that is not relieved by over-the-counter headache remedies. Other symptoms that indicate problems include slurred speech, a stiff neck, double vision, difficulty seeing, pupils of unequal size, weak limbs, fluid or blood draining from the nose or mouth or a slowed rate of breathing.

If you see an obvious wound, dent or fracture in your child's skull—and some bleeding—you should take immediate action. But you should take the following precautions *any* time you suspect that your child has a serious head injury.

- Call for emergency medical help.
- While you wait for the ambulance, do not move your child unless absolutely necessary.
- Do not shake or pick up your child.
- Do not remove any object that is stuck in the wound or protruding from the skull or head area.
- Check the ABCs—airway, breathing and circulation. And, if necessary, begin rescue breathing, CPR and/or bleeding control.
- Try to keep your child calm and still.
- If you suspect your child has a fractured skull, do not apply direct pressure to any bleeding wound in the head area.
- If your child vomits, lean her forward and support her head so she does not choke. Do not sit her up if you think her neck is injured; instead, support her head and neck and roll her to one side.

- Apply ice to areas of swelling.
    Caution: Ice should be wrapped in a cloth or towel—not applied directly to the skin—as it may cause frostbite.
- If your child is dazed or unconscious, assume that she may have a spinal injury. It is essential that her head and neck is kept immobile. Place your hands on both sides of her head, and keep the child's head and neck in the position in which you found them. If the child vomits, roll the child as a unit (head and neck immobile) onto one side to prevent choking and to allow breathing. But otherwise, the child should not be moved at all. Wait for medical help.

Poisoning

If you suspect that your child has swallowed, inhaled, touched or injected some kind of poison, it's important to stay calm to avoid alarming your child. Quietly question your child about what he took and how long ago. (You need this history to be able to respond appropriately.)

Keep the child as quiet as possible while you do the following.

- Look in your child's mouth. If he has chewed on pills or bitten a poisonous plant, remove any bits of pills or plant parts that remain in his mouth.
- Your child should stay with you when you go to the phone to call for help.
- If your child has swallowed a poisonous product or medication, also take the container with you when you go to the phone. Call the local Poison Control Center. If there is no Poison Control Center, call your doctor, a hospital emergency department or Emergency Medical Service (EMS) and follow instructions. Whoever you call will probably ask you to read product information from the container.
- Give specific information about your child's age and weight, and a description of the product or substance

that he swallowed. You should also try to estimate the amount swallowed and exactly when it happened.

- When medical instructions are given to your over the phone, follow the instructions exactly. Never give any poison remedy (even ipecac syrup) without getting medical advice.

Snakebite

Although snakes are plentiful in the United States, only four types are poisonous—the copperhead, rattlesnake, water moccasin and coral snake. Most bites by poisonous snakes require immediate treatment with antivenin, which is available in hospital emergency departments in areas where there are poisonous snakes. If you're not sure whether or not the snake was poisonous, you should call your local Poison Control Center or promptly get your child to the doctor.

Meanwhile, here are some immediate measures you can take while you're on your way to the hospital or waiting for an ambulance to arrive.

- Keep your child still. If he's moving around, the venom will move more quickly into and through his system.
- Wash the wound, but do not apply ice or a cold compress. Don't cut the wound or try to suck out the venom—it does little or no good.
- If the snakebite is on an arm or leg, make a splint out of a stick, tying it with a jacket or the straps from a backpack—anything that will keep the limb from moving around.
- Lower the bitten area below the heart.
- Use a constricting band, if you know how. (This is taught in first-aid courses.)

  Caution: Do not use a tourniquet, which cuts off all blood flow.
- If the snake is dead, take it along to the doctor's office or emergency department. Snakebite can be treated most effectively if the doctor knows exactly what kind of snake bit your child.

Index

Note: <u>Underscored</u> page references indicate boxed text. Brand names of prescription medications are denoted by the symbol Rx.